Protecting Your Potential for Breastfeeding

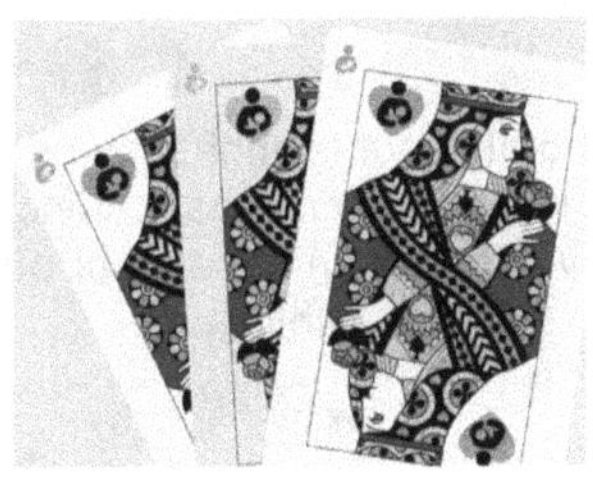

Kelly M. Durbin, M.Ed., IBCLC

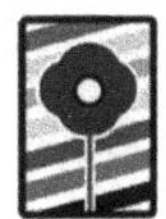

Praeclarus Press. LLC

www.PraeclarusPress.com

Praeclarus Press, LLC

2504 Sweetgum Lane

Amarillo, Texas 79124 USA

806-367-9950

www.PraeclarusPress.com

ISBN: 978-1-946665-66-9

Cover Design: Ken Tackett

Developmental Editing: Kathleen Kendall-Tackett

Copyediting: Chris Tackett

Layout & Design: Nelly Murariu

Contents

Introduction: Protecting Your Potential for Breastfeeding

The Lactation Puzzle

Many people believe that because breastfeeding is natural, it should be easy. After all, the human body grows a baby with relative ease following conception, so how hard could it be to make milk? The answer for many people is: *it depends.* For some people, it can be easy, but for others, making human milk can be challenging because there are (in the modern world) many factors that must align properly to develop and maintain the milk supply and the infant-feeding relationship.

Think of breastfeeding and milk production as a puzzle. Multiple distinct pieces must fit together in just the right way to create a coherent picture. When one element is out of line, it will likely not significantly impact the whole puzzle, but when several pieces are missing or misaligned with the rest of the puzzle, the picture does not come together coherently.

Breastfeeding requires some effort, knowledge, and skill for both parents and the family. The factors that make up the puzzle pieces of lactation extend far beyond the breastfeeding couple and immediate family. We have come to a point where the influence of infant formula and the industry's aggressive marketing tactics, over-management of labor and birth, deficient professional and communal support, lack of basic knowledge of lactation, and negative social factors can come together to create obstacles for the natural process of human lactation. Why is this happening? How can parents cope with these challenges? In short, how can new parents successfully put together their puzzle pieces for breastfeeding?

The purpose of this book is to highlight essential pieces of the puzzle, both positive and negative, that impact breastfeeding. These pieces include a range of critical factors that promote lactation, the maintenance of breastfeeding, and a range of negative factors that may hinder (or harm) the lactation process. Some of the most significant factors for lactation support include:

- Partner support
- Evidence-based care during pregnancy, labor, and childbirth
- Lactation management
- Breastfeeding knowledge and education
- Supportive primary care, pediatrician, and family care with knowledge and training in lactation
- Family support
- Community support
- Breastfeeding support in the workplace

These pieces of the puzzle are critical. In addition, these lactation promotion factors serve as the foundation for breastfeeding throughout the book. Therefore, I dedicate Part I of the book to discussing these elements of lactation in detail.

It is equally important to identify and understand factors that create a perfect storm to negatively impact lactogenesis, the process of making human milk, and the breastfeeding relationship. Those factors show up in many aspects of our lives.

- The negative influence of artificial infant formula and its cultural impacts destroyed generations of breastfeeding wisdom. Unfortunately, few people (if any) in the Western Hemisphere have not been impacted by living in a formula-feeding culture and by exposure to aggressive marketing tactics.
- In the context of birth, factors that negatively impact lactation are often perceived through the lens of managed care and are called *routine birth interventions.* In general, routine birth interventions are rarely presented as interference for lactation. Furthermore, outside of the lactation field, there is little awareness that routine birth interventions can negatively affect milk production.
- In the context of healthcare, we speak about unsupportive care, misinformed doctors, or lack of evidence-based care, but we have no name for how unsupportive care interferes with lactation.

- Family members may share bad or outdated advice from a social or cultural perspective or express their displeasure with breastfeeding. Again, these negative social expressions of breastfeeding have no name.
- An unsupportive or uninformed supervisor may not provide appropriate accommodations for expressing milk in the workplace. This kind of lactation sabotage has no name.

In this book, I cover many of the distinct pieces of the lactation puzzle, giving emphasis and a name to those that negatively impact breastfeeding. In the context of human milk production and infant feeding, I group these factors as *lactation interference factors*. These are the pieces of the puzzle that should be minimized or avoided.

It is essential to acknowledge that these lactation interference factors will not impact every person. Some elements have a greater impact than others, and some people will interact minimally with this constellation of challenges. Each of us is an individual. Although we can discuss risk in general terms, *your* risk concerning any of the factors presented in this book will depend on your circumstances. That said, the more lactation interference factors you encounter, the more likely it is that there will be some challenges in making human milk or sustaining the breastfeeding relationship.

How Do Lactation and Breastfeeding Go Wrong?

There are several points along the breastfeeding continuum from birth to weaning that can negatively impact the process of feeding your baby human milk. Unfortunately, many social factors are in place long before pregnancy and parenting. Some of these factors are:

- Lactogenesis itself
- Inherent maternal factors
- Inherent infant factors
- Birth-related factors
- Lack of skilled care
- Poor lactation management and advice
- Social and cultural pressures

- Cultural influence of living in a formula-feeding society
- Challenges while working, pumping, and storing milk
- Lack of knowledge
- Lack of access to resources and support

One can categorize these breastfeeding challenges in several ways (e.g., maternal factors, infant factors, societal factors, and birth-related factors). To simplify things, two categories can function as the umbrella for all issues: 1) primary lactation interference factors and 2) secondary lactation interference factors. Think of a card game to better understand what these terms mean in relation to breastfeeding challenges. You are dealt a hand of cards at the outset of the game. These cards are your primary issues; you pick up new cards as you play the game, and these are your secondary issues.

It might be easy to think that a person dealt a perfect hand for breastfeeding will experience smooth sailing with no challenges from birth to weaning. It might also be easy to assume that a person dealt a poor hand with several bad cards will quickly lose the game. However, these assumptions are not valid when it comes to making milk and breastfeeding. Yes, there may be challenges, but one can overcome them with the proper support. Likewise, when there appear to be no maternal or infant anatomy obstacles, breastfeeding can still falter because of secondary factors like misguided advice or lack of support.

One key to managing your breastfeeding cards is understanding the nature of your hand. For example, were you dealt a good hand with few primary issues? Or were you dealt a poor hand with several primary issues?

Primary Lactation Interference Factors

Keep in mind that this is not an exhaustive list. There could be others. With that in mind, did you encounter any of these?

Maternal Factors:

- Prior breast surgery (chest surgery, reduction, augmentation, implants, explants)
- Inverted nipples

- Hypoplastic breasts (underdeveloped breasts with insufficient glandular tissue)
- Never been exposed to breastfeeding, lack of knowledge
- Not part of a breastfeeding culture
- Low milk supply resulting from a primary issue
- Diabetes
- Polycystic Ovary Syndrome
- Metabolic impairment (such as insulin resistance)

Infant Factors:

- Premature baby
- An infant who is small for gestational age
- An infant with low birth weight
- Genetic conditions that affect breastfeeding (Down syndrome, Pierre Robin sequence, and others)
- Oral anatomy issues (tongue-tie, cleft lip, cleft palate, and others)
- Poor or uncoordinated sucking skills due to primary issues
- Other health conditions that affect infant feeding

If you have any of these primary factors that interfere with breastfeeding, you will likely need immediate support and guidance as you work your way through the first weeks. While it is possible to overcome some of these factors, other situations may require supplementation with donor milk or infant formula. All is not lost, however; feeding your baby some human milk is better than none. In addition, parents can still develop a strong bond with their babies through partial breastfeeding and/or through the practice of Kangaroo Care (covered in a later chapter).

Once you know the primary issues you are dealing with, it is possible to move forward with breastfeeding management. In life, as in cards, we continue to encounter new situations, experiences, and challenges. For example, to play poker, you occasionally need some new cards. However, you have no control over the cards you pick up when you blindly select from the deck. Similarly, when breastfeeding, you will continue to encounter new experiences that could factor into breastfeeding success or failure. However, unlike poker, these new experiences (i.e., cards) *can* be managed or prevented.

Is Race a Primary Factor?

The Deck is Stacked

Most people can make human milk but there are varying degrees of difficulty. Different cultural and social obstacles, as well as racism and bias, pose real challenges for some people more than others. Aside from the primary factors you bring to breastfeeding (e.g., prior breast/chest surgery), it is critical to note that there are social factors built into the fabric of our current society that stack the deck against minorities and people of color. The differing rates of breastfeeding along ethnic lines in the U.S. tell a complex story but one factor that is apparent in studies of breastfeeding disparities is the lack of breastfeeding support for minorities. The racial disparities surface in many ways: inherent bias and assumptions on part of the perinatal caregivers, lack of family support, lack of culturally appropriate community support, and lack of available community resources for breastfeeding in minority communities.

A recent study examining the breastfeeding experiences of 1,636 people showed that Black parents were offered infant formula as supplementation at a rate nine times higher than white parents (McKinney et al., 2016). Supplementing in the first few days of breastfeeding has known risks and outcomes, including shorter duration of breastfeeding. In this book, we cannot begin to answer questions about the injustice of this scenario, but we can start to peel back the curtain on where race and ethnicity play into our personal and collective breastfeeding outcomes. In Part II, I discuss some of the lactation interference factors that affect minorities in the U.S. in disproportionate ways.

Secondary Interference Factors

Secondary issues that affect breastfeeding are not inherent to the breastfeeding dyad. Instead, one encounters these secondary factors through experience. Think of these as optional (but not always). These are the cards you pick up as you play the game. Not everyone will encounter these issues, and even when one does experience a secondary lactation interference factor, it may not affect breastfeeding or have only a minimal negative impact.

When reading this list, do not be alarmed if you can identify more than one of these lactation interference factors in your experience. One or two of these factors will not likely cause major obstacles for breastfeeding. Remember that breastfeeding success is a compilation of positive and supportive factors over time. Likewise, breastfeeding failure can result (but not always) from the cumulative nature of negative or unsupportive factors over time.

Secondary Lactation Interference Factors

Much like the previous list concerning primary interference factors, the list of secondary interference factors is not all-inclusive. Did you encounter any of these factors?

Maternal Factors:

- Birth by cesarean birth
- Epidural during labor
- Narcotic pain relief during birth
- Long second stage of labor
- Excessive exposure to IV fluid during labor
- Excessive postpartum hemorrhage
- Retained placenta
- Outdated breastfeeding advice from primary care physicians, pediatricians, or others
- Separation from the baby in the early postpartum period immediately after birth
- Delayed breastfeeding initiation (beyond the first few hours)
- Low milk supply (resulting from a secondary issue)
- Fewer than eight breastfeeding/pumping sessions in 24 hours (in the early weeks and months)
- Lack of nighttime feeding or pumping
- Poor lactation management in the early weeks

Infant Factors:

- Intubation
- Heavy suctioning of infant airway
- Jaundice (from bruising and birth trauma)
- Poor latch
- Early use of a pacifier for non-therapeutic reasons
- Supplementation

Societal Factors:

- Pressure from partner, family, or friends to avoid or stop breastfeeding
- Lack of evidence-based lactation management from a pediatrician/caregiver
- Bad or outdated advice from family and friends
- Lack of support for the family's infant-feeding goals
- Lack of access to pumping while working
- Lack of skilled instruction for lactation in the perinatal period

Again, one or two of these factors will not likely cause major obstacles for breastfeeding. Furthermore, over time, these interference factors can be counter-balanced with a range of positive and supportive factors.

Playing Your Lactation Cards

One strategy to managing your hand is to avoid picking up crappy cards, which is not always easy when you are selecting from the deck, and you cannot see what your choices are. In terms of breastfeeding, you *should* be able to make more educated choices because you can factor in the known breastfeeding consequences most of the time. In theory, this *should* allow for the chance to make *informed choices*. Suppose it is true that people can make informed decisions about secondary issues (the cards you pick up during the game). If that is so, why are so many people having difficulty breastfeeding in our society?

Here is where several significant challenges for breastfeeding emerge. First, because the United States is essentially a formula-feeding culture, breastfeeding is not always factored into lifestyle choices. Second, to the untrained eye, the choices that people face (during birth, for example) do not appear to interfere with breastfeeding. Third, the facts about how a choice affects breastfeeding are not well known without doing prior research. Finally, sometimes (many times, really), the facts about lactation interference are not presented at the right time by healthcare professionals. For example, when administering an IV to deliver the fluids that accompany Pitocin, are caregivers informing parents about the potential downstream effects of breast edema and its impact on lactation?

One additional confounding factor is that many people decide about labor and birth on the fly without fully researching the risks and knowing how the procedure or intervention can impact breastfeeding. This scenario is like blindly selecting your cards from the deck because you have no idea how the next card will affect your hand.

There are many complex reasons why modern society sometimes makes it difficult to get lactation flowing positively and productively. However, the short story behind modern-day lactation difficulties is simple; we (in the U.S. and many other places around the world) are coming off a long period of primarily using infant formula. As a result of formula domination, we nearly lost the wisdom of lactation and human milk feeding. Consider this: most adults alive today in the U.S. were fed infant formula at some point during their first year of life. Because of this, many people no longer have the wisdom of breastfeeding in their families and their communities. One other significant factor is that healthcare research largely excluded women from study until recent times. This historical gender bias has created a disproportionate focus on men's health issues.

Fortunately, gender bias in research is decreasing, and studies of human milk are more prevalent than ever. However, while human milk is making a huge comeback, its rise in popularity must be accompanied by an equivalent increase in lactation knowledge, care, protection, and management. This is slowly happening, but we are not yet near the goal of living in a supportive breastfeeding society with breastfeeding-friendly care for all people.

How to Use This Book

This book is a two-part examination of the factors associated with breastfeeding success and breastfeeding challenges or failure. In Part I, we will take a deep dive into the lactation promotion factors, all the elements that come together to create and support successful breastfeeding. Then, in Part II, we will examine some of the most common factors for lactation interference, breastfeeding challenges, and breastfeeding failure. I will also provide you with strategies for preventing those challenges or improving outcomes if you are already dealing with difficulties.

The key to breastfeeding success is not to avoid every single obstacle. That would be nearly impossible in today's world. Instead, the key is to minimize the lactation interference factors and maximize the lactation promotion factors. Encountering one or two negative factors is unlikely to derail your goals. Breastfeeding can be challenging, especially when the interference factors accumulate over time. However, knowing the risks and how to minimize them can help keep milk production and breastfeeding on track for success.

Use this book as your guide for creating your own successful approach to breastfeeding. Since we all come to pregnancy, parenting, and infant feeding with our own unique set of primary and secondary interference factors, the recipe you use for success will likely be different from the recipe that other families use for success. Therefore, it can be helpful to remember that what works well for you may not work well or be necessary for others. In addition, not all the ideas presented in this book will apply to everyone. Use your best judgment to make sound, informed decisions for your family.

If you are currently pregnant and are hoping to maximize your chances for breastfeeding, you have an amazing opportunity *right now* to evaluate the list of secondary issues. You may already be aware of the hand you were dealt initially. Labor and birth will present opportunities to pick up new cards, but unlike poker, *you will be able to choose* the cards you pick up. You can go into labor knowing that some of the choices you encounter might affect your ability to readily produce milk. You may choose them anyway, and that is fine, as long as you know the potential pitfalls and how to get good support if things go awry later on.

If you are reading this book with one hand while holding your baby at the breast with your other hand, you may have already (and perhaps unknowingly) encountered some of the factors that can sabotage breastfeeding and your milk supply. Maybe the hand you were dealt was acceptable, but you picked up some new cards during or after birth that are now interfering with milk production or feeding. Perhaps it seems like the lactation interference factors are giving you insurmountable problems. However, with good support, some hard work, and steadfast conviction to your breastfeeding goals, it is likely you can still make human milk and feed it to your baby.

My Intentions for This Book

I hope you will gain knowledge, confidence, and skills by using this book as a guide to breastfeeding. In this book, I intend to present human milk as a powerful health agent and to portray the breastfeeding relationship as the basis for forming bonds with others.

While I aim to praise human milk and human lactation as the gold standard for first food, I do not intend to criticize infant formula and its users. In fact, it is because of infant formula that I am alive today. My mom chose infant formula during a time when society had a poor understanding of human milk, and reliable lactation support did not exist in many places.

Although I hope that all people have access to evidence-based lactation care and excellent community support, I know by firsthand experience that this is not always the case for some families. Therefore, my hope for this book is that it will help expand your knowledge of lactation and human milk, and that your understanding of lactation eventually contributes to a better communal knowledge of infant feeding.

You may be surprised by what you read in this book, but I promise you, I am presenting nothing new here. All of this information is already out in the world in one form or another. I intend to collect this information, synthesize it, and make it accessible to individuals and communities to help them reach their true potential for making the powerful, mighty force that is human milk.

PART I
Lactation Promotion Factors

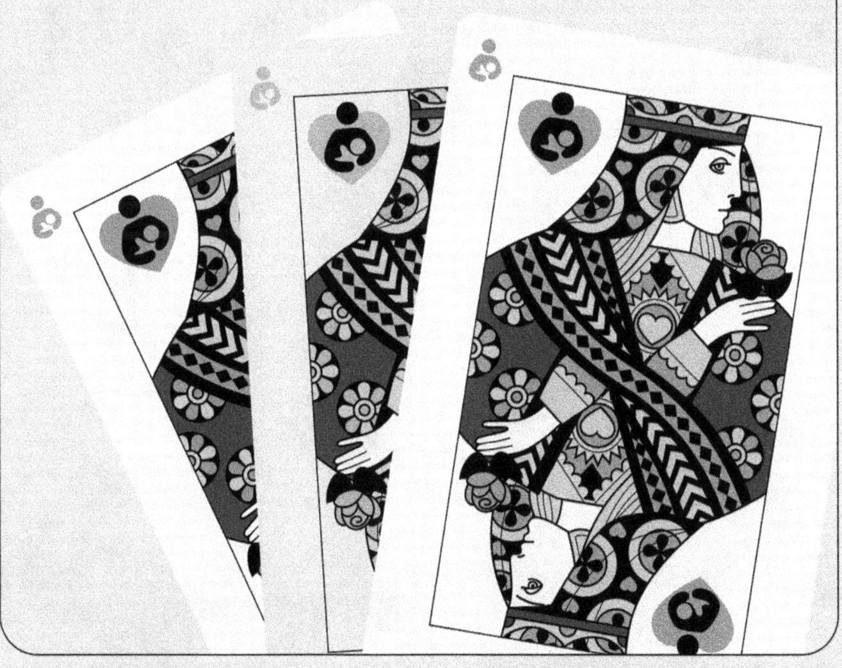

CHAPTER 1

Breastfeeding: What Makes Lactation Work?

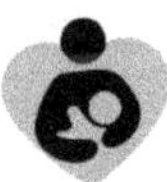

So, you are interested in breastfeeding? Let me be the first to say congratulations! Choosing to breastfeed your baby is not just a choice about an infant-feeding method or where the necessary calories will come from for your baby. Choosing to feed your baby human milk is, indeed, one of the most critical choices you will make about your baby's infancy, attachment, wellbeing, *and* long-term health. While it may seem like a trivial detail to some, infant feeding, especially breastfeeding, is sometimes more about a personal relationship than it is about the calories. Yes, the baby needs to eat; that's rule number one! But during the baby's first year, human milk feeding is much more than a source of calories. It is a personal relationship with important outcomes and experiences for both parent and baby.

People rarely consider what breastfeeding is really like until it is time to choose an infant feeding method. In societies where formula has dominated for many years, breastfeeding is a learn-as-you-go experience because we do not see it. We generally do not face lactation before adulthood, and we do not even discuss it unless we are well into pregnancy. As teens and young adults, we (here in the U.S. and other formula-feeding cultures) scarcely ever see people breastfeeding in public. There is no exposure to breastfeeding education in high school health classes. There are no lactation courses to take as college students (except for the few studying human lactation). Most medical schools do not teach human lactation to doctors-in-training. Some medical schools teach no lactation at all. In addition, people often seek private spaces for breastfeeding, when they are away from home. Breastfeeding can be a hidden part of parenting, something done privately (for many people). When lactation is a hidden, it is quite difficult to learn from others. Finally, most of us have little reason to learn about lactation before having a baby.

Like many aspects of pregnancy, birth, and parenting, choosing to breastfeed is a very personal choice, and one family's pathway through breastfeeding will be different from others. There are many distinct choices to make and ways to do things while breastfeeding. You and your sister or friend may both choose to breastfeed but go about it in two different ways, and that is okay. Before we even get started, I would like to validate your right to choose an alternative path, one that is not necessarily mainstream. It is up to you to make decisions about infant feeding. Most of the time, you can make these decisions or at least consider them before your baby arrives.

What Is Your Milk-Making Potential?

The word *potential* comes from the Latin word *potentia,* which means *power, might, or force*. However, our modern use of the word *potential* is more related to the meaning of the word *possibility,* which focuses on forthcoming prospects, those yet to be revealed. I intend to combine the two ideas for our discussion of lactation and human milk feeding. It is only fitting that the word *potential* also relates to power; human milk and breastfeeding are, indeed, powerful. This book is about protecting the powerful possibilities within the breast to create milk and nurture life with it.

To realize the powerful possibilities of human milk synthesis and sustaining life with your milk, we need to look at what factors support and promote your potential, and the lactation interference factors that are associated with diminished potential.

Each of us has the capacity to make milk, provided that a few necessary factors are present: 1) a functioning pituitary gland, 2) healthy and sufficient mammary tissue, 3) important hormones: oxytocin and prolactin, 4) efficient milk removal system (infant, hand expression, or pump). When these factors are present and in good working order, in theory, there is a high potential for producing human milk.

Why is it, then, that we so often hear about how breastfeeding presents challenges for so many people? How have breastfeeding and human milk sustained people worldwide for centuries but fail in modern society? Why should it be that an entire country, like the U.S., has suboptimal breastfeeding rates at three months and six months of life? Is there something inherent in modern people that diminishes our true potential for breastfeeding? Is there something present in the environment that inhibits our capacity to produce milk? Is there something in the water?

While these questions sound slightly far-fetched, there is a kernel of truth here. *There is something*, many things, in fact, that are present in modern lifestyles that can prevent us from reaching our true milk-making potential.

The potential for making human milk in modern society is truly a balancing act. First, you must be aware of the factors that can tip the balance toward lactation success or lactation failure. Then, you must choose wisely which factors you will interact with and how much interaction you will have. The difficulty that arises for many people is knowing what factors in our lives negatively affect breastfeeding.

This book aims to provide readers with a practical guide for becoming more aware of factors that promote and protect breastfeeding. More importantly, this book will highlight interference factors to minimize (or avoid altogether) because they may sabotage your breastfeeding efforts. Like many things in life, one interaction or exposure to something on the lactation interference list will likely *not* cause harm. However, repeated exposure to such factors is cumulative and may ultimately sabotage your potential to make milk.

What Is Successful Breastfeeding?

What does success mean for lactation? Is it the ability to make milk? Is it the ability to express milk? Is it defined as direct feeding at the breast (no use of bottles)? Is successful breastfeeding equal to exclusive breastfeeding, using no supplements? Is success defined as encountering no feeding challenges? Is it breastfeeding for two weeks? Two months? Two years? Or is it something else?

LACTATION

Total Failure ◄——————————————► **Total Success**

When we consider breastfeeding as a spectrum, most people do not experience the extremes of total success or total failure. Most people who set out to feed their infants human milk would describe their experience as being somewhere in the middle of the spectrum. The good news is that you are the judge of your own success[1]. You are the one who gets to decide what success is for you and how that plays out in your infant feeding journey.

What Makes Breastfeeding Work?

Effective breastfeeding includes several key components, but it is helpful to remember that you and your baby act as a team. Therefore, some factors apply to the infant only; some apply to the parent only, and others are team factors. Without these factors, breastfeeding function may be compromised.

Maternal Factors Necessary for Lactation

- Healthy, functioning pituitary gland
- Oxytocin and prolactin (hormone release and hormone receptors)
- Sufficient glandular tissue
- Intact nerves to the breast and nipple
- Effective milk removal (baby or pump) 8-12 times in 24 hours (teamwork)
- Recognizing feeding cues and responding promptly
- Providing unrestricted access to the breast
- Achieving a comfortable position that facilitates easy feeding (teamwork)
- Achieving an effective latch (teamwork) and assessing the latch during feeding

1 The concept of determining success in breastfeeding is explored in depth in the context of breastfeeding after reduction surgery in the brilliant book called *Defining Your Own Success: Breastfeeding after Breast Reduction Surgery* by Diana West.

- Assessing the infant's satisfaction after the session
- Assessing the baby's urine and stool output
- Mitigating issues with latch, position, forceful let-down, or fast flow
- Recognizing when things are not going well
- Getting help

Infant Factors Necessary for Feeding and to Sustain Lactation

- Demonstrating feeding cues
- Using innate breast seeking and feeding behaviors
- Latching effectively (teamwork)
- Effectively coordinating suck-swallow-breathe sequence
- Transferring milk effectively

When these factors are present, there will be a higher likelihood of effective breastfeeding and milk transfer. Each of these factors noted above makes its own contribution to effective breastfeeding. Let's briefly examine how these elements contribute to effective lactation.

Maternal Factors

Pituitary Gland

The pituitary gland is a small endocrine gland in the brain, about the size of a pea. It releases oxytocin and prolactin in response to nipple stimulation and suckling.

Oxytocin and Prolactin

Oxytocin acts quickly to cause contractions of the alveoli, facilitating the release of milk already in the breast into the milk ducts. In turn, the breast expresses milk through the nipple pores.

Prolactin is also essential for milk making. During pregnancy, estrogen and progesterone inhibit prolactin. These two hormones, which are high during pregnancy, stop the action of prolactin. Once the placenta is delivered, prolactin levels rise and facilitate milk secretion. Prolactin works more slowly than oxytocin. The body releases prolactin in response to suckling, and it promotes milk production by the alveoli (at the cellular level within the breast). Prolactin levels are highest about 30 minutes after the suckling begins, making more milk for the next feeding. Because prolactin governs milk production and the body releases it in response to suckling, the baby must have ample, unrestricted opportunity for breastfeeding in the early weeks.

For either of these hormones to act on the breast, the tissue must have hormone receptors there. The receptors are key to the lactation process. Receptors are laid down in the breast tissue during the early weeks, and they are the landing site for oxytocin and prolactin. Without the receptors, the hormones have no place to "plug in" and cannot act on the breast tissue.

Induced Lactation

Early developmental changes in the breast are a response to the hormones of pregnancy, but pregnancy is not necessary in order to lactate. Using specific protocols, herbs and always medication, people can induce lactation without any pregnancy at all. One of the more commonly used induced-lactation protocols is called the Newman-Goldfarb Protocol, which has several approaches to inducing lactation. In fact, one does not even need ovaries or a uterus to lactate, which means that postmenopausal people and those who have undergone hysterectomy can initiate lactation via an induced lactation protocol. This is important information for families choosing to adopt and wishing to breastfeed their babies. For the record, lactation can be induced in females, males, trans, and nonbinary individuals. In other species, male lactation has been observed. For example, males in the Dayak fruit bat species have functional mammary glands.

Mammary Tissue

Human lactation is a complex, multifactored system that develops at different stages of life, from fetal development to puberty, and finally, during pregnancy. The mammary gland is the only body part not developed at birth. There are distinct times for mammary growth in the human life span: in the embryonic stage with the formation of the milk line and cells that will become the nipple (in both males and females);

the infancy stage with the development of ducts and the mammary fat pad; and later, in puberty with development of structural tissues and more adipose tissue. During each menstrual cycle, the breast is preparing for growth as it anticipates the possibility of pregnancy. The cells grow and then regress each month unless or until pregnancy occurs. During pregnancy, there is aggressive growth and proliferation of the cellular structures responsible for the milk-making process. Most people notice distinct breast changes, and these are associated with structural and hormonal transformation. Common breast changes during pregnancy are:

- Tender breasts, often a first sign that pregnancy has occurred
- Darkening of nipple and areola
- Changes in breast size
- More prominent veins due to increased blood flow
- Leaking colostrum toward the end of pregnancy

By mid-pregnancy, the breast is ready to make milk. This readiness accounts for leaking colostrum (for some people) and ensures that milk will be available if the infant arrives early. In addition, pregnancy hormones are not the same as lactation hormones. This difference helps keep the mature milk on hold until after the placenta is delivered, signaling the end of pregnancy and the beginning of lactation. (It's important to note that the placenta and its hormones are responsible for inhibiting lactation. I discuss this again with regard to placenta encapsulation in Part II of this book.)

Very rarely, during the timeline of mammary and breast development from the embryonic stage through pregnancy, there are cases in which the mammary gland does not develop sufficient tissue structure to create and support a full milk supply. This underdevelopment is called insufficient glandular tissue (IGT). People with IGT can often make milk but may be less likely to bring in a full milk supply. Even so, people with IGT who wish to produce milk and feed their babies at the breast can do so using a supplemental nursing system, also called an at-breast supplementer. If at any time during lactation you feel you are not making enough milk, do not panic. It is unlikely that insufficient glandular tissue is the cause.

IGT is a rare condition, affecting only a small number of people. In addition to low milk supply, several other signs accompany IGT[2]:

- Widely spaced breasts
- Lack of symmetry, one breast is larger or shaped differently
- Long, tube-shaped breasts; lack of round shape
- Lack of breast changes during pregnancy and early postpartum

Intact Nerve Function Serving the Breast and Nipple

Lactation cannot proceed effectively unless the fourth intercostal nerve is intact and functioning well. This functionality is a critical part of milk production mechanics. It is responsible for sending sensory signals from the breast (in response to your baby's suckling or the pump) to the pituitary, triggering the release of oxytocin and prolactin. If prior chest or breast surgery caused any injury to the nerves in the breast, there is the possibility of compromised lactation. However, nerves can and do regenerate. If you had any chest or breast surgery in the past, your nerve structure serving the breast would likely be more functional now than directly after the surgery. The elapsed time since the surgery (or nerve injury of any kind) will allow nerves to heal and regrow. The more time between surgery and lactation, the better.

Effective Milk Removal

Milk removal is one of the essential lactation promotion factors. In the first hours of lactation and milk secretion by the breast, hormones govern milk production. The body establishes local control as the baby begins breastfeeding (or milk is pumped from the breast) over the first days and weeks. Local control is the real-time, baby-driven control that drives milk production; it is the removal of milk that gives the breast the stimulation to make more milk. This signal means that the breast will make milk only when milk is removed from the breast. An empty breast tells the body to produce more milk[3]. A full breast tells the body to slow or stop milk production. Interestingly, the amount of milk removed in the first three to four weeks of lactation influences

---

2 For more information about IGT, see *Finding Sufficiency: Breastfeeding With Insufficient Glandular Tissue* by Diana Cassar-Uhl

3 Empty breast? The breast is never truly empty. But it can be substantially less full.

the volume of milk you will be making for the future. This is because your body lays down hormone receptors as milk is removed from the breast in the early weeks.

Effective milk removal has several essential elements: 1) the baby has a good suck reflex and tongue mobility, 2) the baby can create a good seal during the latch, 3) the baby can create and maintain vacuum pressure in the oral cavity, and 4) one allots enough time for milk removal. Pumping with a double electric hospital-grade pump is standard for milk removal immediately after birth if the baby is not ready or available for direct feeding. Hand expression of colostrum is also possible. Milk removal must be timely, with 8-12 full breastfeeding or pumping sessions in a 24-hour period. Long stretches between feedings or pumping sessions trigger a slowdown in milk production.

Recognizing Feeding Cues and Responding Promptly

In the last section, I stated that you should remove milk from the breast 8-12 times in 24 hours. This general recommendation means that feeding or pumping should occur every two to three hours throughout the day and around the clock. However, watching the clock is *not* the best way to know when to feed your baby. The feeding recommendation for every two to three hours is a broad guideline, given so that people know what to expect for a breastfed baby. Watching your baby is, by far, the best way to know when it is time to bring the baby to the breast. Healthy babies display feeding cues when they are ready for feeding. As a parent, it is your job to recognize the feeding cues and respond quickly before the baby's gentle cues progress into more aggressive cues and agitation. It is much more difficult to initiate feeding with a frantic or actively crying baby. Later in the book, I provide a more detailed discussion on feeding cues in the RELAX Method chapter.

Providing Unrestricted Access to the Breast

Unrestricted access. This term can seem complex or even extreme at first glance but do not let this fool you. It simply means that there are no arbitrary boundaries in place that could limit the baby's time at the breast. For most families, unrestricted access means feeding the baby when you see the feeding cues. Furthermore, this also allows the baby the time they need to get enough milk (some babies take longer than others, especially preemies or other special needs infants). Think of it as an all-access pass to the front row!

Achieving a Comfortable Position That Facilitates Easy Feeding

Contrary to what you may have seen or heard, there are many positions that one can use to breastfeed a baby (e.g., sitting, reclining, lying down). The keys to choosing a position are comfort and alignment. Be sure you and your baby are comfortable; no straining or leaning over. Be sure the baby is aligned – ear, shoulder, and hip are in line. The baby should not be turning their head to reach the breast. It is a great idea to learn and master several different positions so that you have a variety of options. A good position to start learning breastfeeding and latch techniques is the laid-back position. After learning laid-back breastfeeding, try other positions as well. I provide more detail on positions later in the book.

Achieving a Good Latch and Assessing the Latch During Feeding

The latch is another critical piece of successful breastfeeding. In reality, the baby is the one to manage the latch, but you as the parent must know how to provide the proper position and timing to allow him the best chance of latching well. You also need to develop skills to assess the latch. For example, how do the baby's lips look? How about the position of his chin and nose? What is your comfort level with the latch? These and more indicators are discussed in detail later.

Assessing the Baby's Satisfaction After Feeding

How will you know when the baby is satisfied? How will you know that the baby has had enough milk? This evaluation is sometimes more complex than it sounds, but it does not have to be. There are several ways to determine if the baby feels satisfied immediately after feeding. First, watch the baby's fists. When the feeding begins, the baby is likely to have closed fists. As the feeding continues, the whole body, including the fists, will relax, and his hands will open. Next, look for milk at the corners of the mouth or drool that looks milky. Does the baby spit up? Do not be alarmed; many infants spit up. At the very least, it helps indicate the transfer of milk from the breast to the baby. Assess his mood. Is he now more relaxed or even sleepy? Many people refer to this as *milk drunk*. These signs indicate how the baby feels after one feeding session, but they are not absolute indicators of sufficient milk intake over time.

Assessing the Baby's Urine and Stool Output

To know if your baby is getting enough milk over time, not just at one session, you will need to track urine and stool output. What goes in must come out. If the baby is getting enough high-fat milk to help him feel satisfied and have the energy to grow, he will pass stools. This is your main indicator that things are going well. Another way to tell if the baby is getting enough milk is assessing weight gain. **This method is not for everyday assessment**, as it requires a highly sensitive scale and tracking over time. You can use apps for your smart phone to track urine and stool production or print out a chart and keep track with paper and pencil. Track your baby's weight gain over time at your doctor's office or with a lactation consultant. I recommend being cautious with infant tracking apps. Generally, watching your baby is better than using tools (more on this in Part II).

Mitigating Issues and Recognizing When Things Are Not Going Well

Breastfeeding can reach a stage where things seem to be on autopilot, but this is not the case for newborns. You must perform a mental check-in for yourself and your baby to assess whether things are going well in the early months. How do you feel about breastfeeding? Is it going well overall? Are there things you would like to change about your breastfeeding relationship? Do you need help or support? Are you experiencing any pain? Does the baby appear happy and healthy? Use the PACMAAN Breastfeeding Assessment Tool in RELAX Method chapter to help you assess your current situation.

Getting Help

A critical part of success in any endeavor is the ability to realize when you need help and support. In fact, knowing this is essential for successful breastfeeding. There are several types of breastfeeding support available in the U.S. and beyond. For example, breastfeeding support may be available at your baby's pediatrician's office. Ask if they provide on-site lactation care and find out who provides the care. Does the care provider have formal training in lactation? If highly-qualified lactation support is not available at the pediatrician's office, they may have outside resources for breastfeeding. Ask about their lactation support services before your baby is born. In addition, the hospital where you give birth may have breastfeeding support groups or clinics. In the United States, free-standing birth centers often have breastfeeding classes and support groups. Free peer-to-peer breastfeeding support groups are perfect for coaching people with the normal course of breastfeeding and for troubleshooting low-level and some mid-level concerns. Although these groups cannot offer clinical care, they are often knowledgeable about finding higher-level care.

There are additional sources for community support too. For instance, in the U.S., La Leche League has in-person groups in every state, along with phone, text, and online resources. Breastfeeding USA is another organization that offers breastfeeding support. They are growing steadily and adding new resources every month. They provide in-person meetings, text, online, and phone support. Baby Café USA is also a free resource for parents, but peer counselors or leaders do not facilitate the meetings. Group leaders for Baby Café are lactation consultants. There are many organizations outside of the U.S., including the Australian Breastfeeding Association, the Breastfeeding Network (UK), La Leche League International (groups worldwide), National Childbirth Trust (UK), Canadian Breastfeeding Foundation, and many others. Check out local and online resources in your area.

Infant Factors

Demonstrating Feeding Cues

A healthy full-term baby is adept at displaying feeding cues. Feeding cues are the baby's non-verbal behaviors that indicate when she wants to come to the breast. Many people think that crying is the universal signal that indicates infant hunger. However, this is a myth. Infant crying can be a signal for many things, but in terms of feeding cues, crying is usually the last indicator that a baby will use to call for food. Initially, feeding cues are gentle and sometimes subtle. For example, your baby will likely open and close her mouth, display tongue movements or lip-smacking. To the untrained eye, one might interpret this as endearing newborn behavior, but in reality, the baby uses sophisticated innate reflexes to signal her need for food. I discuss feeding cues in more detail in the RELAX chapter.

Using Innate Breast-seeking and Feeding Behaviors

Newborn skills and competence for breastfeeding are usually highly underestimated. Not long ago, the prevailing assumption was that newborns were helpless creatures who needed extensive coaching and assistance at the breast. In reality, infants are acutely aware of the feeding process, how to use innate skills to seek their food source and accomplish the task of feeding all on their own. The most fundamental input infants need from parents is placement in the proper environment, between the breasts. The baby's location determines her behaviors. When she is in the proper environment, she can use innate reflexes to position herself for feeding correctly. I outline these reflexes and the fascinating process of the breast crawl in the RELAX chapter.

Latching Effectively

Indeed, latching is an infant skill, but developing an effective latch requires teamwork. For the baby to latch effectively, she must be in a good position or able to move herself into a good position. If you are familiar with the breast crawl, you already know that infants placed on their tummies (ventral surface) between the breasts right after birth can use innate stepping and crawling reflexes to achieve an optimal position for latching and feeding. In this scenario, an infant can then perform the latch herself. Our job as parents is to provide the optimal environment and then monitor to ensure that the baby's latch is comfortable and effective.

If the latch occurs while the newborn is in a cradle hold, effective latching is possible. However, one needs more teamwork when the parent is upright and seated. In the cradle hold, the baby approaches the nipple from the front. Sometimes, the baby is working against gravity and is not high enough or stable enough to achieve a comfortable latch. Sometimes, the nipple is not aimed toward the juncture of the hard and soft palates. In the cradle approach, the baby cannot effectively use all the breast-seeking behaviors, and as a result, the latch can be suboptimal. As I said above, it is possible to achieve a good latch with a cradle hold, but for a newborn who is learning to latch and transfer milk effectively, the more laid-back position (with the baby on top) is often superior.

Effectively Coordinate the Suck-Swallow-Breathe Sequence

Infants learning to breastfeed must manage to take in milk, swallow the milk, and breathe in a comfortable sequence. This process is relatively straightforward for most healthy babies, but this can be challenging for some premature infants or those with special needs.

Transfer Milk Effectively

A baby can appear to be latched well and even spend ample time at the breast, but that is only part of the equation for effective feeding. Another essential part of effective feeding is the infant's ability to transfer milk from the breast into her mouth and swallow effectively. Effective milk transfer relies on several factors – achieving and sustaining a good latch, maintaining a tight seal without gaps, and creating the intraoral vacuum necessary to help facilitate milk transfer. Effective feeding only occurs if the baby can transfer milk from the breast. Sometimes, oral anatomy abnormalities or oral dysfunction can play a role in problems leading to suboptimal milk transfer.

Making Lactation Work for Society

In addition to the maternal and infant factors (listed above) that help facilitate effective breastfeeding, societal factors play a major role in our collective breastfeeding experiences and outcomes. When society values maternal and infant health outcomes, human milk and breastfeeding become a priority. This outcome will be evident at all levels of society. Some of the ways that societies promote and protect breastfeeding include:

- Signing and enforcing the World Health Organization (WHO) Code for the Marketing of Breast Milk Substitutes
- Adopting nationwide hospital policies that support breastfeeding-friendly labor and birth practices

- Enacting legislation to provide all families with paid maternity/ paternity leave (for birth or adoption)
- Establishing laws to protect break time for all workers who express and store human milk during the workday
- Establishing laws to protect nursing in public spaces
- Normalizing and protecting lactation by having lactation-informed healthcare workers at all levels of physical and mental healthcare
- Ensuring that all healthcare workers have adequate lactation training and that they present a similar message to new parents who are learning to breastfeed
- Establishing breastfeeding recommendations at the professional level (from pediatric associations and societies) that go beyond 12 months

Maternity Leave

As you may already know, we here in the U.S. are still climbing out of a long history as a formula culture, and we have many steps to take to become a breastfeeding culture. Although all of the elements of a supportive breastfeeding culture listed above are important, paid maternity/paternity leave stands out as a critical factor to promote and protect breastfeeding. With guaranteed paid leave, parents can recover from birth and establish breastfeeding without the stress of losing valuable family income or having to go back to work too soon. Establishing paid leave for new parents in the U.S. would likely boost our breastfeeding rates overnight. At present, the U.S. is the only developed nation to offer zero paid leave.

Consider this:

- Estonia offers a year and a half of paid leave at full pay after the birth of a child.
- Austria offers eight weeks paid maternity leave before birth and eight weeks after. Parents can take parental leave following this period until the child reaches 24 months.
- Sweden offers ten weeks of paid leave at full pay, followed by 480 days of leave between the parents.

- Chile requires maternity leave for six weeks before birth and 12 weeks after birth. After that period, an additional 12 weeks is optional and can be transferred to the other parent.
- Mexico offers 12 weeks of paid leave, some of which can be taken before birth. (This paid leave policy only covers people in the formal work economy. Unfortunately, many people in the informal economy remain without guaranteed maternity leave.)
- Canada offers 15 weeks paid maternity leave, followed by 35 weeks of parental leave at variable pay.
- Israel offers 15 weeks of paid leave at full pay.
- The United States offers zero weeks of paid leave. Many individual companies offer paid maternity leave, but there is no national policy in place that guarantees paid leave for every employee.

Current Breastfeeding Recommendations

Many professional pediatric societies and child health organizations worldwide have breastfeeding recommendations in place as guidelines to help people set their own goals for the duration of human milk feeding. However, goal setting is not the only outcome of these policies. They also help set a reference point for what people expect as the normal duration for lactation. So, for example, if the breastfeeding recommendation from healthcare professionals is about 12 months, people may believe that 12 months is all that is needed.

I work with many different people each month who tell me about their goals for breastfeeding. Sometimes, these are arbitrary time limits, but many times, their goals reflect the recommendations from healthcare professionals. Breastfeeding duration is a personal decision that every family makes based on cultural norms, current recommendations, and perhaps their family experience. What is the optimal amount of time for babies to breastfeed? Is there an appropriate time for weaning for all infants?

Katherine Dettwyler's research suggests that a human's natural age for weaning is between 2.5 – 7 years (Dettwyler, 2004). This calculation uses many factors as compared to other primates, including 1) timing of tooth eruption, 2) length of gestation, 3) reaching a multiplier of birth weight, 4) reaching 1/3 of adult body weight, 5) and a few other characteristics. According to the CDC Breastfeeding Report Card, only about 1/3 of babies in the U.S. are breastfed beyond one year. Based on Dettwyler's research, current breastfeeding duration in the U.S. is quite low.

In 2022 the American Academy of Pediatrics (AAP) changed their current breastfeeding guidelines. Previously, the AAP was recommending that infants be exclusively breastfed for about six months and breastfed in conjunction to complimentary foods for about 12 months and beyond. Now the guidelines from the AAP have expanded to recommend that breastfeeding continue for two years and beyond. As I mentioned in other sections, it can take years for individual doctors to change their own recommendations, even though the professional organizations have released updates. Watch for outdated advice on breastfeeding duration in the coming years. It may take a decade or more for some people to modify the advice they give to breastfeeding families. In the following paragraphs, I list the current recommendations from the WHO and professional organizations around the world.

The World Health Organization (World Health Organization, 2021)

As a global public health recommendation, infants should be exclusively breastfed for the first six months of life to achieve optimal growth, development, and health. After that, to meet their evolving nutritional requirements, infants should receive nutritionally adequate and safe complementary foods while breastfeeding continues for up to two years of age or beyond. Exclusive breastfeeding from birth is possible except for a few medical conditions, and unrestricted exclusive breastfeeding results in ample milk production.

The American Academy of Pediatrics (adapted from Meek & Noble, 2022)

The AAP recommends exclusive breastfeeding for the first six months. The AAP supports continued breastfeeding, along with appropriate complimentary foods introduced at about six months as long as mutually desired for two years or beyond.

Canadian Paedatric Society and Health Canada (Government of Canada, 2015)

Breastfeeding exclusively for the first six months and sustained for up to two years or longer with appropriate complementary feeding is important for infants and toddlers' nutrition, immunologic protection, growth, and development.

Australia Department of Health (Australian Government Department of Health, 2019)

Australia's infant feeding guidelines recommend exclusive breastfeeding of infants to around six months of age when solid foods are introduced and continued breastfeeding until the age of 12 months and beyond, if both mother and infant wish.

Making Lactation Work for You

Before your baby arrives, it is a great idea to do some prep work. If you are pregnant while reading this book, you will find a wealth of information to help you plan and prepare. If your baby is already here, congratulations! You can use this book as a guide to help you plan for the infant feeding journey you are already on. There are several important decisions to make during your first year of infant feeding. Think about the following questions for short-term and long-term breastfeeding goals.

Goal Setting - Plan for Breastfeeding Before Baby Arrives

- Why is breastfeeding important to you? What is motivating you to choose human milk for your baby? I recommend writing down a few key reasons and discussing these with your partner. It would be best if you shared what drives your choice to breastfeed so that your partner knows exactly where you stand. Then, encourage your partner to share their thoughts about infant feeding as well.
- What kind of breastfeeding class will you take? In-person or online? Some people skip this but finding a good breastfeeding class truly pays off. You most likely found a birth class already. Remember, childbirth lasts for one day. Breastfeeding can last for months or years. Preparation has rewards.

- Have you talked to your partner and important family members about your decision to breastfeed? Are they on board? Involve your key players early on and set goals together.
- Are you going to need any supplies for breastfeeding? It is a good idea to get a few items before your baby arrives but be realistic about your needs. There are many superfluous breastfeeding items available, and you will not likely need everything in the baby aisle!
- Do you need to speak to your employer about breastfeeding? (Hint: The answer is probably yes.) Learn about the laws for breastfeeding in your state, province, or local area. Also, determine what you may be entitled to at your place of employment. Speak to your manager or boss about breaks for pumping milk and necessary accommodations (private room, electricity, a place to store expressed milk). Finally, find out if your employer offers any benefits for lactating employees. For example, some businesses provide lactation rooms, places for milk storage, and even access to lactation support.
- Have you created a breastfeeding-friendly birth plan? You may have a much better idea about how to plan for that after reading Part II of this book. Keep in mind that less is more when it comes to the birth plan.
- Have you thought about who you will include on your breastfeeding support team? You will need a few key people to support you and provide assistance, information, and guidance for breastfeeding. Your partner may not know anything about breastfeeding, but your partner is likely the person with the most potential to influence your breastfeeding journey, one way or the other. Other people on your support team might be friends, siblings, cousins, aunts, your mother, or mother-in-law (if they support breastfeeding). You may also have a local breastfeeding support group as part of your team, as well as your pediatrician (breastfeeding-friendly, of course), a lactation counselor or consultant, if necessary, a midwife, or other knowledgeable professional. Most of the time, the support team does not consist of professionals. Instead, your

team will likely be other people in your life who have experience with lactation and emotional support for new parents.

- Have you thought about meal planning for after your baby arrives? Taking time to plan a few meals (something you can freeze or have friends drop off) will be essential in the first week or two. This support can help when you learn the ropes of infant feeding because many people find it difficult to find a daily rhythm until a week or two after birth. Your "schedule" will be filled with infant care, often leaving little time for cooking. This period of adjustment applies to those feeding babies human milk or formula.
- Have you found a breastfeeding-friendly pediatrician? Talk to family and friends for recommendations. In addition, local online breastfeeding groups can be a wealth of information about local doctors.
- Have you investigated what lactation services your insurance will cover? For example, some insurance plans cover the cost of a breast pump. In addition, some plans offer a few visits with a lactation consultant, but sometimes these visits are only covered in the first few weeks of the baby's life. Check with your plan to learn more.
- Have you thought about how long you want to breastfeed? This goal is likely difficult to determine before you have any experience with breastfeeding. Because breastfeeding is an all-encompassing life experience involving you and your new baby (and your partner), it is tricky to make assumptions about how you will feel about it before your baby is born. In this case, it may be good to have some ideas about your goals for breastfeeding (in terms of months or years) but remember that you are free to change your plans later on.

If you are still thinking about many of the questions listed above but don't have answers, you may want to read this book thoroughly first. Then, go back over this list of questions. You will likely have a much better idea about approaching your breastfeeding experience after you finish this book.

CHAPTER 2

Move the Needle: Improving Worldwide Breastfeeding Rates

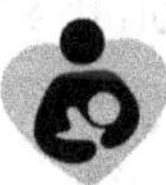

In the 1940s and '50s in the United States, Canada, and other Western countries, breastfeeding rates were in steep decline, and lactation wisdom was in jeopardy. The popularity of artificial baby formula was on the rise, and breastfeeding support was in short supply. A set of interesting circumstances converged over roughly 30 years to bring breastfeeding to its low point in the U.S. by 1970 or 1971.

By the early part of the twentieth century, childbirth had been steadily transitioning away from the home birth with midwives into the domain of managed care found in the hospital setting in the U.S. There were exceptions, especially for urban and rural families living in poverty. The transition to hospital birth created several arbitrary routines and practices that did not support breastfeeding, including infant nurseries, scheduled feeding, immediate separation of parent and child, along with formula supplementation, and extended hospital stays. In addition, as early as the 1930s, formula manufacturers were already marketing their products directly to physicians, a practice that remains common today (Wambach & Riordan, 2016). Despite the strong and contradictory research available at the time, formula manufacturers and physicians alike began equating the quality of infant formula with that of breast milk. Eventually, the social and cultural context of breastfeeding also began to change in the U.S. and elsewhere, particularly in the 1960s and '70s. Many women were seeking employment outside of the home and infant formula played a large part in facilitating the early return to work.

Interestingly, around this same time, the contraceptive pill was introduced in the U.S. In 1957, the FDA approved the pill for menstrual irregularities, and in 1960, it was available for contraception. People who chose to use estrogen-containing birth control pills were advised *not* to breastfeed for fear that the hormones from the contraception would pass into breast milk (Wambach & Riordan, 2016).

In the U.S., these factors fully converged in the early 1970s, nearly flatlining breastfeeding initiation rates. In 1971, only 24.7% of families chose to initiate breastfeeding on the first day of life (Ryan et al., 1991). Of that 24.7%, some may have also intended to use formula in conjunction with breast milk. The Ross Mothers Survey did not differentiate between exclusive breastfeeding or any breastfeeding (including mixed feeding). In addition, in 1971, most people who did choose to start breastfeeding eventually abandoned it in favor of infant formula long before their baby was six months old. In fact, by six months of age in 1971, the Ross Mothers Survey reported only 5.4% of people were still breastfeeding, and again, this might have included mixed feeding with formula too (Ryan et al., 1991). That means that more than 94% of infants in the U.S. were formula-fed during that year. Although breastfeeding initiation rates began to climb in 1972, the overwhelming use of infant formula continued throughout the 1970s.

Since then, breastfeeding has experienced a dramatic resurgence. This growth includes a major expansion of governmental and non-governmental organizations supporting a more breastfeeding-friendly agenda. As a result, today's breastfeeding initiation rates suggest that many new families in North America and worldwide are choosing human milk. Since 1971, breastfeeding rates for the *first day of life* in the U.S. have increased dramatically. Statistics from 2019 show that the U.S. national average rate for breastfeeding on the first day of life was 83.2%. While that seems like a huge improvement over the 24.7% initiation rate from 1971 (and it is), we are still lagging in breastfeeding rates for 3, 6, and 12 months. The chart below shows the U.S. states with the highest and lowest breastfeeding rates in 2019.

Table 2.1: Highest and Lowest Breastfeeding Rates in the United States, data from infants born in 2019

Highest Rates	Ever Breastfed/ Initiated Feeding	Exclusive Breastfeeding 3 months	Exclusive Breastfeeding 6 months
Alaska	92.9%	57.6%	30.9%
Colorado	94.0%	62.8%	32.1%
Idaho	93.5%	57.6%	30.4%
Minnesota	91.9%	57.5%	36.5%
Washington	93.7%	57.0%	29.5%
Wyoming	92.4%	55.3%	27.2%
Lowest Rates			
Alabama	71.1%	38.0%	21.0%
Florida	71.0%	32.4%	18.2%
Louisiana	71.1%	38.0%	22.2%
Mississippi	69.4%	31.1%	15.6%
West Virginia	59.8%	28.0%	13.8%

Source: Adapted from the CDC (2020b) Breastfeeding Report Card Using 2019 Data

While these statistics indicate substantial progress, celebrating these achievements would be premature. Consider the lowest rates on this chart for exclusive breastfeeding at six months (i.e., LA 22.2%, AL 21%, FL 18.2%, MS 15.6%, WV 13.8%) compared to the national average of breastfeeding at six months in 1971 (i.e., 5.4%).

This modest growth reflects only a 10.2% increase in exclusive breastfeeding rates at six months in Mississippi and an 8.4% increase in exclusive breastfeeding rates at six months in West Virginia *over a period of 48 years*. Worse, we are comparing exclusive breastfeeding in 2019 to the national average for any breastfeeding during 1971. Of course, the exclusive breastfeeding rate in 1971 could have been lower, but there is no way to know with the absence of exact data.

It is clear that, despite all the good work that continues to turn the tide for breastfeeding initiation and duration, there is room to improve breastfeeding rates in the U.S. and elsewhere. Yet, given this quick overview, one nagging question remains: *why?* Why do we need to improve our breastfeeding rates? To put it another way, why should we decrease our dependence on artificial infant formula?

According to UNICEF (UNICEF, 2021), only 42% of the world's infants were breastfed exclusively from birth to five months in 2018 worldwide. This rate represents a major gap in optimal infant feeding for 58% of the world's children. The lack of optimal infant feeding has swift and detrimental ramifications for everyone. In fact, the effects of suboptimal infant feeding are far-reaching, impacting multiple factors, including:

- Infant and childhood growth and development
- Maternal health and wellness
- Environmental health

Suboptimal infant feeding gives rise to suboptimal outcomes for infant health, child health, maternal health, and the environment. Clearly, we need to *move the needle* to change our infant health, maternal health, and environmental health outcomes.

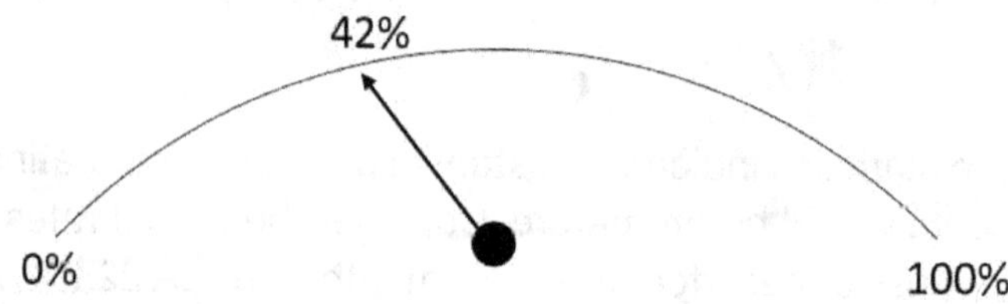

Figure 2.1: Rate of Exclusive Breastfeeding for Infants 0-5 months, Worldwide, 2018

Moving the Needle for Infant and Childhood Health, Growth, and Development

If health is the interaction between our genes and environmental input, we must consider the infant's diet as one of the most significant parts of the environmental input. Human milk and artificial human milk substitutes impact infant health and childhood health dramatically. In this chapter, we examine the known outcomes of breastfeeding and using formula.

Before we begin, I want to remind readers that my aim in including this material is not to criticize infant formula and formula users. Truth be told, I was fed formula exclusively as an infant in the 1970s. As a lactation consultant, I know many clients who have used formula in addition to breastfeeding because they have experienced issues with milk supply. I never judge others for making infant feeding choices. More importantly, it is impossible to know exactly what leads to a family's decision when choosing infant formula. Therefore, I do not judge, and I cannot claim to understand someone else's circumstances.

I do know that for many people who intend to breastfeed, the perfect storm of lactation interference factors can derail one's best intentions. I also know that many people who want to breastfeed often resort to formula, not because they want to, but because factors in their experience or lifestyle can sabotage breastfeeding. Rather than villainizing the people who use infant formula and blaming them for creating or perpetuating our dependence on artificial milk substitutes, I see this as a much larger problem associated with the aggressive and unethical marketing of infant formula and its legacy, societal attitudes toward the breast as more sexual than nurturing, and highly-managed labor and birth. These outcomes can also result from manipulative and unscrupulous marketing tactics in the infant food sector, some healthcare professionals still buying into the old model, and a lack of equitable community lactation support for every person.

Today, we are fortunate to have a viable substitute for human milk when it becomes necessary. Unfortunately, we radically overuse this alternative, which has detrimental effects on our entire society's short-term and long-term health.

Risks of Using Artificial Human Milk Substitutes - What Does the Research Say?

Many people in developed nations think of infant formula as comparable to human milk or approximately as good as human milk. However, the composition of artificial baby formula and the outcomes of the large-scale use of formula show that it is not comparable or even approximately as good as human milk. Examining the components of human milk compared to formula is beyond the scope of this book. Instead, our discussion will focus on infant and childhood health risks and outcomes associated with artificial infant formulas versus the outcomes for breastfeeding.

Infant Mortality

Infant feeding and infant mortality have a closely-linked relationship. Before the development of modern infant formulas, feeding an infant anything other than human milk usually meant certain death for the baby. While this is no longer the case, infant formulas are still associated with an elevated risk of infant death. Consider the evidence. In a recent systematic review that includes infants from all over the world, Sankar et al. (2015) compared infant mortality rates between breastfed babies and formula-fed babies. This study revealed higher *all-cause* mortality rates for formula-fed infants. The mortality rate was 14.4 times higher for formula-fed infants from birth to five months when compared with exclusively breastfed infants (Sankar et al., 2015). This research also shows the protective effect of partial breastfeeding. Specifically, infants who were partially breastfed (while receiving formula) had better outcomes than infants fed formula-only diets. In these cases, mortality rates for partially breastfed infants were 4.8 times higher than exclusively breastfed infants, an improvement over the higher mortality rates of exclusively formula-fed infants (Sankar et al., 2015). Interestingly, the higher relative risk for all-cause mortality persisted into the second year for formula-fed infants. Exclusively breastfed children, ages 1-2, had half the risk of dying compared to the formula-fed children (Sankar et al., 2015).

Breastfeeding provides infants with protection from all-cause infant death. When breastfeeding rates are low, infant mortality rates are higher than average. In other words, when formula use is dominant, infant death rates are higher. Consider this: in the United States, our highest formula feeding rates (lowest breastfeeding rates) are in the very same locations where infant mortality rates are highest. For 2019, the U.S. average for exclusive breastfeeding at three months was 45.3%, and the U.S. average infant mortality rate was 5.58 deaths per 1,000 live births. Compare those numbers with the chart below. Generally speaking, as the breastfeeding rates decline, infant mortality rates rise.

Table 2.2: Infant mortality rates and breastfeeding rates from 2019 for six U.S. states

States	Exclusive Breastfeeding Rates at 3 months	Infant Mortality Rates per 1,000 live births
U.S. National Average	45.3%	5.58
Alabama	38.0%	7.71
Arkansas	42.0%	7.0
Louisiana	38.0%	7.97
*Mississippi	31.1%	8.71
Oklahoma	43.1%	7.0
West Virginia	28.0%	6.12

Source: Adapted from Ely et al., 2021, & CDC Breastfeeding Report Card, data from 2019

*In 2019, Mississippi had the highest infant mortality rate and the second lowest exclusive breastfeeding rate at 3 months. Obviously, infant feeding is not the only factor impacting infant mortality rates, but it is an important element of the complex infant mortality puzzle.

Racial Disparities, Infant Mortality, and Breastfeeding

No discussion of breastfeeding and infant death rates can exclude mention of the stark racial disparities in the U.S. In the introduction, I note that the deck is stacked against some minority groups regarding breastfeeding. For numerous and complex reasons, many minority groups in the U.S. have depressed breastfeeding rates. Not surprisingly, the groups with the lowest breastfeeding rates, including African Americans, Native Americans, Alaskan Natives, Pacific Islanders, and Native Hawaiians, all experience higher infant mortality rates than the national average. The infant mortality rates for these groups are also higher than mortality rates for Hispanic people, non-Hispanic white people, and Asian Americans. Of these three groups, Asian Americans have the lowest infant mortality rates. Not surprisingly, this group exhibits high breastfeeding rates in many U.S. states. Again, this does not suggest that lack of breastfeeding is the only factor in the increased risk for infant death. Still, it is indeed one part of the picture. For Mississippi in 2017, the mortality rate for the entire state was an alarming 8.73 per 1,000 live births (Centers for Disease Control, 2020). For the Black infants born in Mississippi in 2017, the mortality rate was 11.9 (MDH, 2018). To be clear, the infant mortality rate for African Americans in Mississippi was more than double the national average in 2017. To put this in perspective for world health, Japan's infant mortality rate in 2017 was 1.9, and that same year, Finland reported an infant mortality rate of 2.0. In the U.S., our current lowest infant mortality rates are just over 3 per 1,000 live births in places like New Hampshire and Massachusetts (Ely et al., 2021). Mississippi and other places with low breastfeeding rates and alarmingly high infant mortality rates would benefit dramatically from reducing the use of infant formula by supporting breastfeeding for all people. This effort should include a focus on supporting lactation in culturally competent ways from birth to weaning for groups with high infant mortality rates.

Sudden Infant Death Syndrome (SIDS or cot death, crib death)

Although infant mortality rate statistics include Sudden Infant Death syndrome (SIDS), it is worth mentioning here because of the clear relationship between infant feeding methods and SIDS. Specifically, there is an increased risk of sudden infant death that is not explained by other causes when infants receive artificial baby formula. Breastfeeding offers protection from SIDS (Ip et al., 2009; Moon & Hauck, 2016; Vennemann et al., 2009). One study showed that infants fed formula had double the risk of dying from SIDS compared to infants who were breastfed (Vennemann et al., 2009). Other studies highlight breastfeeding as protective and indicate that breastfeeding has a dose-response effect on SIDS risk. In other words, more breastfeeding offers more protection, and the protection is stronger when there is no use of formula (Hauck et al., 2011). Many voices promoting the Safe to Sleep campaign (known initially as Back to Sleep), which seeks to reduce SIDS, want to focus on infant sleep arrangements, sleeping environment, bed-sharing practices, and other related factors. However, it is essential to remember that breastfeeding is a significant and modifiable element of SIDS risk factors (Moon & Hauck, 2016), reducing the SIDS risk by about 50% (Vennemann et al., 2009).

A 2017 study of more than 2000 SIDS cases published in the journal *Pediatrics* compared the use of breastfeeding versus formula with SIDS deaths. The authors of this study found that limited breastfeeding (two months of breastfeeding or less) did not protect infants from SIDS (Thompson et al., 2017). However, this study found that the duration of breastfeeding (length in terms of weeks or months) impacted the incidence of SIDS. Specifically, a longer duration of breastfeeding provides better protection from SIDS (Thompson et al., 2017).

Infant Illness and Infection

Infant mortality is not the only outcome linked to the overuse of artificial infant formulas. Formula feeding influences a variety of additional infections and illnesses. The discussion below highlights many of these illnesses, but this is not an exhaustive list.

Respiratory Illness

One of the leading causes of hospitalization of infants and young children is respiratory infections. There are many respiratory infections and ailments that are common among infants and children. For example, upper respiratory illness includes throat, ears, nose, and sinus infections. Lower respiratory infections include the windpipe, bronchial tubes, and the lungs. Respiratory illness can manifest as the common cold, cough, sinus infection, runny nose, sore throat, tonsillitis, laryngitis, nasal congestion, ear infection, bronchitis, pneumonia, and influenza. These can be life-threatening conditions for some infants, especially immunocompromised, small for gestational age, low birth weight, and premature infants.

Studies show that infant formula use is significantly associated with an increased risk of upper and lower respiratory infections. For example:

- A study of over 15,000 infants in the UK who were either exclusively breastfed, partially breastfed, or not breastfed showed that *not* breastfeeding increased the risk of hospitalization in the first eight months of life for lower respiratory infections (Quigley et al., 2007).
- Infant formula use in the first year of life is associated with a significantly increased risk for lower respiratory infections later in childhood, but breastfeeding reduces the risk for such infections. In fact, one study found that breastfeeding during the first six months of life was significantly associated with a reduction in the risk of lower respiratory infections four years later (Tromp et al., 2017).
- Exclusive use of infant formula is associated with higher rates of ear infections. For example, Frank et al. (2019) found that exclusive breastfeeding lowers the risk of ear infections, even after breastfeeding has stopped, up to 4 years of age.

- A study of premature infants of low birth weight found that not breastfeeding increased the risk of hospitalization due to respiratory illness for infants with low birth weight (Miller et al., 2012)burden of illness, and risk factors for human rhinoviruses (HRVs.

It is important to note that breastfeeding is not the only variable factor that can greatly impact infant risk for respiratory illness. For example, research indicates that prenatal and postnatal exposure to smoking increases the risk of respiratory illnesses and complications for infants.

Diarrhea and NEC

Infant formula raises the risk of diarrhea among babies. In addition, because powdered infant formula requires mixing with water, there is a chance that contaminated water can introduce pathogens into the infant's gut. For this reason, powdered infant formula is considered unsafe for infants under the age of two months, infants of low birth weight, premature infants, and those who are immunocompromised. In addition, bottles that are not properly cleaned or sanitized (if necessary) are also vehicles for introducing pathogens to an infant.

In addition to the risks posed by contaminated water or equipment, there is a risk of contamination in the powdered formula, including *cronobactor sakazakii*, a pathogen that can cause a severe infection in infants. Cronobactor, formerly called *enterobacter sakazakii*, can cause necrotizing enterocolitis (NEC). NEC causes bowel tissue inflammation and tissue death. NEC is a serious concern for any infant, especially those immunocompromised, extremely low birth weight, or premature. There is a greater risk of NEC for infants of low birth weight when breastfeeding is absent (Kair & Colaizy, 2016).

Crohn's Disease and Ulcerative Colitis

Breastfeeding is protective against Crohn's disease and ulcerative colitis, with the protection being dose dependent. Studies show that breastfeeding for 12 months offers more protection, especially for Crohn's disease, when compared to breastfeeding for shorter durations (Xu et al., 2017).

Childhood Cancers

Leukemia and lymphoma are two childhood cancers affecting the function of blood cells and the lymphatic system, respectively. Large meta-analysis studies show that lack of breastfeeding increases the risk of these cancers.

- A large meta-analysis study indicates that breastfeeding for six months or more lowers the risk for childhood leukemia by 19% (Amitay et al., 2016).
- Breastfeeding accounts for a modestly lower risk of childhood Hodgkin lymphoma (Wang et al., 2013).

Type 1 Diabetes

Type 1 diabetes (formerly called juvenile diabetes) is a chronic condition of the pancreas, causing reduced insulin levels, which leads to high levels of blood glucose. There is evidence that breastfeeding lowers the risk of type 1 diabetes in children.

- A large study of 155,392 Norwegian and Danish children showed a twofold increased risk of developing type 1 diabetes among children who had never breastfed (Lund-Blix et al., 2017).
- An extensive systematic review initiated by the U.S. Departments of Agriculture and Health and Human Services also showed that less human milk feeding or none at all raises the risk for type 1 diabetes (Güngör et al., 2019).

Asthma

Asthma is a condition that involves the chronic inflammation of the airway, causing difficulty breathing. According to the CDC, asthma is increasing among children and adults in the U.S. each year. There are several theories about the increasing rates of asthma, including 1) exposure to air pollution, 2) the role of genetics and family history of asthma, 3) lower vitamin D rates, 4) higher overweight and obesity rates, 5) higher cesarean delivery rates, 6) overuse of antibiotics, 7) less exposure to childhood illnesses, 8) exposure to smoking and secondhand smoke, and 9) exposure to dust mites and mold.

Breastfeeding can reduce the risk of childhood asthma.

- Formula-fed infants have lower gastrointestinal bacterial diversity, which is associated with a greater risk of developing asthma (Oddy, 2017).
- No breastfeeding or short duration of breastfeeding is associated with a greater risk of asthma (Güngör et al., 2019b).

Obesity

Childhood obesity is a substantial public health concern in many developed countries, including the United States. The CDC defines obesity by using the Body Mass Index (BMI), a ratio of weight to height. The CDC defines overweight individuals as having a BMI at or above the 85th percentile. The CDC defines obese individuals as having a BMI at or above the 95th percentile. Data from 2015-2016 reveals alarmingly high rates of childhood obesity in the U.S.; obesity among children ages 2 to 5 was 13.9%, and obesity among children ages 6 to 11 was 18.4% (Hales et al., 2017). Obesity is a danger for children (and people of any age) because it is associated with other problematic health conditions like sleep apnea, high blood pressure, diabetes, cardiovascular disease, joint disorders, kidney disease, liver problems, and early puberty. According to UNICEF, from 2000-2016, the percentage of children ages 5 to 19 worldwide who were considered overweight or obese rose from 10% to nearly 20% (UNICEF, 2019).

Obesity and overweight conditions are not limited to children over age 2. There are situations where infants might be obese. Studies show that children diagnosed as obese at 24 months were more likely to have been obese at only 6 months of age (McCormick et al., 2010).

Consider these research findings on breastfeeding and obesity.

- Breastfeeding helps prevent childhood obesity and thus, contributes to preventing a host of other non-communicable diseases associated with obesity in later life (Uwaezuoke et al., 2017).
- Several theories exist on the nature of how breastfeeding prevents obesity. One theory suggests that the composition of infant formula, contributing to higher protein intake, accounts for the greater risk of obesity (Taylor et al., 2005). Other studies suggest that the hormone *leptin* (found in human milk) inhibits

obesity. Leptin is responsible for energy balance and satiety, which signals the body to turn off hunger cues (Miralles et al., 2006; Palou & Picó, 2009).

- Another theory suggests that infants who feed at the breast can self-regulate their own intake with internal cues. Interestingly, research shows that bottle-fed infants (early in life) were more likely to finish a bottle or cup in later infancy (Liu et al., 2010). If so, perhaps family feeding patterns of encouraging an infant to finish the bottle in early infancy persist and supplant the internal cues of satiation.
- Other theories suggest a strong link between overfeeding infant formula and obesity. A fascinating study investigating the overuse of formula among infants revealed that overfed infants (who received more than 30ml at one feed) during the first day of life were significantly more likely to be characterized as overweight or obese four years later (Watchmaker et al., 2020). This study suggests that feeding babies with an inappropriate volume in the first 24 hours of life is associated with excess weight gain over time. Interestingly, breastfeeding solves this riddle because colostrum, the human milk available on days one and two before the transition to mature milk, is only available in tiny amounts. Some estimates suggest that in the first 24 hours of life, a healthy, full-term breastfed infant only takes in 2-5 ml of colostrum per feeding (Kellams et al., 2017). In the study mentioned above, some formula-fed infants took 30 ml at a single feeding on the first day of life (Watchmaker et al., 2020). The study reports the overfeeding of 93% of infants, at least once, during the first 24 hours after birth. Similarly, the study reports the overfeeding of 71% of infants during three of their first seven feedings (Watchmaker et al., 2020). In other instances, there were reports of *overfeeding at each feeding on the first day of life*. The study results suggest that overfed infants (at each of their first seven feedings) were seven times more likely to be classified as overweight or obese four years later (Watchmaker et al., 2020).
- Bottle size is also an issue with increased human milk or formula intake among infants. Those who use bottles for pumped human

> milk find that paced bottle feeding with small volumes of milk and slow flow nipples helps normalize the amount of milk an infant takes in when bottle feeding. For example, in a study of formula-fed infants, larger bottle size correlated with larger formula intake, on average four ounces more per day than infants using smaller bottles (Wood et al., 2016). The authors state that this risk of overfeeding may put some formula-fed infants at risk of obesity (Wood et al., 2016).

Obesity is a complex issue, and it seems intuitive that one factor alone is not the single cause of childhood (or adult) obesity. However, what is clear is that there is mounting evidence that exclusive breastfeeding for the first six months of life puts in place many factors that help to prevent overweight and obese conditions in childhood and later life (Twells et al., 2012).

Maternal & Family Health Outcomes

Breastfeeding is optimal for infant growth and development, but it is equally advantageous for maternal health. The positive effects of breastfeeding are not only for those who commit to a long-term breastfeeding path. In fact, valuable impacts of lactation begin for maternal health moments after birth, immediately when breastfeeding begins. Let's examine some of the most important maternal and family health outcomes.

Preventing Postpartum Hemorrhage

Postpartum hemorrhage (PPH) is one of the leading causes of maternal death following childbirth. PPH is increasing worldwide and may be related to the increasing use of obstetric interventions (Rossen et al., 2010). PPH is defined as blood loss of more than 500 ml following a vaginal birth and 1000-1500 ml following cesarean delivery. The risk of hemorrhage is high in the period between the birth of the baby and the birth of the placenta. However, hemorrhage can occur any time in the first 24 hours after birth (primary hemorrhage) or the weeks following birth (secondary hemorrhage).

There are several risks factors for PPH. Uterine atony (failure of the uterus to contract) is the leading risk factor for hemorrhage following childbirth. Risk of atony, loss of tone or strength of a muscle, increases with labor induction, long labor, and administration of Pitocin (synthetic oxytocin) during labor. Breastfeeding and immediate skin-to-skin care with your newborn can reduce the risk of postpartum hemorrhage (Saxton et al., 2015). It also promotes maternal oxytocin release (endogenous oxytocin made by the body), which helps the uterine muscle contract, forcing blood vessels in the uterine wall to close.

Other treatments for PPH include administration of Pitocin (through IV or injection) and active management of the third stage of labor with cord traction (gentle pulling on the umbilical cord). Unfortunately, despite these practices being widespread and standard care, PPH continues to increase.

Diabetes

Diabetes is a complex chronic condition in which blood sugar levels are abnormally high and are not controlled well by the body. Type I diabetes can be autoimmune-related, whereas type II diabetes is closely related to obesity and lifestyle factors. Type I and type II diabetes can occur in any person, male or female, of any age. Gestational diabetes mellitus (GDM) is a type of diabetes that manifests only during pregnancy. The worldwide incidence of GDM is increasing, and people with GDM have an increased risk of developing type II diabetes later in life (Much et al., 2014). In fact, the risk of developing type II diabetes is seven times higher for those who experience GDM during pregnancy versus those who do not (Much et al., 2014). Breastfeeding reduces maternal diabetes risk later in life. Consider the following:

- A recent meta-analysis revealed that breastfeeding for more than 12 months can reduce the risk for maternal diabetes by as much as 30% (Rameez et al., 2019).
- People with a history of gestational diabetes have a lowered risk of developing type II diabetes later in life after breastfeeding, and a longer duration of breastfeeding offers more protection (Ley et al., 2020).
- People who give birth but do not breastfeed have a 50% greater risk of developing diabetes when compared to people who have not given birth (Liu et al., 2010). However, breastfeeding lowers the risk significantly.

- For people with type I diabetes, breastfeeding can lower insulin requirements (Davies et al., 1989; Riviello et al., 2009).

Female Cancers - Breast, Ovarian, Endometrial

Of all cancers, breast cancer is the most frequently diagnosed. Men can also develop breast cancer. Despite relative improvements in breast cancer treatments over the last few decades, breast cancer remains a leading cause of death among women in the U.S., Canada, UK, and Australia. Endometrial cancer, cancer of the uterus lining, is not as common as breast cancer but remains a leading cause of death among women. Endometrial cancer is associated with obesity and diabetes, which may account for the increasing incidence of this cancer in recent decades. Ovarian cancer forms in the ovaries, often with no symptoms in the beginning stages of the disease. Ovarian cancer is associated with more menstrual periods over a lifetime. The links between breastfeeding and cancer are multifaceted. Consider the following evidence:

- *Not* breastfeeding increases breast cancer risk (Holm et al., 2017).
- Exclusive breastfeeding offers more protection from developing breast cancer than non-exclusive feeding (Unar-Munguía et al., 2017).
- Knowledge of breast cancer risk reduction influences the decision to breastfeed for some people. Still, one study showed that only 16.6% of patients received this information from their healthcare provider (Ganju et al., 2018).
- No breastfeeding or abrupt cessation of breastfeeding (resulting in involution, pruning back the milk-making cells) raises inflammation. It also increases cell proliferation and other known risk factors for the development of breast cancer (Basree et al., 2019).
- The World Cancer Research Fund, the CDC, and the American Cancer Society recognize that *not* breastfeeding is a risk factor for breast cancer. All of these organizations recommend that people breastfeed their children if they are able.
- The mechanism by which breastfeeding protects against breast cancer is not well known. However, some researchers theorize

that breastfeeding reduces lifetime exposure to menstrual cycles (via lactational amenorrhea), promoting healthier breast tissue.

- Breastfeeding reduces the risk of invasive ovarian cancer by as much as 24% (Babic et al., 2020; Sasamoto et al., 2019). In addition, a longer duration of breastfeeding is associated with lowered risk of ovarian cancer compared to shorter durations of lactation (Sasamoto et al., 2019).
- Breastfeeding provides at least an 11% reduction in risk of endometrial cancer, and longer durations of lactation provide further reduced risk (Jordan et al., 2017).

Cardiovascular Disease and Hypertension

Cardiovascular disease (CVD) is the leading cause of death in the U.S. and Australia. It is the second leading cause of death in the U.K. and Canada. Cardiovascular disease is a catch-all term for describing a group of conditions related to the heart, blood vessels, and circulatory system. Examples of cardiovascular conditions include stroke, coronary artery disease, heart failure, carditis, etc. Hypertension, also called high blood pressure, is related to cardiovascular disease and is a known risk factor for CVD. According to the CDC, hypertension affects half of all adults in the U.S. Breastfeeding reduces the risks for CVD and hypertension. Consider the following:

- In a large study of over 63,000 people, any breastfeeding (mixed or exclusive) for at least four months or more was associated with a risk reduction for CVD and hypertension from 20-30% compared to those who breastfed for less than four months (Kirkegaard et al., 2018).
- People who encounter pregnancy complications (e.g., high blood pressure, gestational diabetes, preterm delivery) experience lower cardiovascular risk factors after six months of breastfeeding (Yu et al., 2019). This finding is significant because there is a known link between pregnancy complications and maternal CVD risks later in life (Armeni et al., 2019).
- Breastfeeding decreases the risk for maternal hypertension (high blood pressure) after pregnancy, and the effects are long-term, lasting for decades (Bonifacino et al., 2018).

- Breastfeeding impacts for maternal hypertension in later life are dose-dependent like many other maternal health outcomes. In other words, the duration of breastfeeding can impact the intensity of health outcomes and protective effects. For example, a large meta-analysis of over 444,000 people showed a substantial protective effect against hypertension for people who breastfed for greater than 12 months versus those who breastfed for less than 12 months (Qu et al., 2018).

Lactation as Birth Control

Exclusive breastfeeding for the first six months of life can suppress ovulation and provide effective birth control. This approach to birth control is known as the Lactational Amenorrhea Method (LAM). It is temporary birth control for the first six months postpartum.

Three conditions must be in place to consider using LAM as birth control (98-99% effective).

1. The infant is exclusively breastfed on demand around the clock and receives no other supplements, water, or food.
2. The baby is not yet six months old.
3. After the lochia (postpartum bleeding) has stopped, menstrual periods have not returned. This includes spotting or any type of breakthrough bleeding.

If one meets these conditions, LAM is effective as birth control. Once any of these conditions are no longer in place, backup birth control is necessary. Lactational Amenorrhea Method is sensitive to abrupt changes in breastfeeding patterns and can be disrupted by lengthening out time between feeding sessions, such as when an infant under six months of age unexpectedly sleeps longer stretches at night.

LAM has several advantages over hormonal birth control. First, LAM is available and effective immediately after breastfeeding begins. In addition, it is free, and no prescription is necessary. Best of all, it is non-hormonal and will not interfere with your milk production as many hormonal types of birth control can. Be aware that while this may be an effective approach to birth control, it will not protect against sexually transmitted diseases.

More Optimal Child Spacing

Child spacing refers to the time interval between the birth of one child and the next child for the same person. Due to the natural way lactation suppresses ovulation, children born before the advent of infant formula were typically spaced at least two years apart (Jackson, 1988)1988. However, during the transition to infant formula and abandonment of breastfeeding in the U.S., 1930-1960, the length of child spacing decreased by about one year (Jackson, 1988). Shorter intervals between births can have negative impacts on maternal and infant health.

When infants are born closely following the birth of an older sibling, they are at risk of adverse neonatal outcomes (Conde-Agudelo et al., 2006). Children born with shortened birth intervals (generally 18 months or less) are at greater risk of these complications:

- Small for gestational age
- Preterm birth
- Low birth weight

Each of these conditions is associated with increased needs for observation, care, and attention, especially when it comes to infant feeding. Depending on the severity, these complications can greatly impact breastfeeding and early infancy (e.g., very low birth weight, preterm birth). Exclusive breastfeeding for the first six months of life (and gradual addition of solid foods after that) can help suppress ovulation. Some people may experience lactational a menorrhea for more than 12 months following childbirth. Although LAM should only be used as birth control when an infant is under six months of age, *ovulation may not resume precisely at six months postpartum.* Ovulation and regular menstrual periods may not return until later in the first postpartum year or even later for some people. It is this effect on fertility that naturally creates longer birth intervals. It is worth mentioning here that ovulation can occur before the return of the first postpartum menstrual bleeding. Do not assume that because your period has not returned, you cannot conceive. Abrupt changes in breastfeeding patterns can bring on ovulation. Be aware of your fertility signs throughout the first postpartum year and use backup birth control if necessary.

Maternal health is also impacted by shorter birth intervals. Consider these outcomes:

- Shorter birth intervals are associated with precipitous labor (speedy labor, which has its own risks).
- There is more risk of maternal obesity with the subsequent pregnancy if the length between one birth and the next is short (Hutcheon et al., 2019).
- Short birth interval increases the risk of gestational diabetes in the subsequent pregnancy (Hutcheon et al., 2019).
- With shorter birth intervals, the risk of uterine rupture is greater for people attempting a VBAC (vaginal birth after cesarean) (Conde-Agudelo et al., 2007).
- Other complications include placenta previa, placental abruption (Conde-Agudelo et al., 2007), anemia, and a greater risk of maternal death (Conde-Agudelo, 2000).

Environmental Impacts of Unsustainable Infant Feeding

Sustainability is an incredibly important topic, but people rarely consider the issue of sustainable infant feeding. This is not simply an infant health or maternal health issue that affects a person for some finite amount of time in the childbearing years. Instead, sustainable infant feeding and the risks of unsustainable infant feeding are global health issues, climate issues, natural resource sustainability issues, and food security issues that affect every single person on earth whether they choose human milk feeding or not. There is a steep cost to pay for unsustainable infant feeding for every person on the planet, even those who are childless.

Before we dive into the details of unsustainable infant feeding, I need to address one myth that consistently comes up in breastfeeding versus formula feeding discussions, especially concerning sustainability. Many have promoted breastfeeding as more sustainable because it is *free*. But is it really free?

After several years of feeding my own children at the breast, I can say for sure that breastfeeding is most certainly not free. Every part of the production and delivery of human milk has a cost. For me (and many people who have chosen to breastfeed), most of the cost was associated with my time and energy, neither of which are "free."

Let's consider the factor of time. The total time it takes to nurse a newborn is quite different from the time spent nursing a 12-month-old. It is intense during the early months and changes somewhat over time and after introducing complementary foods. Nonetheless, it is a substantial investment of time over the first 12 months. One person calculated and posted on Instagram a rough estimate of the time spent feeding her baby at the breast for one year. Her 12-month breastfeeding time logged in as 1,825 hours. If this were equivalent to a 40-hour week full-time job, it would equal slightly more than 45 weeks of work. There is more time involved if you are occasionally pumping in addition to nursing at the breast because this requires a few extras like milk storing, cleaning, and maintaining the pump and bottles.

Strictly speaking, in terms of time, 1,825 hours of infant feeding in the year following birth is quite an investment. But that is not the whole story. Parenthood itself (in the U.S. and anywhere, paid maternity leave is not a guarantee) brings with it a penalty of lost wages and missed opportunities. No matter if people breastfeed or choose formula, statistics show that in the year following the birth of a child, American mothers suffer wage losses (Glauber, 2018) due to a variety of reasons. Researchers refer to this phenomenon as the "motherhood wage penalty." Interestingly, some subtle nuances regarding the motherhood wage penalty are curiously aligned with the infant feeding method. For example, research shows that people who breastfeed longer often have more earnings loss in the year after childbirth than people who breastfeed less or not at all (Rippey & Noonan, 2012). This outcome may be due to longer periods of maternity leave taken by those who intend to breastfeed longer, but that is undoubtedly not the only factor. Of course, paid maternity leave for all people in the U.S. would likely solve that issue, but we do not have guaranteed paid maternity leave for all workers.

Whether calculated as wages or not, the value of your time is not the only factor to consider. Energy is yet another matter. Many estimates claim that a person making milk needs an additional 400-500 calories per day. The actual amount of extra energy required to produce milk will differ depending on several variables: degree of exclusive breastfeeding, amount of body fat stores available as an energy reserve, and whether tandem feeding (toddler and newborn or multiples) or not. The extra energy required for milk production translates into extra calories for the one's diet, increasing the weekly grocery bill slightly. So, although the infant's meal appears to be free (because there is no need to purchase milk), it costs slightly more to feed a nursing parent than one who is not nursing.

In addition, breastfeeding for many parents usually involves extra supplies. The gear for breastfeeding often includes nursing bras, nursing shirts, breast pumps (electric and manual), nipple ointment, nursing pillows, milk storage containers, bottles, breast pads, nipple shields, vitamins, teas, and so on. Although some of the lactation gear can be considered optional and even unnecessary, much of it is helpful, and some gear is not optional in certain circumstances. Consider the breast pump. Some people can nurse a baby from birth to weaning and never need a breast pump (people have done this for millennia). Others rely on a high-quality pump five days a week and could not make use of human milk without it. Other parents find that they are exclusive pumpers, using the pump to express milk every single session! The reality is that most people who choose to breastfeed will encounter the need for some extra gear, even if it is the most basic (bras, breast pads, breast pump). The cost of breastfeeding gear will vary widely from family to family but none of it is free.

Finally, there is a cost for breastfeeding education and support. For breastfeeding to work well, people must learn the basics of human milk production. Face-to-face and online classes are good options, and most are fee-based. Buying an informative breastfeeding book is also a great option, but this too has a cost. Additionally, it is equally important to have access to skilled care for breastfeeding, which can sometimes be expensive if not covered by insurance. Ironically, it is precisely because of the dominance of infant formula for many decades that communal knowledge of lactation nearly disappeared. This is, indeed, why people today spend money on breastfeeding books, breastfeeding classes, and skilled lactation care.

Consequently, while breastfeeding is sustainable, it is not sustainable because it is free. We usually place a high price on our time, physical resources, and energy. Why devalue that by saying that breastfeeding is free? I look back proudly on the years I spent making milk and feeding it to my children. It took a hell of a lot of information, skill-building, time, energy, and support for me to achieve my breastfeeding goals. There is no way that I am looking back at that experience and calling it "free." If we truly respected the actual work, time, and energy parents put into infant feeding, we would never refer to it as free.

Sustainable Infant Feeding

We have established that producing human milk does have costs but the costs do not include directly using environmental resources to create the final product. Aside from the costs associated with adequate food and drink to fuel the lactation process, there is no cost for agriculture, manufacturing and processing, packaging, transportation, marketing, and sales. So, consider this: instead of using valuable natural resources in its production, *human milk is a valuable natural resource.*

Let's briefly examine the environmental costs associated with artificial formula.

- Companies create most infant formulas with powdered cow's milk. As a result, the dairy industry is the foundation of formula manufacturing. The dairy industry is well known for overusing natural resources and contributing pollution to the environment.
- The dairy industry has a huge water footprint and creating powdered cow's milk is particularly water intensive. Some estimates say it takes several thousand liters of water to produce one kilogram of powdered milk, which serves as the base for formula's recipe.
- Dairy production requires land for cattle grazing and the growth and harvest of other food additives that create formula, such as palm oil, other vegetable oils, corn syrup, etc.
- The dairy industry contributes an alarming 30% of the world's greenhouse gas in the form of methane, produced when the

cows pass gas. (Yes, infant formula would not be possible without cow farts.) Unfortunately, methane gas is highly effective as a greenhouse gas, contributing substantially to climate change.

- The world's infant formula manufacturing occurs in 40-50 facilities, which means the formula must travel long distances to be sold at retailers worldwide. These transportation and fuel costs add to the unsustainability factor of artificial infant formula. In addition, the supply chain disruptions of 2021 and 2022 revealed the fragile nature of distribution for infant formula, contributing to its unsustainability.
- Formula packaging creates waste. Companies routinely package powdered formula in metal containers, while ready-to-feed formula arrives in single-use plastic containers. 2009 estimates suggest that consumers threw 550 million cans of infant formula into landfills that year, and since then, the formula industry has more than doubled in size (Joffe et al., 2019). This industry growth means the waste produced at every level of manufacturing and packaging has also more than doubled.
- People who use formula exclusively do not benefit from lactational amenorrhea, which means there is no break from menstrual periods following childbirth. This contributes to the use of menstrual products, and collectively, the waste produced each month from the feminine hygiene industry is staggering. About 3.5 million singleton babies were born in 2020 in the U.S. If only 25% of these parents breastfed exclusively enough to prevent ovulation, that would equate to 875,000 people with lactational amenorrhea after childbirth and thus, reduce waste from pads and tampons. Consider this; if the average person uses about 20 tampons per month, lactational amenorrhea (absent periods due to breastfeeding) saves approximately 17,500,000 tampons per month that otherwise would be in landfills. At this same rate, we could save 210 million tampons from arriving in landfills annually.

Human milk uses none of the earth's natural resources. There is no packaging required. There are no transportation costs. There are no supply chain disruptions. It creates no waste. Lactation does not produce greenhouse gases. Lactational amenorrhea saves millions of tampons and pads annually from going into the landfill. Human milk is the only truly sustainable infant food choice.

What is the Formula for Change?

We need to move the needle to increase our dependence on human milk and decrease our reliance on artificial formula. The world is ready for the long-overdue shift back to human milk feeding and the minimization of commercial infant formula. But how do we get there? How can we move forward when there are clear and present barriers to breastfeeding for so many people worldwide?

The answer to shifting the balance away from formula and back to breastfeeding is so complex that it could fill an entire book of its own. There are no easy solutions or "magic bullet" tactics that will quickly counterbalance years of formula feeding. The hurdles we need to overcome are significant but not insurmountable. In her 2011 Call to Action statement, former U.S. Surgeon General Dr. Regina Benjamin compiled a comprehensive list of strategies to help improve breastfeeding rates and support nursing mothers and their families. Here are five critical steps, some echoing Dr. Benjamin's recommendations, that could accelerate the move to embrace human milk feeding.

1. End the marketing of infant formula.
2. Assure that every person who gives birth has follow-up lactation care, similar to delivering postpartum care. This care should include several lactation visits in the first weeks after birth. Delivering this type of early lactation support is where the U.S. fails.
3. Expand breastfeeding education for new parents, their partners, and grandparents. Through community-based education programs, new parents and family members can get the up-to-date information they need about breastfeeding management and support. Dr. Benjamin outlines the need to educate parents, partners, fathers, and grandparents to provide critical and necessary support for human milk feeding. Remember, the family and social network heavily influence breastfeeding decisions.

4. Expand the breastfeeding education curriculum for every medical professional who works with breastfeeding families. The medical personnel who care for new parents and babies should have a solid education in human lactation and training to support breastfeeding.
5. Guarantee several months of paid leave for all parents following childbirth or adoption.

Decreasing our dependence on infant formula is entirely possible. In fact, most of the infrastructure that will facilitate and enable more people to breastfeed throughout the first year is already in place. Working to eliminate the roadblocks and challenges will undoubtedly reap positive changes if there is significant support from all levels of healthcare, lactation care, and infant care. There are no downsides to improving breastfeeding rates. We simply need to make it our priority and fund the efforts to make it happen.

CHAPTER 3

Lactation Promotion Factors: Protecting Your Potential

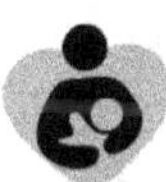

Creating and sustaining a full milk supply is a balancing act, but it is not enough to avoid the lactation interference factors (discussed in Part II). A good approach also incorporates careful attention to the lactation promotion factors. Here, we examine many of the ways you can protect and promote your milk supply from the moment your baby is born (and even before).

Before I get too deep into the aspects of lactation promotion, I want to stress that not every person has to incorporate every last one of these factors into practice to have breastfeeding success. Remember that success is defined differently for each of us because we all have our own specific goals.

As I mentioned in the introduction, breastfeeding outcomes are a compilation of the hand you were dealt and the cards you picked up as experiences. Your breastfeeding outcomes reflect a complex balancing act between your lactation promotion factors and your lactation interference factors. To be clear, you need many more positive factors than negative ones. However, the idea here is not to prescribe that you must do all these things. You can choose to incorporate all of them if you want, but most people cannot or do not because of, well, the circumstances of life.

If you are 100% wedded to the idea that you must have an epidural during labor, even though it could lead to lactation interference, do it. I am not going to say no to that. If you want it, own it and own the potential outcomes. Just know that you must specifically focus on lactation promotion factors to build and maintain a healthy and plentiful milk supply. If you choose to have birth interventions or get to a place in labor where it becomes necessary to use interventions, recognize that you might need extra support to mitigate some of the downstream effects in the days and weeks following birth.

We all choose a different path to parenting and breastfeeding. Most parents do not even choose the same path with their all of their own children because people learn, grow, and change along the parenting journey. We tend to do better when we know better, and for most of us, it is not possible to know everything during our first birth experience, our first attempt at lactation, and our first time as a parent. There isn't one perfect way to feed human milk to your baby; there are hundreds of ways to do it right. Think of this like the *Choose Your Own Adventure* books – you are in charge of your outcomes. I am showing you the options, and you get to choose. No judgment.

Lactation Promotion Factors: The Stuff That Makes Breastfeeding Work

Attention: not all factors are created equal. Some of these will have a much greater impact on lactation and breastfeeding than others. I indicate the high impact factors with this notation: **High Impact!**

Before birth:

- Take steps to plan a low or no intervention birth. Many "routine birth interventions" can harm lactation, and most of the time, caregivers do not discuss the downstream effects of birth interventions as they relate to lactation. One minor birth intervention may not derail your breastfeeding efforts but be cautious. Usually, one intervention leads to another. There is a reason why it is called t*he cascade of interventions*. (I discuss the impacts of birth interventions in Part II of this book.) **High Impact!**
- Be sure to get good prenatal care.
- Take a good quality childbirth class – one that will teach you natural coping techniques for labor. This course is likely not the class offered by the hospital. I am not criticizing the hospital or their courses in any way but think about it; what

they want and what you want during your birth experience are likely to be different things (aside from a healthy baby). Your need for a low stress, low intervention birth is usually in direct opposition to their agenda. They want speed, cooperation, and predictability. None of these things come with a more natural approach because birth takes time and is highly variable from one person to the next. With the addition of Pitocin and pain medications, birth can and does often become more predictable. As you will see, the predictability that Pitocin and epidurals provide comes with a price. To some people, these interventions may be nice for labor, but those same interventions and drugs do have consequences for breastfeeding. Therefore, it pays to prepare for a low or no intervention birth. This type of birth usually does not simply *happen,* especially in the hospital setting. One has to plan for it. You will need some skills and support for this type of birth experience.

- Let go of the fear model of childbirth. Don't let fear get the best of you, and do not let it drive your plan or choices. If your worries stem from the idea of coping with labor, seek alternative skills that can help you cope. I am not advocating that we must suffer through birth. Some people find that natural coping techniques are enough. Some people find that they plan a drug-free birth but change their minds during labor after trying natural coping techniques for a time. Some people need to know that they can get pain relief as soon as they need it. All of these are okay; there is no reason to suffer, but drugs do not have to be the first choice for comfort measures. They can be the last resort if you plan for that. Remember, for some people, labor and birth are exhilarating. Think of it as climbing a mountain or doing a triathlon. Of course, there are some difficult parts, but people choose to do these challenges because they are also exhilarating. Birth is similar, but you have to listen to your body and follow your own cues and instincts. These actions can be tough to do if you're confined to a bed, lying on your back, unable to feel or follow your instincts.

- Read about and talk to people who have had positive drug-free birth experiences. This information can go a long way to expanding your view of what is possible during labor and of your own abilities. Have you ever heard that labor and birth can be positively life-changing? Many people discover their true power and potential for the first time in their lives while giving birth.
- In the days leading up to 39 weeks, your caregiver may raise the topic of labor induction. Be wary of inductions and even the do-it-yourself natural labor-inducing techniques that you can do at home or away from the clinical setting. These techniques are *not guaranteed* to bring on labor. In fact, even with medical interventions at the hospital, your labor is more likely to start only *if the time is right*. Unless there is a compelling reason, buy yourself more time. Avoid elective induction at all costs. **High Impact!**
- Learn to clearly communicate when care providers confront you with an ultimatum or an unfavorable recommendation. These communication skills are no joke. You need to have resources, skills, and strategies on board before you enter the hospital so you will be confident in communicating effectively with caregivers. You must know what you want and you must be an advocate for yourself. Many people report that they were coerced into birth interventions and even unnecessary cesarean surgery by a caregiver. Do not let caregivers bully you into interventions you do not want or need. (Remember, part of this is solved when you choose the best caregiver and the best location for your birth with low rates of intervention and cesarean deliveries. Consequently, select your caregiver and birth location wisely.) Effective communication is an important part of advocating for yourself, but these are skills that require practice. **High Impact!**
- Learn how breastfeeding works by taking a high-quality, comprehensive breastfeeding class. Nothing can truly prepare you for the reality of living with an infant and the constant demands of infant feeding, no matter which method of infant feeding you choose. If you learn the ins and outs of breast-

feeding and what it takes to make it work, you will set yourself up for success. Just remember that most of the physical learning you will do is on-the-job training after your baby is born. **High Impact!**

- Get several nursing bras and nursing shirts. The right clothing makes a world of difference because regular bras are not advantageous for breastfeeding. Most people recommend buying nursing bras at the end of pregnancy and then remember that once your supply transitions to mature milk at full volume, your breasts will likely be a little bigger.
- Select a breastfeeding-friendly birthplace. Investigate cesarean delivery rates for your local hospitals, ask about intervention rates, and talk to people who have delivered at local hospitals. Find out if there is a Baby Friendly Hospital in your area.
- Consider out-of-hospital birth. This option is real and gaining traction. Once upon a time, all births were out of the hospital. Discussing the history of hospital birth and why or why not deliver at a hospital is outside the scope of this book. However, this is a valid and healthy choice for new families and babies. Options include standalone birth centers and home births.
- Select a breastfeeding-friendly pediatrician. This choice is huge! Talk to friends, family, neighbors, and other breastfeeding parents. Interview a few pediatricians in your area and ask specific questions about breastfeeding. Ask about their resources for breastfeeding families. They may have a lactation consultant on staff, a breastfeeding book list, a list of local support groups, a nursing room in their office, a list of phone numbers for breastfeeding phone support, or they may offer none of these. Ask about their breastfeeding credentials. Do they have any current training in lactation (beyond medical school where lactation training is minimal or absent)? Ask about their guidelines for starting solids. At what age do they recommend solid food? Anything before six months is not in line with current recommendations. What foods do they recommend for six and seven-month-old babies? Rice cereal is an outdated concept for infant food. Whole foods are best: avocado, sweet potato, banana. Ask what growth charts

are in use at their office. The WHO growth chart normed for breastfed babies is appropriate for infants receiving human milk. Finally, ask about their recommendations for nursing beyond 12 months. This information is especially important as many people still believe that nursing beyond one year is useless (which is totally false). **High Impact!**

- Enlist the help and support of your partner or from your family and social networks. Research shows that partner support can have a substantial impact on breastfeeding outcomes. Infant feeding decisions and information are not just for the maternal domain. It may seem like breastfeeding is heavy on the maternal parenting workload, but this child is your partner's child too. So, share the load when you can. For example, the partner can be a breastfeeding advocate, provide emotional support, facilitate a breastfeeding-friendly environment, be a good listener, research breastfeeding-friendly pediatricians and birthplaces, head off or deal with unsupportive comments about breastfeeding from family or friends, encourage and investigate other support avenues (e.g., find local lactation support meetings and maybe help get there if needed), or provide a snack, drink, or meal while the baby is at the breast. **High Impact!**
- Watch breastfeeding videos before your baby arrives. Long ago, people used to see breastfeeding in family and community contexts. In some parts of the world (USA included), breastfeeding in public is rare because of social taboos. Watching videos of babies at the breast can help expose you to another level of understanding (beyond what you can read in a book or learn in a class). Stanford University has good lactation videos. Dr. Jack Newman's website is a good resource as well.

During labor:

- Rule 1: **AVOID INDUCTION.** According to Lamaze International, the first thing you can do to maximize your chances of having a low or no intervention birth is to avoid induction (Lamaze International, 2007) unless it is 100% medically indicated. Low amniotic fluid and a big baby are two of the most cited reasons for induction, but both are widely known for being inaccurate. Also, many practitioners like to induce at 39 weeks. As you may have guessed, this practice has many flaws, and there is no rigorous, evidence-based research to support it. Henci Goer, medical writer and author of *The Thinking Woman's Guide to a Better Birth,* analyzed every angle of the ARRIVE study, which concluded that a 39-week induction is safe and advantageous for parents and babies (Goer, 2019). However, her conclusions raise some fundamental questions about the study's validity. (Dig into the study if you like or read Henci Goer's analysis on the Lamaze International blog called *Connecting the Dots*). In short, allow the baby to start labor when the time is right, *not* to accommodate arbitrary (39 week) deadlines. **Very High Impact!**

- Advocate for yourself (sometimes this is difficult to do in labor). Hire a labor/birth companion. Have a focused and vocal partner accompany you into birth to help advocate for you. **High Impact!**
- Avoid routine interventions by avoiding the bed. Birth is an upright endeavor, not meant to be accomplished while lying supine (on your back). Work with gravity, not against it. Stay upright, keep moving; when necessary, use a squat position, use the squat bar, sit on a birth stool, change positions frequently, lean over the peanut ball, kneel on all fours, and kneel next to the bed while leaning over the end of the bed. Stay as upright as you can. Upright positioning is Mother Nature's way. The pelvic outlet is open more while upright. Your body will tell you which position is most comfortable, not your caregiver. **High Impact!**
- Use natural comfort measures first. Use epidural as a last resort after trying other options, including physical support techniques, emotional support, and other comfort measures.
- Do not give away your power during labor and birth. *You* are the one having your baby. This power means you get to choose what interventions you want to interface with and which ones you do not. Problems arise when the parent's goals and caregiver's goals are not well-matched. Find a caregiver who aligns with you and your goals for birth. **High Impact!**

Postpartum:

- Immediate skin-to-skin (Kangaroo Care) with your new baby promotes bonding and enhances opportunities for breastfeeding. **High Impact!**
- Keep your baby with you at all times. Room in with your baby at the hospital after giving birth. When the baby is not with you, breastfeeding cannot happen. If separation must occur for several hours, request a double electric pump and begin pumping as soon as possible or within the first two hours after birth. **High Impact!**
- Provide the baby with the opportunity to accomplish the first feed within 60-90 minutes after birth. No delays unless it is medically necessary. **High Impact!**
- Feed frequently during the first 72 hours; this milk, called colostrum, is highly beneficial for your baby. It is packed with antibodies and immune factors. In addition, colostrum helps to seal the infant's gut. The more babies nurse in the first 72 hours, the earlier meconium is passed, and the sooner colostrum transitions to mature milk. In the first 72 hours, frequent feeding also protects the baby from excessive weight loss. **High Impact!**
- Delay the first bath for 24 hours, if possible.
- Dry the infant after birth but leave the hands as they are. The smell and taste of the amniotic fluid on the infant's hands help the baby remember the scent and look for it at the breast. (The small glands around the nipple give off a similar scent.)
- Sleep with your baby close to you. This positioning could mean that you share the same bed or the same room. Solitary sleep (infant alone in a room by herself) is a risk factor for SIDS and is not conducive to breastfeeding. Practice Safe Sleep if you share the same mattress surface with your baby.
- Most guidelines recommend that infants nurse 8-12 times in 24 hours. This recommendation is a suggestion but does not tell how much *your baby* will need to nurse in 24 hours. Generally, new babies need frequent trips to the breast, and many new parents can attest that some newborns require

more than the recommended minimum. Therefore, I suggest that you aim for **ten feedings in 24 hours with a new baby.** Remember, this situation is exceedingly temporary. You won't be nursing a newborn for long because your baby will grow rapidly, and her feeding patterns will change. Every month, I meet with several new parents who are experiencing low supply because they are not breastfeeding enough, especially overnight. Remove milk as frequently as you can in the first few weeks. **High Impact!**

- Use a responsive feeding approach instead of scheduled timing for bringing your baby to the breast. Responsive feeding (also called feeding on-cue or on-demand) means that parents respond when they see the baby display feeding cues each and every time. It may sound a little silly at first, but in reality, this is a major factor in determining whether you will bring in a full supply or not. Feed your baby every time you see feeding cues. Wake the baby if he is too sleepy to display feeding cues (preemie, jaundice, other conditions). *Feeding on demand could be one of the best ways to protect your potential for making human milk.* **High Impact!**
- Learn to recognize feeding cues. See the discussion in the RELAX chapter for full details about early, active and late feeding cues. Both you and your partner must learn to recognize feeding cues. Respond every time your baby displays feeding cues. **High Impact!**
- Be aware of the daily rhythms of human milk production, like high tide and low tide at the beach. Humans experience a peak milk production time in the morning, generally between 3 am and 6 am. Conversely, our low milk production occurs between 3 pm and 6 pm. While this seems counterintuitive because we want to sleep from 3 am-6 am, when milk production is at its highest, it might be genius in a way. Specifically, it is dark and Mother Nature plans for us to be in low-activity mode during the overnight hours. In other words, work and our daily routines are not occupying us in any way. Most of us have nothing to do (but sleep), which means we are with our babies during the nighttime hours – perfect for peak milk production. Yes, it

is tough! I know it is. But as I said above, this is a short period in your baby's life. Nighttime nursing will *not* go on forever. Also, a low tide of milk production does not mean that your milk has disappeared. Remember, during low tide, there is still water on the beach. You still have milk, and you are still making milk. There is just more of it during high tides. Take advantage and nurse a lot during peak production times. Morning is an excellent time to add an extra pumping session if you seek to boost supply. Otherwise, nurse when you see your baby displaying feeding cues.

- Meet all sucking needs at the breast. Infants have an intense sucking reflex. It must be so to ensure they survive. Therefore, you must meet their sucking needs at the breast in the early weeks, not with pacifiers, dummies, or other artificial teats or nipples. This accomplishes several things. First, it helps promote the earliest transition to mature milk. Second, it helps promote the best milk supply volume. Third, it ensures optimal milk intake for the baby, and allows the newborn to practice with the right equipment (instead of using artificial nipples, which are quite different). Avoid pacifiers (dummies) until you and your baby establish a strong breastfeeding connection and a good milk supply. Some recommendations state this could be about six to eight weeks, but some people who breastfeed avoid pacifiers altogether. As a side note, pacifiers can also be used for therapeutic purposes to help some babies improve their suck reflex. If your baby needs this kind of therapy, it will be designed to help your baby with breastfeeding, not negatively impacting your experience. Otherwise, allow the baby to meet all his sucking needs at the breast. Be aware that pacifier use is associated with a shorter duration of breastfeeding (Buccini et al., 2016). In addition, for breastfed infants who use a pacifier, the incidence of ear infections increases after the first six months of life (Sexton & Natale, 2009).
- Kangaroo for 72. One of the best ways to promote a healthy milk supply is to stay close to your baby and nurse frequently. There probably is no better way to accomplish this than to

do continuous or intermittent Kangaroo Care (skin-to-skin) for the first 72 hours (first three days) of life. In this way, you will be meeting all your baby's needs for warmth, food, love, attachment, security, comfort, and body system stability (heart rate, breathing rate, blood pressure, and body temperature). Kangaroo Care also ensures access to the breast, which is now your highest priority. **High Impact!**

- Allow your baby to establish the length of feedings. Some pediatricians tell new parents to feed the baby for eight minutes (or ten, twelve, whatever) at each breast. This recommendation is extremely suspicious. Numerous factors can impact how long a baby may take to nurse. Your baby may need extra time, or she might be sleepy at the breast, which means slightly longer nursing sessions. Perhaps your baby was born at 37 weeks gestation – not quite a preemie but acts like one. This baby may need *plenty of extra time*. Don't watch the clock or set a timer. Let the baby come off the breast when he is ready. **High Impact!**
- Offer both breasts during a single nursing session.
- Use comfortable positions that allow for gravity to assist. For example, no leaning over to bring the breast to the baby; bring the baby to the breast. Be sure there is no space between your bodies. I will discuss this in more detail in the RELAX chapter.
- Wake an excessively sleepy baby for breastfeeding. This baby might be a preemie, might be jaundiced, could have been an early full-term baby (born during 37-39 weeks), or have other conditions. People used to say, "Never wake a sleeping baby." This is terrible advice for a breastfed baby who has trouble waking for feedings or staying awake at the breast. Many people find that they must undress their baby, tickle him, or provide other wakeful stimulation to help their newborn stay awake at the breast. Sometimes, it helps to compress and massage the breast so that milk is immediately available. This strategy can help a sleepy baby become more interested in waking to nurse.

- Monitor your mental health. Taking care of your newborn regardless of feeding method is extremely intense. For some people, especially those with a history of anxiety and depression, the early postpartum period can tip the balance toward depression. The key to achieving a better balance with mental health (at any point in life) is to identify your needs and get help without delay. There is a short period of sadness or blues after giving birth for many people. If this seems to linger for you or you feel familiar feelings of anxiety and depression, get help immediately. It can be overwhelming to try to care for your newborn when experiencing any type of postpartum mood condition. If you are unsure about what to do, find a trusted family member or friend to help you. Speak to your physician, OB, the baby's pediatrician, or other caregivers. All of them should be able to point you toward appropriate resources and care in your community. In my opinion, mental health screening should be standard care for new parents, but this is not standard practice in the United States, which means that too many people fall through the cracks and never receive the care they need. Don't let that be you. It can be helpful to keep in mind that becoming a parent is incredibly challenging and requires support. There is nothing wrong with getting support for your mental health, even if you do not characterize your mental state as a postpartum mood disorder.

TRUE STORY

A co-worker and I were discussing the stress of parenting during the transition from one child to two children. Years later, she told me that she cried every day, usually while she was alone in the shower, for the first six or eight months after her second child was born. I asked if her partner had been available for support at that time, and she revealed to me that she never told him that she was not mentally or physically coping with the stress of parenting. Instead, she had a glass of wine or two every night after dinner and kept her misery to herself. She did not want to burden her partner, so she suffered for most of that year alone. It's such a shame that she felt she had no one to turn to for support.

Plan in advance to speak to your partner about parenting stress and the possibility of depression. Please note that anxiety, stress, and depression are not strictly reserved for those who give birth. Parenting and infant care can be stressful for either partner, whether giving birth or not. Adoption can bring on the same host of stressors concerning parenting. Be open to having a conversation about this with your partner or trusted friend if you feel yourself sliding into postpartum depression.

- Nurse your baby every time you see her display feeding cues. As mentioned above, don't wait to see feeding cues if your baby is sleeping too much; wake the baby and offer the breast.
- Achieve a comfortable latch. Before latching, the baby should have a wide mouth and take in plenty of breast tissue, not just the nipple. Therefore, aim your nipple for the roof of the baby's mouth, back toward the soft palate. For many newborns, this can be accomplished by using the laid-back breastfeeding position. I discuss this in more detail in the RELAX chapter.
- Become aware of how your breasts feel before and after breastfeeding. Before feeding, you may feel full, especially after day three or four. After feeding your baby, your breasts should feel noticeably less full. This indicator is good for estimating effective milk transfer (removing milk from the breast). If your breasts ever become engorged, they may feel very hard and painful. This condition can occur due to the transition to mature milk, or it can be edema, which results from swelling and sometimes excess fluid. If feeding does not resolve the issue or if feeding is not possible because the breasts are too full for effective latching, *immediately* begin techniques to resolve swelling and edema. Try Reverse Pressure Softening, cabbage leaves, cool compress for 20 minutes on, 20 minutes off (avoid heat in the case of edema because heat can increase inflammation). It is never advantageous to allow the breasts to become too full. After ruling out edema, breasts that are too full could indicate that breastfeeding is ineffective (poor milk transfer) or that breastfeeding is not frequent enough. Begin remedies immediately to remove milk.

This effort will also help prevent plugged ducts and possibly mastitis. Professional help is usually necessary in the case of resolving edema.

- Monitor wet and dirty diapers (nappies) during the first two weeks. Use a diaper tracker app or write down the diaper output on paper. During the first one to two days, you should see one or two wet diapers and at least one stool. This first stool is called meconium. Meconium is made of material that the baby ingests (amniotic fluid, cells, bile, mucus) while in the womb. Meconium looks black or dark green. It's thick, sticky, and does tend to stain. On day three, look for three wet diapers and three transitional greenish-black stools. By days four and five, you should see the transition to yellow, seedy stools (three to five stools per day) and five to six wet diapers. More breastfeeding in the first hours and days of life means faster elimination of meconium and return to birth weight.
- Monitor your baby's weight gain *at your pediatrician's office*. All infants lose a little weight after they are born. At birth, they hold onto fluid from their liquid environment in the womb. As they transition to life on the outside, they shed some weight. Your baby should regain birth weight by ten days to two weeks. More frequent nursing can help prevent excessive weight loss and help hasten the return to birth weight, even before day ten. If you were exposed to excess fluid during labor (IV fluids that accompany Pitocin and epidurals), your baby was also exposed and could have more weight on board than he would have otherwise. In this case, some researchers suggest using the 24-hour weight instead of the birth weight to account for the excessive weight loss (Noel-Weiss et al., 2011). This strategy can help avoid unnecessary and potentially harmful formula supplements during the first days of life.
- Find local breastfeeding support groups. Many groups are run by trained volunteers and offer lactation support and education. In addition, meeting with other people who are also breastfeeding can help to normalize breastfeeding and give you a source of emotional support. If you find no in-person groups in your area, join online groups. There are hundreds of them.

- Birth control. Although initially, you may not feel ready to think about sex and birth control, it may be necessary at some point. The good news is that you can learn how to use lactation to suppress your fertility. The not-so-good news for those who prefer to rely on birth control methods you may have used in the past is that estrogen can suppress lactation. **Therefore, avoid any birth control in the early weeks and months that contains estrogen.** Traditional combination birth control pills use estrogen, but there are some options for progestin-only pills. This medication is known as the mini pill. It is not risk-free, however. Some people report that the mini pill impacts milk supply. In addition, it may be wise to avoid using anything that cannot be immediately stopped, for example, four times yearly injectable birth control. Once you receive the injection, there is no way to remove it or eliminate the influence of this birth control. If your milk supply is affected by this, you cannot stop or reverse it until it runs its course, which can take months. This limitation also includes the birth control implant, which might also affect your milk supply. Avoid any long-acting birth control that is offered in the immediate postpartum period.
- If caregivers recommend formula supplements for slow weight gain, too much weight loss, failure to thrive, or a similar situation, see if it is possible to express your own milk and feed that to the baby (or donor milk if it is available) instead of using formula. Anytime there is a recommendation to interrupt breastfeeding or stop breastfeeding and use formula, it may be best to investigate why breastfeeding is not going well. First, investigate. Then, fix or correct the issues. If breastfeeding is supported and managed well, supplementation becomes unnecessary. Another choice for supplementation is donor human milk. According to the Academy of Breastfeeding Medicine's protocol for supplementation, "When supplementary feeding is medically necessary, the primary goals are to feed the infant and to optimize the maternal milk supply while determining the cause of low milk supply, poor feeding, or inadequate milk transfer" (Kellams et al., 2017). If you find that your baby's pediatrician recommends formula supplements, consider speaking to a

lactation consultant (LC) right away to determine the cause of breastfeeding problems. If supplementation is essential, your LC will help you develop a plan to protect and preserve your milk supply and discontinue the supplements when the time is right.

Choosing Your Path: Build an Effective Breastfeeding Plan

After reading through the Lactation Promotion Factors above, you might be thinking, "Wait, what? I thought this was natural and straightforward! There are too many variables! I cannot possibly do all that!"

First, regarding the lactation promotion factors, you do not have to put them all into practice at once. Some of them only happen one time. Some of them are out of your way by the time the baby is born – no need to consider those factors again.

Second, most of these factors are things that you will begin to master in the first four weeks of breastfeeding, and once you have a good grasp on the concept or technique, it will become second nature to you. These skills are why many LCs tell new parents that there is a reasonably steep learning curve for breastfeeding. However, after you get your approach mastered and learn the skills, it becomes much easier than bottle feeding with formula (which never gets any easier because it is always the same process).

Your first strategy is to develop an effective breastfeeding plan. Essentially, you must choose which lactation promotion factors you plan to incorporate into your strategy. I highly recommend giving more weight to those I denote as **High Impact!** These are important parts of effective breastfeeding for every person. I flagged these particular factors because they have the power to have a substantial impact on your milk-making potential. In essence, think of these as the non-negotiables and the others as somewhat optional. For example, breastfeeding ten times per day is labeled **High Impact!** and delaying the bath is not. While delaying the first bath is a good idea for various reasons (discussed in detail in Part II), it is not crucial to getting lactation off to a good start. Frequent breastfeeding in the early days and weeks, on the other hand, has a major potential to impact your breastfeeding experience and infant health. These outcomes are why I highly recommend incorporating this and other **High Impact!** factors into your plan.

To begin, use the matrix below as a guide. Feel free to fill in additional factors that are important to you. Use this as your guide and timeline to help you stay on top of your breastfeeding goals. You can also take the few items that relate to birth and weave them into your birth plan. Although, I always recommend using the most concise birth plan that you can. In recent years, there has been some pushback with parents who arrive in labor with a two- or three-page plan, explaining their wishes in exact detail. Less is more for your birth plan. My friend, Jackie Kelleher, teacher and author of *Nurturing the Family: A Doula's Guide to Supporting New Parents*, taught me about a straightforward but comprehensive approach to the birth plan. This birth plan has only three elements:

1. Request a labor and delivery nurse who is supportive of the use of natural comfort techniques during labor. Keep in mind that if you don't connect with your nurse, you can request a different person.
2. Be active decision-makers.
3. Ensure that you have informed choice throughout the process.

Part of making a simple birth plan work well is choosing the right birth attendant (OB or midwife) and the right location (for example, a hospital with low intervention rates). In addition, the person who attends your birth should have similar beliefs and expectations about birth as you do. If there is a mismatch, you could experience some trouble putting your birth plan into practice.

Creating your breastfeeding plan is different. Remember that you are the end user of this plan, and it will pay to be as detailed as you can. This information is your guide to protecting your potential for breastfeeding, created by you for your own use. If something does not apply to you or your circumstances, cross it off. Add what you need to make this your own plan. Visit my website to print this breastfeeding plan (www.protectingyourpotential.com).

During Pregnancy	During Labor & Birth	First Month Of Life	Second & Third months	Fourth, Fifth & Sixth months
Take a comprehensive breastfeeding class	Avoid induction of labor unless 100% medically indicated	Kangaroo for 72 hours after delivery	Continue following feeding cues and nurse on demand	Continue following feeding cues and nurse on demand
Take a comprehensive childbirth class	Use drug-free comfort measures first	Room in with your baby during the hospital stay	Learn several positions especially laid back and side-lying	Learn about starting solids and WAIT until about six months
Plan a no or low intervention birth with drug-free coping methods	Advocate for yourself or have a partner with you to advocate for you	Learn BF cues and BF your baby on demand around the clock	Continue nursing during overnight hours	Develop several responses to critical comments in advance
Learn and practice communication strategies for talking with caregivers	Give birth in a more upright position, not on your back	Breastfeed your baby about ten times in 24 hours, during daytime and nighttime	Monitor your mental health	Learn about teething patterns
Get your partner on board and make decisions together	Place the baby on the chest after birth. Accomplish the first feeding within 60-90 mins after birth	Be sure your baby achieves a comfortable, deep latch	Get comfortable breastfeeding in public spaces	
	Use expressed breast milk before using formula supplements	Postpone the use of birth control with estrogen	Be skeptical of questionable advice	
	Try the laid-back position for newborn nursing	Find local breastfeeding groups or online support		

Table 3.1: An outline for a breastfeeding plan

To summarize some of the most important lactation promotion factors:

1. **Low intervention birth.** Avoid unnecessary interventions and procedures. Research your alternatives. Take a birth class that teaches labor coping strategies. Hire a labor companion.
2. **Milk must move!** Producing milk is facilitated by removing milk. Begin breastfeeding or pumping within 90 minutes of birth. Then, remove milk from the breast around the clock, about 8 -12 times in 24 hours.
3. **Nurse on cue.** The baby sets the schedule, not the clock or another person. No doctor, lactation expert, book author, sleep consultant, blog writer, or friend knows when your baby is hungry or needs comfort at the breast. Only your baby knows. Watch for feeding cues and respond every time.
4. **Let comfort be your guide.** If you experience nipple pain, get help and find the source of the pain. Pain while breastfeeding is a sign that something is not quite right.
5. **Create your team.** Know who you will be able to rely on for breastfeeding support. Have the contact information written down, or better yet, add team members to your phone now. Research local lactation services and check them out before the baby arrives.

Beyond the Breastfeeding Plan - What Does the First Week Look Like?

Sometimes, even with all the information from a breastfeeding class or a well-written lactation guide, people still feel like they need a road-map showing exactly what to do when the new baby arrives. Because we rarely live in multi-generational close family communities anymore, most of us did not grow up helping our aunts, cousins, and extended family with immediate postpartum infant care and breastfeeding care. In other words, we did not get to see the early days of postpartum and breastfeeding close up. Most of us encounter a newborn baby for the first time in life when we give birth the first time. Because of this, many people lack a realistic reference point or context for how life goes with a newborn, especially one who is breastfeeding.

During the first week of life, breastfeeding has dramatic shifts from the moment of birth through day seven postpartum. These general outlines of each day will provide you with some context for caring for a newborn and breastfeeding during the first week. Remember that there is some wiggle room here. For example, sometimes, the events of day one happen a little later, depending on the time of day your baby was born. This delay is especially true if your baby is born later in the day. Also, remember that this is not an exact science because all births and babies are different but generally, look for the patterns discussed below throughout the first week.

Day One (or first 24 hours)

After birth, your most important priority in lactation is to move milk out of the breast. Many people think that your milk is not available until about day three, when milk "comes in." Do not fall for this outdated idea. You already have milk. In fact, your body has been ready to release milk since mid-pregnancy. In the first hours of your baby's life (and even before birth), your body is making colostrum. This early milk is available in small amounts, which is convenient because your baby's stomach is so tiny (only about the size of a big marble) and cannot expand as an adult stomach can. During the first 24 hours after birth, the baby will take small but frequent feedings. The *frequency* is critical. Infants who take in more colostrum during day one move meconium out of the intestines faster, lose less weight, and hasten the transition to mature milk. There is no schedule for day one, but you should feed the baby no less than (about) ten times, which means that your baby will likely come to the breast every two to two and a half hours. While breastfeeding can be more frequent than every two and a half hours, it should not be longer than every three hours. In fact, aim for only one long three hour stretch in the whole day, most likely while your baby is asleep. In other words, your baby may take one long period of three hours between feedings, but the others throughout the day will likely be shorter. To calculate the interval, count time from the start of one feeding to the start of the next. It might look like this:

8am – Breastfeed on the right side

8:20 – Switch sides and offer the left breast (this is still considered part of one feeding session)

8:35 - Diaper change, the baby goes to partner; you use the bathroom, get food, a drink, self-care, take a shower

9:00 - Baby naps or baby is held in Kangaroo Care

10:30 - Baby wakes and displays feeding cues

10:35 - Another feeding begins; breastfeed on the side that has the most milk/feels the fullest (and repeat the cycle above)

In the scenario above, the interval for breastfeeding is two hours and 35 minutes, from 8 am to 10:35 am. Your actual times will likely be different, but this helps you see what a small portion of your day will look like. This interval could be shorter as well. For example, the baby could nurse at 8 am and then display feeding cues at 10 am. Be sure to respond to the feeding cues even though only two hours have passed since the start of your last feeding. Infants do not know any type of routine or schedule. Remember, they are just transitioning from continuous nutrition provided during pregnancy to intermittent feedings at the breast.

Many people advise new parents to sleep when the baby is asleep. This advice is good but be sure that the baby naps on a safe surface for infant sleep near where you will sleep. This will allow you to get rest too. Do not plan to sleep while holding your baby skin-to-skin in Kangaroo Care. Any adult holding a baby skin-to-skin should remain awake for the entire Kangaroo session.

Day Two

Today will look much like day one. You are likely to be learning about umbilical cord care, breastfeeding cues, diaper changes, postpartum self-care, and calming techniques for your newborn. Be sure to bring the baby to the breast at least ten times today, whether you *think* you see feeding cues or not. Watch for at least two wet diapers and two stools. Today, the stool will likely look blackish green. It takes a few days to transition from passing all the meconium to passing stool. Stool color will change every day this week until you see a yellow, mustard-like texture. Spend time holding your baby skin-to-skin, even if you only plan for one or two 90-minute Kangaroo sessions today.

Day Three

Things may start to shift today. Your milk is transitioning now from early milk (colostrum) available in small amounts to mature milk secreted in a much higher volume. Continue to nurse on demand whenever you see feeding cues. Be sure you are feeding the baby about ten times today. If you are experiencing any type of nipple pain, get help right away. Do not let this fester. Your baby should produce at least three wet diapers and three stools. The stools should be larger than just a small stain in the diaper, and the color is transitioning today to green. Continue with Kangaroo Care. It will help stabilize your baby's body systems, meet all the baby's needs, and provide excellent access to your milk.

Day Four

You likely woke up this morning (or yesterday for some people) feeling like your breasts are full of milk! You may have tender, sore breasts due to the expanded milk volume. Nurse the baby early and often to keep the milk flowing. Milk stasis (stopped-flow, milk is not moving) is no friend to a person who is lactating. Your baby's stool is now turning more yellow, and you may begin to see the seedy mustard texture that is relatively typical of breastfed infant stool. Today, you should see at least four or more wet diapers. I have heard some people call day four the "wet day." This reference suggests that everything is flowing! Your baby should be producing a more significant amount of urine than the past few days. By day four, your milk supply amplifies, and you may feel that your breasts are leaking, even when you are not feeding your baby. You may feel a little sad today and overwhelmed, so tears may be flowing as well. Be kind to yourself and rest your body. Practicing skin-to-skin care with your baby is a great way to get the rest your body needs while still meeting all of your baby's needs for warmth, comfort, food, and body system regulation. Resist the urge to do something other than self-care and baby care. Your body is only beginning a long recovery process from birth, and you need lots of rest.

Day Five

Today, your breasts may still feel tender and larger than usual. In the coming days and weeks, milk volume will be regulated by the amount of milk that your baby takes from the breast. Over time, you will begin to feel less full even though you will be making plenty of milk. In other words, you will not continue to experience the extreme feeling of fullness throughout your breastfeeding experience. Today, look for at least five wet diapers and about five stools that are yellow and seedy. Remember, the stool indicates that your baby is taking in sufficient amounts of milk. If you have not experienced a rapid increase in milk volume sometime between day three and day four postpartum, consider this a red flag. Continue to put your baby to the breast every two to three hours but get help immediately. See a breastfeeding-friendly pediatrician, midwife, and talk to a lactation consultant. No delays. Read in Part II about Delayed Lactogenesis to find more information.

Overnight Feedings

The baby will continue a cycle of awake, alert, feeding, and sleeping throughout the day and the night. Babies, especially newborns, do not have any sense of nighttime the way adults do. Therefore, they will need nighttime care and feeding followed by short sleep intervals. The first few nights after birth can be a wild free-for-all, no matter how you feed your baby. It takes some time to get used to being up frequently at nighttime. There are many strategies to help you cope with nighttime parenting and feeding. Here are a few. Pick what appeals to you for now. You may try a few of these strategies now and postpone some until later. Be flexible.

- Set up sleeping arrangements for your baby in your bedroom. It has taken years, but even healthcare professionals (who have a good working knowledge of lactation) realize that breastfeeding works best when the breastfeeding dyad is together during the nighttime hours. While this does not sound revolutionary, for some, it is. The American Academy of Pediatrics has come around to promote room-sharing for parents and infants in recent years. (They will not go as far as promoting bedsharing, but many others {including me} do promote bedsharing – but it is your choice.) The Canadian Paediatric Society also recommends that infants sleep in the same room with their parents. Having your baby close by at night allows for better maternal recognition of infant waking, feeding cues, ease of nighttime feedings, more sleep for parents and babies, and less worry about your baby in solitary sleep in another room. Imagine a primate animal mother (gorilla, chimpanzee, orangutan) in the wild; would she ever make a lovely nest for her newborn in one place and then walk away to put herself to sleep in another place? This would not happen because the maternal-infant pairing is inherently protective for the newborn. Infants cannot survive without their parents/caregivers. In addition, solitary sleep (infant sleeping in a separate room) is a risk factor for SIDS.

- Learn about Safe Sleep if you do plan to bedshare. Dr. James McKenna's books are two outstanding resources, as is *Sweet Sleep* by West, Wiessinger, and Pitman.

- Learn to nurse your baby while lying down. Sometimes, this position is hard to do with a fresh, tiny newborn. It may take four to six weeks of mastering breastfeeding while in a more upright or laid-back position before attempting the side-lying position. During that first month, you can get the hang of breastfeeding in other positions, and your baby will get bigger, both of which will make side-lying easier. Some newborns are able to get the hang of the side-lying feeding position so it may be worth trying.

- Consider a side-car arrangement for having your baby's bed directly next to your bed. Some infant beds are designed to be co-sleeper cribs or bassinets. These are placed close to the adult bed so that the baby sleeps in her own space with three sides. One side is open to the adult bed. This setup gives the baby her own space but allows for incredibly easy access when it is time for feeding or snuggling.

- Keep lights low or off for nighttime feedings. Use only the lowest light for diaper changes or for taking yourself to the bathroom. Exposure to evening light, especially blue light emitted from TVs, computers, laptops, tablets, phones, and LED lighting, can disrupt our brain's interpretation of night and day. Promote good nighttime sleep routines by eliminating all light from night lights, screens, and LED bulbs in the evening. Instead, use soft light bulbs and cover all clocks or other sources of light. Remember that incandescent bulbs are nearly impossible to find these days now that LED bulbs are popular. Some LED bulbs emit harsh lighting. Instead, you may need to find soft or warm LED bulbs.

- Expose your baby to natural sunlight in the early morning hours after she wakes up. Humans use this cue from the sun to set the circadian rhythm for our diurnal schedule. It helps the brain run the daytime waking program while low or no light in the evening helps the brain run the nighttime sleep program. Bright morning sunlight is great for your baby, and it is good for you as well.
- One of the best pieces of advice I ever got during the first eight weeks with my oldest child came from my sister, Andi. I called her one day, near tears, complaining about the fact that my baby woke to nurse at 10 pm, midnight, 2:30 am, and again at 4:30 am before "waking up" for the day at 7 am. I was exhausted and near the end of my ability to cope. Her advice was simple; throw away the clock (or put it in another room temporarily). Stop looking at the clock! Part of the reason I was so tired and mentally tapped out was that I was obsessing over the fact that I had been up so much. My sister explained that if I would just wake with the baby, nurse, and go back to sleep without worrying about what time, how many times, how long we were up, and so on, that I would not be so distressed about it in the morning. Of course, she was right. I eliminated the clock and felt so much better. I was still tired but no longer anxious about it.

Remember, feeding your baby (or removing milk by pumping) is your first lactation priority today. A close second is skin-to-skin time with your newborn. Get as much skin-to-skin contact with your baby during the first three days as you can. Kangaroo for 72!

Final Thoughts

The lactation promotion factors are truly important. Indeed, these factors make up the pathway to success, no matter how you envision that for your family. Although I have noted many of these as **High Impact!**, you may have other priorities or needs that I fail to mention here. Think about your needs and your breastfeeding plan before your baby arrives. Incorporate all the positive breastfeeding elements that you can in the early weeks because that is when you are laying the foundation for your milk supply. It is a lot of work initially, and there are many balls to juggle but after the first month or two, this gets infinitely easier. You will become an expert on feeding your baby, and your baby will become an expert feeder. These are learned skills, and they take time to develop. Stick with it and be proud of the valuable work that you do as a parent!

CHAPTER 4

Introduction to the RELAX Method

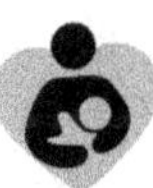

The RELAX Method for learning to breastfeed your newborn is a simple five-step approach that recognizes the roles of both the parent and baby in the feeding process. The RELAX Method focuses on a keen awareness of infant behaviors and responses, sensory input, advantageous body positions, self-assessment of breastfeeding, and of course, relaxation. Breastfeeding is a learned skill and using the RELAX Method can help you master the skills needed to feed your baby effectively.

Who Can Use the RELAX Method?

The RELAX Method is for people new to breastfeeding. This group includes new parents and new babies. If you are expecting your second or third new baby, you may not be new to breastfeeding, but your baby is. Use the RELAX Method in the newborn phase, even if you are already skilled with breastfeeding. This approach can help your baby make the most of early attempts to latch and hopefully pave a smooth path for your journey into lactation. The RELAX Method allows your baby to use innate breast seeking and feeding skills in the most favorable position. Later, once your baby masters the latch process and effectively transfers milk, try other positions.

When to Use the RELAX Method

If you're currently pregnant, you can learn the steps of the RELAX Method and use this approach right from the start after your baby is born. You can use this process in the moments after birth at the hospital, at a birth center, a home birth, or even birth in an unplanned location. You can also use this approach in the early weeks of your baby's life, as you both adjust to your new infant feeding skills.

If you have already had your baby and you are interested in trying the RELAX Method, you should absolutely do so. The skills involved in the RELAX Method are not reserved only for newborns. Any parent-baby pair can try the RELAX Method, but it is especially useful for young babies. You can successfully use this method with infants and small babies in the first months of life, even if you did not start breastfeeding this way. Innate skills for breastfeeding do not become extinct quickly in the first year. Dr. Christina Smillie, lactation consultant, and pediatrician has observed innate breastfeeding skills well beyond the first months of life (Smillie, 2008).

Where Does RELAX Breastfeeding Happen?

This approach, especially with the laid-back latch position, is best accomplished while reclining somewhat. You recline enough so that gravity, not your arms, supports the baby's entire body weight. In other words, you can recline enough to enable the baby to rest on top of your body comfortably. Lying flat back is not advantageous because the baby should still make eye contact with you while the baby is seeking the breast and feeding. Think of the position you might use to read or watch TV while reclined. Your head and chest are somewhat elevated. At first, you may think that this position requires you to recline fully, but you can achieve similar results by sitting in a chair or couch with your butt and legs moved as far forward as you comfortably can. If you're seated in a chair or on a sofa, you may want to use a pillow behind your lower back. Once you and the baby have mastered the RELAX process and the latch, you can modify the body positions for both partners.

Why is the RELAX Method Important?

The steps of the RELAX Method are not new. I did not *invent* anything about this process, but after more than a decade of helping people achieve effective breastfeeding, I (and many other LCs) have found that many breastfeeding dyads are not approaching feeding and latching in an optimal way. People often skip over or minimize genuinely essential parts of the process. Over the years, I began to note what set successful nursing couples apart from those who struggle. Those who are successful are more likely to practice certain aspects of effective breastfeeding consciously. As I said, I didn't invent successful breastfeeding. I am simply giving the essential steps a name so that it's easy to learn and remember the process. While some methods of teaching parents to breastfeed focus on effective latching, the RELAX Method takes a different approach. RELAX recognizes the essential steps that must occur *before* latching can occur and the use of an effective latch position for newborns. The RELAX Method also incorporates self-assessment of breastfeeding, establishing the parent as an expert. In addition, no discussion of this approach can ignore the relaxation factor. Many breastfeeding experts fail to explain that feeding your baby should be a relaxing reprieve, not a stressful event.

To learn more about the RELAX Method, read on. You can also visit my website to print the RELAX steps and the infant feeding self-assessment at www.protectingyourpotential.com.

The RELAX Method

There are five simple steps in the RELAX Method. Hopefully, this acronym will allow you to remember the steps with minimal effort. The RELAX Method steps are:

1. **R**espond
2. **E**xperience
3. **L**atch
4. **A**ssess and Adjust
5. e**X**hale

In the following discussion, I outline each step in detail. First, we look at the process while directly breastfeeding, followed by a short recap of the steps during a pumping session. Each step is essential, but they may seem cumbersome (at least initially). However, over time, you will quickly gain experience and fluency with breastfeeding and move through the steps seamlessly in seconds.

RELAX Method

R - Respond to your baby

The first step in the RELAX Method is to *respond* to the baby when the baby displays feeding cues. Sometimes, this is where people run into trouble, even before they begin to feed the baby. Responding to the baby's early feeding cues is one of the *essential steps* to bringing in a full milk supply and for protecting your milk supply. It is also a way to build trust between parents and babies. When the baby initiates communication with you by displaying feeding cues, your job is to recognize this communication signal and respond promptly. Over time, the baby learns that you will meet his needs when he communicates with his parents in these ways. You can see that the baby and his needs (i.e., food, comfort, warmth, and protection) set the feeding times, not the clock and not an arbitrary feeding schedule.

We tend to think of crying as the universally accepted signal of infant hunger, but this is, in fact, the last (and most desperate) in a long line of cues that babies use to get our attention. Parents can recognize infant feeding cues early in the process, long before the baby begins crying. This recognition makes the feeding process go more smoothly and helps build trust over time. As a result, the baby will trust that you will meet his needs. According to Dr. Nils Bergman, public health physician and perinatal neuroscientist, your baby has several "programs" that help facilitate his neurobehavior. Two of these include a 1) defensive program and a 2) feeding program (Bergman, 2017). These two programs cannot run simultaneously, which is why a baby won't be likely to latch when he is displaying defensive behaviors (e.g., crying, irritated, angry). Instead, when the baby actively seeks food, comfort, warmth, or protection, he will display feeding cues. This display is the baby's gentle way of asking parents to provide food, opportunities for holding, snuggling, warmth, and protection.

What Are the Feeding Cues?

Full-term, healthy infants are competent. Decades ago, there was a prevalent notion that infants were helpless creatures who required intensive assistance and management during the feeding process.

In reality, newer research shows that infants display the proper cues, including behaviors for seeking the breast and locating the nipple. It is our responsibility as parents and caregivers to recognize and respond.

Infant feeding cues represent a small part of a complex sequence of events that initiates the feeding process. Feeding cues are generally characterized as 1) *early*, 2) *active*, and 3) *late*. It is far better to recognize and respond to the early or active feeding cues. This response allows a calm baby to come to the breast to latch on. If your baby is displaying late feeding cues, you will have to spend time calming the baby before attempting the latch. Here is what to look for:

Early Feeding Cues

- Opening and closing the mouth
- Lip-smacking
- Sucking sounds
- Pushing out the tongue
- Waking up from a period of sleep

Active Feeding Cues

- Rooting at the breast
- Hands in the mouth
- Mild vocalizations, happy baby sounds
- Active body movements
- Wiggling, arms and legs moving

Late Feeding Cues

- Fussiness
- Vigorous vocalizations, frantic sounds
- Dramatic, demonstrative arm and leg movements
- Angry crying

Respond whenever your baby displays feeding cues. Sometimes, you may think, "I just fed you an hour ago! It can't be time for feeding again!" Remember that babies come to the breast for many reasons: comfort, warmth, safety, food, help with body system regulation, human connection, loving interactions, and probably others. You may not know why the baby wants to nurse but respond with nursing if he shows feeding cues. In the early weeks, *this kind of timely response* is what builds your milk supply. You are also building trust, teaching your baby through loving interactions, and fostering a sense of compassion.

There is a notion in some parenting circles that once you have fed the baby and changed his diaper, parents should allow the baby to fuss and cry as a means of self-regulation or self-soothing. This is terrible advice. Remember that crying is a signal of the defense program, and it's your baby's way of indicating that something is not right. If you have responded to feeding cues, fed the baby, changed diapers, and your baby is still signaling the need for attention, try holding your baby in an infant carrier or try Kangaroo Care (KC). The details about KC and the "Stability Habitat" are in the chapter on Kangaroo Care. Respond to your baby's cues every time and remember that breastfeeding meets physical and emotional needs. Infants do not self-sooth. That is a myth.

R**E**LAX Method

E - Experience your baby

The second step in the RELAX Method for parents is to *experience the baby*. You may be thinking, "What? How do I experience my baby?" Better yet, "I experienced this baby enough during the birth process!" This step may seem nonsensical or ridiculous at first, but it is crucial to the RELAX process.

To experience your baby means connecting with the baby through *your senses*. Breastfeeding is, indeed, a sensory experience for both parent and baby. When a parent connects with the baby through sound, sight, smell, and touch, amazingly powerful but unseen hormonal processes begin within the body as a direct response to contact with the baby. The maternal response to seeing, hearing, smelling, and touching the baby will result in a profound shift of the hormonal profile. Oxytocin, the love hormone, is released, which helps prepare the breast for milk letdown and the continuation of the milk-making process. Oxytocin also facilitates and promotes nurturing behaviors that allow parents to respond to their babies. This interaction between parent and baby by connecting through the senses "primes the pump" to facilitate milk flow. Your hormonal response to baby pheromones also enhances responsive nurturing behaviors.

How can you experience your baby? Most likely, you are already doing practically all of these things every day. But, in preparation for feeding at the breast, remember to do them with purpose. These actions help shift your hormonal profile just before nursing to support milk letdown and milk making. Here is what to do:

- Smell the baby's head.
- Kiss the baby.
- Touch the baby, give a mini massage.
- Practice Kangaroo Care or skin-to-skin contact.
- Listen to your baby's breath or happy sounds.

Connect with your baby by way of your senses each time you get ready for feeding. Connecting through the senses facilitates milk letdown and hormonal shift that promotes breastfeeding. In addition, the oxytocin release helps facilitate and enhance nurturing behaviors. Even though this step may seem trivial at first, do not skip it. Breastfeeding is a total sensory experience for both parent and baby.

RE**L**AX Method

L - Latch your baby to the breast

The next step is to latch your baby to the breast, or better yet, allow the baby to latch. Many people wrongly assume that the infant needs a lot of guidance or management with latching onto the breast, but that is not true. As parents, in this step, we provide the right environment (think body position) so the baby can use innate skills to locate the nipple and latch on. In this part of the process, we want to focus on position, including 1) position of the parent's body, 2) the baby's body, 3.) the nipple, 4) the baby's tongue and lips, 5) the hands and arms, all of it. Before we begin, let me say that there are loads of right ways to latch the baby. This scenario is one where the parent-baby dyad has to find what works for them. What feels suitable and effective for you may not be right for another dyad. We are all different with different body shapes and sizes. Our babies are different, too, each with varying anatomy and skill ability. Some people with large breasts may need to support their breasts. Some preemies or fragile babies require extra support. Since we are all different and our circumstances are unique, the same old cross-cradle position won't work for everyone. Try different positions until you find *several* that work for you. Remember that there are a variety of ways to achieve a good position. Some positions are better for newborn breastfeeding than others. In this context, do not let someone tell you that you're doing it all wrong. Having said that there are a few guidelines that you should be aware of for positioning.

First, consider body positions for parent and baby:

Parent's body

- Needs to feel comfortable, able to maintain the position for at least 45 minutes
- Needs to be supported (use pillows strategically)
- Must be able to relax
- Should not be in pain
- Should not be hunched over or leaning over the baby to achieve a latch
- Should have complete contact with the infant, no gaps between the bodies

Baby's body

- Must be fully supported
- Should be relaxed, not straining to reach the breast
- Positioned well when ear, shoulder, and hip are inline
- Should be tummy to tummy with the parent, no gaps between the bodies
- Baby's head and neck align with his shoulders, not turned to the side

Nipple

- Aim the nipple at the juncture of the hard and soft palate on the roof of baby's mouth

- It should be deep in the baby's mouth
- The nipple and areola will adapt to the shape of the baby's mouth and tongue
- It should be comfortable, no long-lasting pain

Baby's tongue and lips

- The tongue should be on the bottom of the mouth, covering the lower gum
- The tongue must be free enough to stick out and move all around the mouth (up, down, and side to side)
- Lips flared while the baby is latched (no sucking in the lips with breast tissue, especially the bottom lip. Top lip can be flared or neutral.)
- Tongue and lips must create a tight, stable seal without gaps, clicking, or "sliding down" the nipple

Location

Consider where you will sit or lie down for breastfeeding. You may think sitting down is the natural, normal way to position yourself, but other positions are worth exploring, especially for nursing a newborn.

Choose a chair or position on the sofa or other safe surface that is comfortable (obviously). Remember that your newborn can take quite a bit of time at the breast in the first few weeks and will sometimes fall asleep. If you are in a comfortable chair or lying down comfortably on a *safe surface*, you won't mind sitting or lying there for about 45 minutes. It will become a chore if you are uncomfortable, and you will quickly find that you need to make a change. It is helpful to remember that these tips are for people who are just getting the swing of things, just learning how this works. When you become a pro, you can nurse your baby in any old chair, walking down the street with your baby in a baby carrier, on the bus, or at a restaurant. For now, let's focus on getting the hang of it at home, in comfort.

Finding a position: Chair, Sofa, or Safe Flat Surface

A comfortable chair will support you, and perhaps an upholstered chair is superior to an upright wooden chair. Use a footstool if you have one. Pillows are okay for supporting your arm or elbow. You can also use a small pillow behind your lower back for support. Having a table nearby can be a big help. You will have a place to put down a book, a sandwich, a drink, the remote, or your phone. Using a nursing pillow is fine, but sometimes, they create a surface that is too flat for some infants. (For some babies, being in a more upright position or even diagonal position at a 45-degree angle with bum, legs, and feet lower that the head can be easier.)

You can also breastfeed your baby in a reclined position, which can be advantageous for various reasons that I will explain in just a moment. If you're interested in reclining while breastfeeding, there are a few things to note. First, I recommend *against* sitting with your newborn for nursing or for Kangaroo Care in a recliner chair. Specifically, I recommend against using a recliner that can be upright and then changes to recline or almost flat. I do not recommend sitting in this chair with your baby because of the risks involved should you fall asleep. If you were to fall asleep and the baby could not maintain her position on top of you, she might get trapped between your body and the side of the recliner, putting her at risk of suffocation. You might think this is an exaggeration, but it is not. Please do not nurse your baby in a recliner. Instead, if you'd like to recline while breastfeeding, you can lie back on a safe flat surface with your chest elevated, like a position you'd use to relax and read a book or watch TV. Your baby will lie down on her tummy on top of your upper torso and chest in this position. With the baby positioned on her ventral (front side) surface, this position is advantageous for eliciting innate feeding behaviors from your newborn. Dr. Nils Bergman says that the baby's position and environment will determine her behavior. Think of this position as a trigger for feeding.

Newborn Expectations Before and During Latch

Let's look at what a newborn *expects* to do when approaching the breast. Biologically, humans are mammals. All mammals have innate programming that allows them to seek the nipple, latch onto the breast, and begin to nurse. Human babies are good at this, provided that they are in the right environment, are healthy, and have not been exposed to too many birth interventions.

If placed on the mother's abdomen just after birth, the baby will use stepping motions to crawl up toward the breast. He will use his hands, arms, legs, and sense of smell to guide himself toward the nipple and effectively latch, unassisted. We sometimes refer to this process as the breast crawl or self-attachment. Whatever you want to call it, call it amazing! But how does this help explain what the newborn expects to encounter when approaching the breast? Research shows an eight-step process that a baby will go through in roughly sequential order that will lead him to latch on to the breast. The steps include 1) hands to the mouth, 2) moving the tongue, 3) opening the mouth, 4) visual focus on the nipple, 5) stepping or crawling toward the nipple, 6) hands massage the breast or nipple, 7) licking at the nipple, and finally, 8) latching onto the breast (Ransjo-Arvidson et al., 2001). Of course, the newborn expects to use his innate programming, run through these steps, and get to the breast. These behaviors make the most sense under certain conditions:

- the baby is on his belly (but this is not the position most people use to learn to breastfeed)
- the baby acts primarily unassisted
- the baby's body is stable (using gravity to keep him on top of the parent)
- the baby has free use of his hands, arms, legs, and feet (not tightly swaddled in a blanket)
- the baby has enough time, isn't rushed or hastened along

So, how can you help the baby run through this program? The answer is simple: the parent's position will determine the position of the baby. If the parent is seated upright, the baby will likely come to the breast in the cradle or cross-cradle position. This position happens in *front* of the parent. If you're at the hospital, the infant might come to you wrapped in a tight swaddle, with arms and legs completely pinned to his sides. Let me repeat that there is nothing wrong with nursing this way, and once you and the baby are pros, any position is acceptable. I want to stress that when you try the first attempts at breastfeeding your newborn, both you and the baby are learning what works and, more importantly, how to achieve an excellent latch so that effective milk transfer can occur. Try different positions while you are learning. Your position will determine the position of the baby. If you are seated in a semi-reclined position or the laid-back position, the baby will be approaching the breast from on top of your body. This position allows the baby to be on his belly, fully supported and kept in place by gravity (and a little help on either side by your arms, if necessary). With his arms and legs free, he can use innate skills to achieve an optimal position near the nipple and latch onto the breast. Does it make sense that the parent can help facilitate what the baby expects in the laid-back position? Give it a try. Even if you do not plan to nurse this way all the time, I highly recommend that you try this because, for many babies, this is the best way to achieve a solid latch and effective milk transfer. In addition, your baby already knows how to nurse in this position. Another excellent reason to try the semi-reclined or laid-back positions with your brand-new baby is this: your baby has innate programming that helps facilitate early attempts at breastfeeding. Even though the baby can use innate skills to get to the breast, your baby can also learn new skills. In fact, the infant's ability to learn and modify breastfeeding behaviors is high. Laid-back positions help facilitate effective latch and milk transfer. Why not allow for the first attempts at breastfeeding to be peak performance, ones that the baby will learn from, instead of taking the chance that there may be suboptimal learning with another position?

Here are my final thoughts on body position. First, use the most comfortable, stable position that enables the baby to achieve an excellent latch and efficiently transfer. Second, try several positions, including laid-back breastfeeding. The baby will drive the feeding process with innate breast seeking and breastfeeding skills in this position.

Latch: How to Achieve a Deep, Comfortable Latch

By now, we have considered your body position and your baby's body position. But what about the mouth? What about the breast? How do you facilitate the best opportunity for your newborn to achieve a good latch? Remember when I said that there are lots of positions? That is true for the body position, but when it comes to the nitty-gritty of latching the baby to the breast, there are a few non-negotiables.

Let us consider latching in the cradle or cross-cradle position. First, hold the baby close, with no space between you and your baby. Second, the baby should be at the height of the nipple, not below. The baby's nose and your nipple should be on the same plane. Using a pillow to raise the baby up off your lap is okay. Third, allow the baby free head movement. In other words, support the upper back and shoulders, but don't put pressure on the back of the baby's head. When the nipple contacts the philtrum (skin just below his nose), the baby needs to extend his head slightly. Fourth, brush the philtrum with the nipple. This brushing should cue the baby to extend his head and open his mouth wide. Fifth, when you see the wide-open mouth, bring the baby in close and allow him to latch. The nipple should be aimed slightly upward toward the roof of his mouth, as far back as the juncture of the hard and soft palate. Bring the baby to the breast chin first. Sometimes, to help facilitate his chin in the breast tissue, bring the baby's bottom closer to you. The closer his lower half is to you, the closer his chin should be to the breast. This position also allows his nose to be free, not touching the breast. Sixth, be sure that the baby's lips are flanged outward. Lastly, although it is hard to tell, the baby should extend his tongue over the lower gum ridge. If the baby cannot stick his tongue out over the lower gums, the latch will be uncomfortable, and it could be a sign of restricted tongue mobility.

Some additional tips may help. For example, some people find it helpful to hold the baby with one arm and use the other hand to support the breast. Also, the more reclined you are, the more gravity will help keep your baby in place. Finally, if the latch is uncomfortable or painful beyond the first minute or so, use a clean finger (with a trimmed nail) to break the seal and begin the latch process again.

Consider the following tips for latching in a laid-back position:

1. You recline and position the baby on your upper torso and chest.
2. The baby will approach the nipple from over the top. She may use hands, cheeks, nose, tongue, arms, and legs in the process of getting just the right position to attempt the latch. Allow her the time she needs to achieve her optimal spot.
3. As your baby attempts to latch, she will lift her head and take in a big mouthful of breast tissue (not just the nipple). Her

chin will make full contact with the breast, and her nose will be free.

4. Lips should flare, and her tongue will extend over the lower gum ridge.

Try latching in both upright and laid-back positions. The laid-back position will allow better use of innate newborn skills when seeking the breast and when latching. However, after establishing breastfeeding, any comfortable position is acceptable, as long as it facilitates effective milk transfer.

RELAX Method

A - Assess and Adjust

The baby has latched on to the breast. Now what? There are several things to check for and assess before deciding whether or not to adjust positions or start over. Two of the most important things that we can assess at this point are the baby's latch and your comfort level. You can make this assessment of breastfeeding every time you nurse your baby. It takes only a few seconds to assess latch and comfort level.

How Does the Latch Look?

Take a good look at your baby's mouth while she is latched. Can you tell if the lower lip is fully flanged? Did the baby's mouth look wide open just before latching? It can be tough to determine the position of the tongue. If possible, try to see if the baby has her tongue extended over the lower gum ridge. Remember, while it may be important to know if the baby's tongue is extended and the lips are flaring, the look of the latch is not the most important factor. A good latch also involves comfort and facilitates effective milk transfer.

Is the Latch Comfortable? Are You Experiencing Pain?

For effective feeding to take place, you must maintain the latch for up to 30 minutes at a time. It may not take nearly that long, but breastfeeding can take time for some infants (preemies, babies with low muscle tone, infants with heart conditions, and some other babies).

Feeding will be challenging if you are experiencing discomfort. First, assess for nipple pain. Sometimes, people feel pain when latching during the first few days, but that should not last. In addition, pain during the nursing session should not persist beyond the first minute. Ask yourself, does any nipple pain continue beyond the first 30 to 60 seconds of the nursing session? To assess for pain, you need to be honest about your comfort level with the baby's latch. This seems obvious, but I have encountered many people who went for weeks with a painful latch because the latch "looked good" according to their caregiver. The latch cannot be assessed based on looks alone. If you're experiencing discomfort in the early attempts to get a good latch, do not wait to resolve this issue. Infants can learn and practice poor sucking skills, just like they can practice good sucking skills. Parents have to encourage effective and comfortable sucking skills, and part of the feedback loop is nipple pain.

So, be honest with yourself, even if the lactation consultant at the hospital or your baby's pediatrician said that the latch looked good. *You are the only one who can decide whether it feels right or not.* Essentially, this means that any lactation consultant, nurse, pediatrician, dentist, ENT, or other professional you speak with cannot successfully determine if your baby is latching well, because they cannot feel what you feel. With comfort (or pain) as your guide, you will be able to tell if the baby has a good latch or not. However, if your nipples have any prior damage, trauma, thrush, or anything lingering that has caused pain in the past, the latch can still be uncomfortable until the nipple heals, even if the latch is perfect. A nipple shield can facilitate healing in some cases while still bringing the baby to the breast.

If there is pain with the latch, the first thing to check is whether the latch is too shallow. What is a shallow latch? A shallow latch, simply put, is when the baby does not have enough breast tissue in his mouth, and the nipple does not reach as far back in the mouth as it should. The baby needs to bring the nipple back far enough in his mouth so he can feel it on the juncture of the hard and soft palates. You can locate this spot in your mouth by moving your tongue along the roof of your mouth until you feel the palate turning into soft tissue. It seems far back in the mouth, but your baby's mouth is much smaller than your own and remember that the nipple-areola complex is quite pliable and can stretch far beyond its resting length.

If you have nipple pain while the baby is latched, insert a clean finger along the corner of the baby's mouth to break the seal before attempting to unlatch the baby. Then, you can begin again with the latch steps. Remember to allow the baby to use his face and hands to help with latching, and laid-back feeding may be the thing to try in this situation. Find a comfortable, laid-back position and apply the RELAX Method with the baby on top of you, coming to the breast from over the top of the nipple. This position can often facilitate a much deeper latch. For some infants who have trouble in the cradle positions, this position might enable pain-free feeding and optimal milk transfer. See the picture below showing the ventral feeding/ laid-back position for latching.

A More Comprehensive Approach to Breastfeeding Assessment - PAC MAAN

Remember Pac-Man©? It is an old-school maze video game. The yellow character is nothing more than a circle with an open mouth, moving through the maze, eating up dots to earn points throughout the game. It looks like ancient history compared to today's graphics and video games but for our purposes, think of it as a baby drinking human milk. While you won't earn points with this tool, it will help you determine if breastfeeding is going well, or if you need support. You can use this self-assessment instrument during and after a nursing session. The PAC MAAN tool will give you an excellent idea about how breastfeeding is going for you. It takes a little longer to use this assessment tool than the simple assessment detailed above, but it gives you more detail and includes a few more factors to consider.

The elements of the PAC MAAN tool are: 1) position, 2) attitude, 3) comfort, 4) milk, 5) abundance assessment, and 6) nipple shape. I explain each element in further detail below.

Position - Checking in With Your Body

Are you relaxed? Are you comfortable and able to maintain your position for 30 to 40 minutes? It may not take that long but some babies linger at the breast for a variety of reasons. For example, suppose you have a baby with some challenges (e.g., small for gestational age baby, a preemie or near preemie, an infant with low birth weight, a baby with jaundice, an overly sleepy baby or a baby with some other special needs). In that case, it can take a while for the baby to take both breasts and effectively remove enough milk to feel satiated. It may also take longer for the baby to remove enough milk to stimulate milk production. Be sure you are not leaning over, hunched forward in any way. If you are sitting upright, you can move forward in the chair to help you lean back slightly. Remember to bring the baby to your breast; you are not bringing the breast to the baby. Use pillows if necessary. Use the most optimal position for your comfort and to facilitate effecting feeding.

Attitude - How Do You Feel About This Feeding and Breastfeeding in General?

Are you generally doing well? Or are you feeling overwhelmed? Do you need more help and support than you're getting right now? Are you feeling resentful toward your partner because this is a lot of work on your end right now? Are you doing well, aside from feeling tired? Now is the time to go back to your initial breastfeeding plan and access your support team. Who can you talk to today about how you are feeling? Who will provide you with the emotional support you need? Can you talk to your partner now (or soon) about any feelings of frustration or exhaustion? Negative feelings are common but don't let negative feelings fester. Please take the time to talk to a supportive friend or family member. If you feel isolated but need to speak with someone right now, call a national hotline for breastfeeding support. La Leche League (chapters worldwide) and Breastfeeding USA have trained support people ready to listen and offer help.

Comfort - Let Comfort be Your Guide!

How is your comfort level? We assessed comfortable body position earlier. How about nipple and breast comfort level? If you are experiencing nipple pain or breast pain, take note of exactly where you feel discomfort to explain it to a lactation support person. If nipple pain persists beyond the first minute or two of breastfeeding, consider this a red flag. Most of the time, you can eliminate these discomforts with changes in position. Please do not let pain linger. There is nothing good that will come from "toughing it out." Ignoring nipple pain can lead to nipple trauma and damage. First, try to unlatch and relatch. If your attempt at a deeper latch does nothing for the pain, seek help immediately from skilled lactation care or trained counselors, volunteer breastfeeding support, or peer-to-peer support. Remember that if you are trying to latch and have pain each time, it may be an excellent opportunity to switch to a new or different body position. If you have been nursing in a seated position, try the laid-back position. If you have been using cross-cradle, try the football hold. This repositioning will totally change the way your baby approaches the breast. Further, it will change the nipple positioning in her mouth. Remember, the breast is a circle so the baby can approach it from any side.

Milk - How's it Going? Are You Flowing?

While the baby achieves a proper latch, it will not be easy to see milk flowing unless the baby pops off and milk sprays everywhere during letdown (this does happen). So, what should you look for to see if milk is flowing? First, look for active sucking with pauses. The pauses let you know that the baby is taking in milk and forming a bolus (several gulps of milk combined together) for swallowing. The baby does not suck and then immediately swallow that bit of milk. Instead, he will use the following pattern: suck, suck, pause, swallow. Look for the pause and listen for swallowing. The pattern can change throughout the feeding, especially right after the letdown has occurred.

Watch the baby's chin as he is nursing. You should see movement (especially when using the cradle or cross-cradle position). You may also see milk dribbling out of the mouth if the baby unlatches or see milk in the corners of the mouth. Many babies will burp and sit up a little milk but this is not reliable for checking for milk transfer. Some infants simply do not sit up much. Some do, and it's individual. All babies (when breastfeeding is effective) will suck, suck, pause, and swallow. Look for this pattern or something like it. Also, when your baby is actively nursing, you should see rhythmic sucking for a sustained period of about five to ten minutes. Preemies and other special-needs babies likely won't sustain breastfeeding that long without several breaks.

Assess abundance - Softer Breast Tissue?

After you have offered both breasts and the baby has nursed well, you should feel that your breasts are noticeably softer and less full of milk. In other words, your abundant milk supply should feel less generous after a feeding. When your baby is older, this indicator will be less noticeable. Assessing abundance at the end of a feeding, especially when you feel your breasts are less full, is an excellent indicator of effective milk transfer. Many people can tell that they have a lot of milk in the morning because the breasts feel full (it's high tide). Remember, it is never good to let the breasts get too full. Too much milk in the breast signals the body to slow down milk production. Less full breasts trigger more milk production. That said, many people find they wake up in the morning feeling quite full of milk. Bring the baby to the breast, offer both breasts, and assess whether or not your breasts feel less full after a complete breastfeeding session. If they feel less full, this is a good indication of milk removal. If they do not feel significantly less full, your baby might not be draining the breasts as well as you would like. First, work to find out why milk removal is stalling. Then, you can consider adding hands-on breastfeeding or pumping after feeding to remove more milk. Hands-on pumping is effective in helping remove more milk. Work with skilled care if there are other indicators that the baby may not be getting enough. Watch diaper output and weight gain in the early days and weeks if you're concerned.

Nipple Shape - Natural Shape or Flattened After Feeding?

After your baby has finished nursing, check the shape of your nipple immediately after the baby comes off the breast. You should see a naturally shaped nipple, looking like it did before your baby latched on to the breast. If you see some other shape, consider this a red flag. Sometimes, when the nipple does not get back far enough in the baby's mouth, the nipple compresses. This compression will likely cause pain, and the nipple may come out of your baby's mouth looking flat on one side. Most people compare this compressed shape to a brand-new tube of lipstick. This shape is certainly a red flag, with or without pain. It indicates that the nipple should be further back in the baby's mouth. Try techniques to attain a deeper latch: consider latching more laid back, try the c-hold, and aim the nipple toward the roof of the baby's mouth, watch for a wide-open mouth before attempting to latch, improve your posture (no leaning over), bring your baby up higher, use a different pillow, and use a different position. There are great videos out there for latch but beware! I have seen videos and pictures of people trying to achieve a deep latch, but the parents are leaning over. You already know this is a non-starter for better breastfeeding. Instead, try watching videos for breastfeeding help. Stanford University and Dr. Jack Newman have good breastfeeding videos. Remember, not all videos are excellent quality; anyone with a camera can post a video of "how to get a good latch." Be mindful of where you get your info.

RELA**X** Method

X - eXhale

Part of nature's design of lactation involves a calming response for you and your baby. This response makes sense biologically because infant care can be stressful, especially for new families. It is nature's design for infant feeding to feel calm so that parents and caregivers will continue to care for and feed newborns. Hormones released during a feeding session help create a relaxation response for the parent, which can facilitate stress relief during the day and promote sleep during the nighttime hours. The infant benefits from a relaxation response as well. Beyond the biological aspect of the hormone release, I have included this step to remind parents that infant feeding can be a time for you to relax, restore, rejuvenate, and enjoy a quiet moment with your baby. Of course, this is a little more difficult when your second child is born, so if you're breastfeeding your first baby, take time to enjoy the peace.

Set an intention to relax during your breastfeeding session. Organize your environment to promote relaxation. Choose a cozy spot for nursing; create a calm place where you can sit or lie down in comfort. Set up all the items you might need nearby so that you can grab things at close range. You may need a table, a footstool, pillows, burp cloths, or nipple ointment. You might need your phone or tablet, a good book, a drink, or a healthy snack. You may want to set up a diaper changing station close to your preferred nursing location. If you are caring for older children, you may need a safe place for toddler playtime that allows you to nurse the baby while watching your older child. Plan out your best breastfeeding location before your baby arrives. This planning will allow you to get all the items you need in one place and ready for breastfeeding when the day arrives. Some people need two breastfeeding stations in the house: one for daytime and a separate one for nighttime or nap time. This setup usually equates to one place where you can sit upright while nursing and another where you can stretch out, try laid-back breastfeeding, or side-lying.

Sometimes, infant feeding can be overwhelming, and you may not feel relaxed. You might feel stressed out in the early days while still learning how to meet your baby's needs by breastfeeding. Some people feel isolated while their new babies are tiny because it can feel like breastfeeding and nap times have you tied to your home. You may feel frustrated that other people in your life are still carrying on as usual and you are suddenly trapped by breastfeeding your baby every few hours. Acknowledge your frustrations and reach out to your support team. Talk to your partner about your feelings and try to connect with other people who are breastfeeding. This situation is incredibly temporary, but it can feel overwhelming while it is happening.

Adjusting your expectations can be an excellent way to help prepare for the reality of life with your newborn. However, many people in the modern world have no reference for infant feeding and infant care before their baby arrives. If you were expecting life to be similar to your current life but with a baby around, you may be completely surprised by how much your life will change. Talk to people who have recently had their first child and get a good handle on how much time you will spend doing infant care and how much time you might have free outside of infant care. This balance is different for all of us, but it will help you get a good idea of what to expect.

Darker Feelings of Parenting

Parenting can be incredibly lovely and rewarding, but it is not all roses. If parenting is overwhelming for you and you feel uneasy about the darker side of childrearing, you might consider reading Kathleen Kendall-Tackett's book called *The Hidden Feelings of Motherhood*. Some people feel guilty about their darker feelings, which causes even more stress. Reading about the negative aspects of parenting and strategies for coping with them can help normalize the challenges and balance your feelings. Most people do not feel that their life with a newborn is simple and easy. Sadly, people are not expected to air their negative feelings either. One way to address this is by finding a supportive parenting group or breastfeeding group to connect with others who are in the same boat. Remember, it is okay to ask for help.

Strategies to help promote relaxation while nursing:

- Find a bright, sunny location for your daytime infant feeding location.
- Set up a cozy spot where you will feel relaxed while feeding or practicing skin-to-skin care.
- Get all your supplies ready before the baby arrives.
- Have some resources for infant feeding that you can read while you are feeding your baby.
- Listen to relaxing music, a meditation, or an inspirational podcast.
- Get audiobooks from your library or an online audio service.
- Watch great movies or a TV series you have wanted to see.
- Incorporate a few ways to pamper yourself while feeding your baby during your daily routine. These treats might include your partner providing a shoulder or foot massage, enjoying your favorite herbal tea (no spearmint or peppermint), or simply enjoying the peace and quiet.

It's All About Our Perspective

TRUE STORY

Amy, a teacher, and mother of two, has a busy work life and her kids are active and outgoing boys in middle school. Amy's partner travels several times a month, leaving her with much of the childcare, meal prep, and other parenting duties like driving to soccer games and band practice. As a result, her weeknights are hectic, and she rarely gets free time on the weekends because of her family's active schedule. She recently posted a picture on social media of her boys as babies and commented about how much she missed the days of a simpler life. No doubt, she was overwhelmed and stressed when her boys were small, but two toddlers suddenly seemed easy compared to having two middle schoolers. It's all about the perspective.

RELACS: The RELAX Method for Pumping

One can adapt the RELAX Method for expressing milk and storing it for later use. The steps are similar but adapted for pumping. The RELACS steps for pumping are 1) Respond, 2) Experience, 3) Latch, 4) Assess, and 5) Collect and Store. While most of the process is similar, you will need to know how to adapt them for pumping.

R - Respond

In this scenario, you are going to respond to the clock. If you have had time to establish breastfeeding with your baby at the breast, you will now be pumping milk during the times when your baby would normally be coming to the breast.

Imagine going back to work when your baby is about eight to ten weeks old. In advance of your first day, you will need to pump some milk to have enough for your first day back to work (and probably a little more). You can build up a small supply in the week before you return to work. *It is a myth that you will need a massive freezer stock of milk before you return to work.* In fact, pumping too much while you are also directly feeding the baby can cause some problems once you settle into your work routine. It may lead to oversupply issues.

On your first day back to work, you will nurse your baby just before you are separated, before you leave the house, or at daycare before you leave. Then, you will begin your pumping schedule during (what would be) the next nursing session. Set up a plan that aligns with your work schedule and closely mimics the time intervals you were using to feed your baby before going back to work. Sometimes, it can be challenging to get your work schedule and pump times to match up exactly. For example, if you need to pump at 10:30 am, and your work schedule does not permit you to take a break until 11:30 am, your breasts may start to feel quite full. Not getting sufficient regular access to pumping "on time" can slow milk production. Remember that your body is adaptable. This scheduling does not mean that your milk production is doomed but you may need to add one more direct breastfeeding session (with your baby at the breast) in the morning hours before you leave for work.

Suppose you work in a job with limited set break times (e.g., teacher, nurse, doctor, flight attendant, pilot, food service industry, manufacturing industry). In that case, you may need to proactively discuss with your employer how you can set up break schedules for pumping. Determine your rights and what you are entitled to under your state or local laws. In the U.S., some employees (depending on the company's size) can take pumping breaks under the "Break Time for Nursing Mothers" law. Visit the United States Breastfeeding Committee (USBC) online for more information. The information provided on the USBC website covers the details of the law and answers various questions, including how to talk to your employer about pumping breaks.

TRUE STORY

While running a breastfeeding support group in Phoenix, AZ, I met a new mother who came to our group looking for supportive ideas on reconnecting with her baby after work, and balancing pumping and direct breastfeeding. She worked as a military pilot and was away from her baby for three consecutive days a week. Because her job as a pilot required her to fly for several hours, part of her pumping schedule included expressing milk in-flight in the cockpit. She was able to pump on the three days she was separated from her baby and feed the baby directly at the breast on the other four days each week. After many years of helping people with infant feeding and pumping, I am still amazed by the creative situations and inventive solutions people find for pumping while working.

Pumping from Day One

Another scenario for pumping human milk starts on the first day of life when a baby must be separated from the parent for some reason. In this scenario, follow step one of the RELACS Method by responding to a set schedule. Create a pumping schedule for yourself that allows for pumping or hand expressing milk every two to three hours. Remember, the same core rules apply for bringing in a full milk supply with pumping (instead of direct breastfeeding). Specifically, the more often milk is removed from the breast, the more milk your body makes. Therefore, aim for as many pumping or hand expressing sessions as you can manage in 24 hours, with a minimum of eight. In addition, in this scenario, you *must* remove milk during the nighttime hours.

E - Experience your baby

In this situation, you and your baby are likely separated while pumping. How can you experience your baby while you are separated? Experiencing your baby involves connecting with your baby through your senses. In the RELAX Method, you use your senses (seeing, hearing, smelling, touching) to promote the hormone shift and facilitate milk letdown. You can still do this even when you are separated. For example, have you ever watched a movie and laughed out loud or cried? You could do this because you were taking in sensory information that caused a physical and hormonal reaction within your body. The same principles apply to experiencing your baby when you are separated, but in this case, you will rely more on seeing, hearing, and smelling the baby. Here are some suggestions:

- Smell an item of clothing (a hat, a blanket) that your baby wore recently.
- Look at happy pictures of your baby.
- Watch a happy video of your baby.
- Listen to a recording of your baby making noises or happy sounds.

It's still important (and maybe more so) to experience your baby by connecting through your senses, even when you are pumping. This connection will help you make the mental shift from a work-related mindset to connecting with your baby. In addition, this will help facilitate the hormonal shift necessary to promote milk flow.

L - Latch

This step is relatively straightforward. Connect your pump to the breast and begin pumping. Be sure the nipple is a comfortable fit for the tunnel. Your nipple should be able to move freely in the tunnel while you are pumping. With the pump on, watch the nipple moving in the tunnel. Do you see any areola tissue (beyond the base of your nipple) moving into the tunnel? This movement could mean that the flange is too large. If your nipple is coming in contact with the tunnel and there is friction, this could mean the flange is too small. Having a flange that is too small can lead to nipple pain, swelling, and damage, and uneven or incomplete drainage of the breast. Sometimes, pumps have comfortable inserts that can help with this.

A - Assess

As detailed above, you can complete part of the assessment while pumping (i.e., latch). Another part of your assessment is milk flow and volume of milk. Are you letting down easily to your pump? Some people have to train themselves to letdown for their pump, but if you followed step two (experience the baby), you are likely letting down. If not, revisit step two.

In addition to milk flow, assess the volume of milk that you can pump. Some people find that milk output increases dramatically (by up to 30% sometimes) when using hands-on pumping. Hand-on pumping is simply using breast compression and massage to move more milk while you are pumping. You can use this strategy while your baby is nursing at the breast too. Be sure to move your hands around the breast and even up near your armpit because your body produces milk in all quadrants of the breast. It is important to note that what you can express by pumping is not always a true reflection of the volume of milk that the baby can get from the breast while nursing. If you're only able to pump a small amount, do not be alarmed. Milk volume changes over the course of the day, and people can pump different amounts of milk at different times. In addition, anxiety and stress can influence milk quantities during pumping versus the amounts the baby takes from direct breastfeeding. Sometimes, pumping can be challenging even when infant feeding is going well.

C - Collect

Depending on how you are expressing milk, the collection will vary. When using a pump, collecting milk is straightforward. As you pump, you collect the milk in bottles. If you are hand expressing, you can collect milk in various ways. Be sure to wash hands first before you begin hand expressing or pumping. Use a small sterile cup or sterile spoon to collect colostrum (before birth, if necessary, or on days one to two postpartum). You can store the colostrum in a small syringe if you feed it to your baby soon after expressing it.

Use glass or hard plastic bottles for storing milk. You can also use BPA-free milk storage bags made specifically for storing human milk. Do not use softer plastic bottles, bottles labeled with recycling number 7, or plastic bags not made explicitly for human milk storage. Be sure your bottles (glass or plastic) have tight-fitting lids. Collect and store milk in small amounts, usually the same amount your baby would take in a single feeding. This practice will help reduce the potential for wasting any milk the baby does not drink. Always label the expressed milk with the pumping date (e.g., February 12th).

Storage Guidelines

After you pump or hand express milk, you have several choices about where and how to store the milk. How it is stored will determine the shelf life of the milk. Therefore, please follow milk storage guidelines carefully and check milk storage protocols from time to time. Occasionally, there are updates to these guidelines.

In general, there are three choices for storing freshly expressed human milk.

1. Room temperature (no hotter than 77 F & 25 C)
2. Refrigerator (40 F & 4 C)
3. Freezer (0 F & -18 C)

If you choose to express milk and leave it at room temperature, it can safely last up to four hours before it must be used or discarded. Milk that is expressed and then put in the back of the refrigerator (don't use the door or the front part of the refrigerator) can safely last up to four days before being used or discarded. In the back of the freezer, human milk can safely last up to 12 months. However, it is best to use the milk by six months.

General Pumping Guidelines

- Wash your hands thoroughly or use an alcohol-based hand sanitizer before expressing milk.
- Express your milk in a quiet place where you are not likely to have any disruptions. If your employer suggests using the restroom, calmly but firmly explain that it is not a sanitary place to express milk, collect milk, or prepare it for storage. It is also not legal in the U.S. to ask workers to pump in the bathroom, according to Section 4207 of the Affordable Care Act.
- Simulate your sensory experience with your baby by looking at happy pictures of your baby, watching happy videos, or listening to your baby making happy sounds. Some people like to do a simple hands-on breast or nipple massage before pumping to help stimulate milk flow.
- Invest in a high-quality nursing bra. You can purchase these at stores and online, or you can make your own (search online for simple instructions).
- Get the best pump you can buy to fit your needs. For example, if you work full-time five days a week, you will need a high-quality pump. Look for a highly rated *double electric pump*. You will be using it frequently, so it needs to have a good motor that will last. On the other hand, if you work part-time and have some flexibility, your pump can be a step down from the highest quality. Consider the double electric in both cases because pumping both breasts at once saves time (10-15 minutes versus 30 minutes with a single pump) and helps keep prolactin levels high. Lately, I have heard many stories about people who are having trouble expressing enough milk or believing they have low supply because they are using the wrong pump. Get the heavy-duty pump if you are pumping daily. Wearable pumps and manual pumps may not have the suction strength needed for maintaining a full milk supply if you must pump several days a week.

R RESPOND	Respond to your baby's feeding cues. Attending to early cues makes for easier feeding.
E EXPERIENCE	Experience your baby by connecting through your senses. Hold the baby, kiss her, smell her head, listen to her breathe.
L LATCH	Facilitate the best position that allows your baby to latch well. Be aware of your posture and the baby's posture.
A ASSESS & ADJUST	Assess your comfort level. If there is pain, clicking, or sliding, unlatch and adjust for a more effective latch.
X EXHALE	RELAX. Sit back, recline if possible and relax. Focus on your comfort, listen to relaxing or inspiring music, read a book. Appreciate the peace.

Table 4.1: The RELAX Method

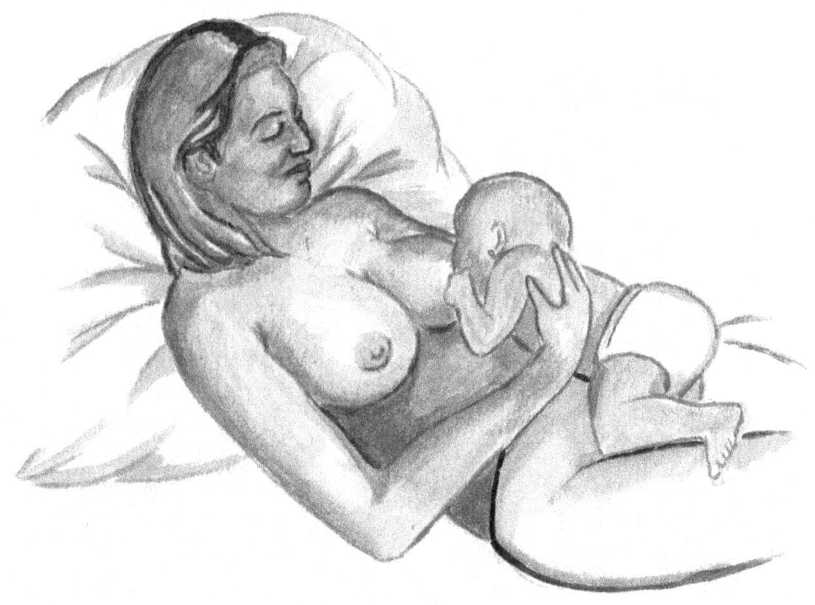

Figure 4.1: Laid-Back

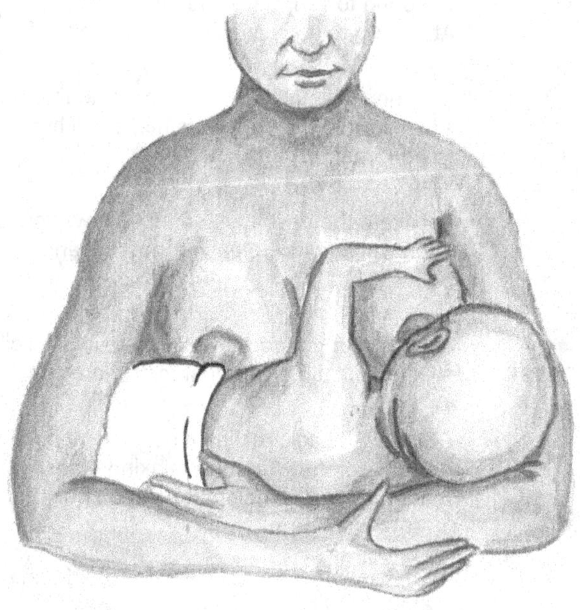

Figure 4.2: Cradle

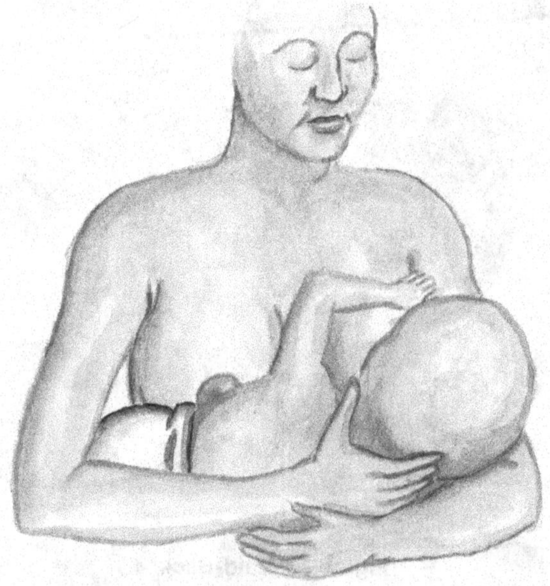

Figure 4.3: Cross-Cradle

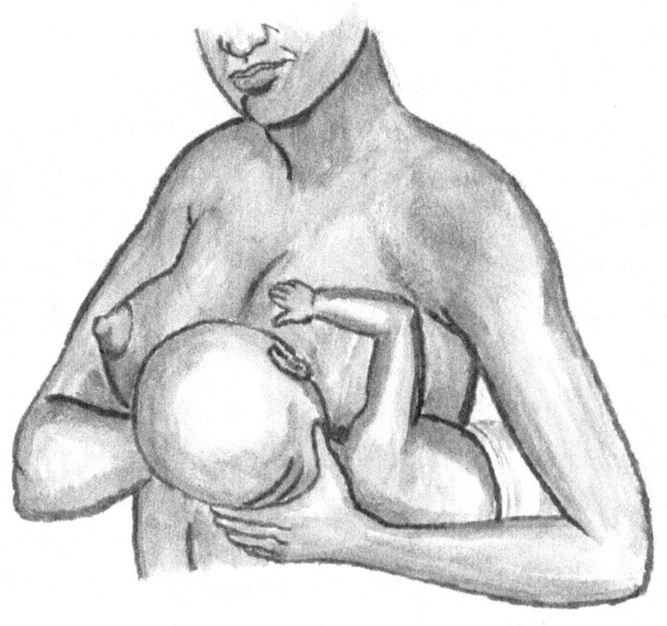

Figure 4.4: Football

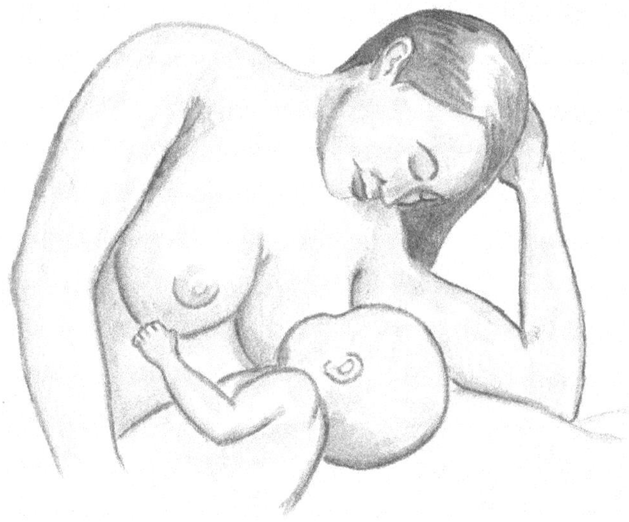

Figure 4.5: Side-Lying

CHAPTER 5

Kangaroo for 72

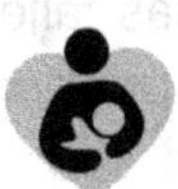

By now, you have likely heard about the benefits of skin-to-skin care, also called Kangaroo Care. This term refers to how kangaroos carry their young in a pouch. You may be wondering why there is so much emphasis on immediate skin-to-skin care directly after delivery. Many people I work with have asked me, "Do I really need to practice skin-to-skin care? I know they didn't do that when I was born. So, what is the big deal?"

What is Kangaroo Care?

Kangaroo Care (KC) or skin-to-skin care is the practice of placing a newborn (or older infant) directly between the breasts, while both the parent and the newborn are free of clothing, blankets, or other fabric. The skin-to-skin aspect of this practice allows for the direct sensory exchange between the parent and the baby. The sensory input that the baby receives in this position drives biological responses within the newborn to help with state stabilization and organization. Stability and organization in this context refer to body system regulation (heart rate, body temperature, breathing patterns, oxygen saturation, level of contentment, and so on). The parent is also getting input from the newborn, which results in hormonal changes that promote bonding, attachment, nurturing, and breastfeeding. Either parent or other caregivers/family members can practice KC, which can be helpful immediately after delivery if one person is unavailable or at other times when two people are sharing the work of KC. Some processes are enhanced when skin-to-skin care is practiced in the maternal habitat, for example, thermoregulation and, obviously, the opportunities for breastfeeding.

Who Invented Kangaroo Care?

The practice of holding a newborn skin-to-skin has likely been a persistent feature in childcare for millennia. It's anyone's guess as to why skin-to-skin care was abandoned in many parts of the world. However, there is evidence of why KC has fallen out of favor in many clinical settings. For example, hospital protocols took precedence over bonding in the twentieth century. In addition, the popularity of infant formula combined with hospital births and central nurseries increased parent-infant separation in the immediate postpartum period. While this may seem harmless, there are real costs associated with these separation periods.

In the 1970s in Bogota, Columbia, there was a severe shortage of equipment necessary to handle premature infants and overcrowding in the central infant nurseries. As a result, the infection rates, infant morbidity, and mortality rates were extremely high. Doctors were facing incredibly difficult decisions on what to do with these babies to ensure their survival. Instead of leaving the newborn preemies to struggle on their own, they were placed skin-to-skin with their mothers. As a result, the infants who benefitted from KC not only improved, but they had lower infection rates, lower mortality rates, and increased breastfeeding rates.

Two of the doctors working in the overcrowded nurseries in Columbia, Drs. Rey and Martinez, published their findings on this innovation in 1979. In time, the practice of skin-to-skin care spread worldwide, and researchers began to study its clinical outcomes. Establishing KC as standard care has taken decades, but we are making continued progress. Ask if your hospital and caregiver routinely recommends 90 minutes of uninterrupted skin-to-skin care immediately following delivery.

The Stability Habitat

Skin-to-skin care with your newborn dramatically affects the baby's biology and behaviors. In terms of the biological responses, skin-to-skin contact between parent and baby drives the *stabilization of infant body systems*. Consider this list of outcomes of Kangaroo Care for your newborn:

- Stabilizes heart rate
- Stabilizes blood pressure
- Stabilizes breathing rate
- Improves infant body temperature
- Improves oxygen saturation
- Improves ***blood sugar levels**
- Improves emotional state (helps your newborn feel secure, content, and organized)
- Helps calm an infant before breastfeeding
- Provides immediate unrestricted access to the breast
- Promotes organized sleeping patterns
- Promotes weight gain for newborns
- Decreases crying episodes
- Decreases apnea episodes
- Decreases infant infection and mortality rates
- Decreases the length of stay in hospitals for preemies

As you can see, Kangaroo Care has an impressive range of positive effects for infants, some of which directly benefit breastfeeding. For example, one of the ways KC helps to protect breastfeeding is by improving infant blood sugar levels. Low blood sugar for infants can sometimes cause problems and doctors are eager to see healthy blood sugar levels, especially in at-risk infants. Consequently, low blood sugar is often the main variable on the road to formula supplementation, and some of which is unnecessary. If KC were standard procedure, perhaps we could dramatically lower rates of formula supplementation in the first two days of life.

One of the infant's main goals is survival. Body system stability facilitates survival. Thus, for the baby to survive, it runs several programs, one of which is the defense program. The defense program is one way of sounding the alarm. When the baby feels overwhelmed or lacks any feeling of security, the body systems begin to become disorganized: blood pressure increases, breathing rate increases, emotional state deteriorates (and can include angry crying, but not always), oxygen saturation decreases, and so on. The infant who is out of his secure habitat will most likely run the defense program in an attempt to alert parents or caregivers. Fussiness and crying are two common ways infants express the need for stabilization. Sometimes, babies can be so overwhelmed that they will experience a system shut down, a coping strategy that helps them conserve energy. This shutdown may look like sleep but is not.

When your baby is in defense mode, it takes time and effort to stabilize again, and babies cannot do this alone. *Their most stable environment is in physical bodily contact with another human.* Fortunately, one of the best approaches to help your baby regain stabilization is to place the baby skin-to-skin. One can practice Kangaroo Care immediately after delivery, but it can also be practiced at other times throughout the first year to help the baby regain body system stability. Think of this as the baby's natural stability habitat. Because skin-to-skin is incredibly effective at helping stabilize a new baby (and promotes a healthy milk supply), I recommend that all parents practice long periods of Kangaroo Care for several days after birth.

Kangaroo for 72

Seventy-two hours is equal to three days. If you have not had your baby yet, you might be thinking that my recommendation to snuggle your baby skin-to-skin on your chest for three solid days sounds absolutely ridiculous. Perhaps this is outrageous, but once you see the benefits and how this works, you may change your mind. If you have already had your baby, you may be open to the idea that you have a stealthy approach for helping your newborn achieve stability, no matter how much time is involved.

There are several variables involved in the practice of Kangaroo Care:

- Those who breastfeed can hold their infants skin-to-skin
- Partners can provide KC, as well as other adults
- KC can be continuous
- KC can be intermittent (now and then throughout the day)
- It is the optimal environment immediately after the baby emerges from birth until the first latch and feeding have

occurred (because this facilitates stable body systems and elicits the breast-seeking behaviors)

- KC can be practiced safely with twins and triplets in Shared KC
- You can practice KC in the NICU with babies who are ill or premature
- You can practice KC after cesarean delivery, but you may have to request this before the birth (be aware that some hospitals may not accommodate KC immediately after a cesarean)
- You can practice KC anytime your baby needs a body system reset, even with older babies

Kangaroo Care frequently occurs between babies and the breastfeeding parent, but this nurturing environment is not limited to the maternal habitat. Anyone with skin can provide skin-to-skin care. This practice is a fantastic way for fathers, partners, or other close family members to bond with the baby and provide nurturing infant care. The maternal stability habitat does have certain advantages, with the obvious one being the availability of breast milk. However, there are others. For example, the infant will likely have more success with precise body temperature regulation in the maternal habitat because breastfeeding parents are highly attuned to the body temperature needs of their newborns. For example, research shows that during the thermal regulation of twins held in KC, each breast can respond to the baby's unique needs on that side (Ludington-Hoe et al., 2006). In other words, one breast can increase body temperature for a twin needing warmth, while the other breast can lower body temperature for a twin needing to be slightly cooled. Other adults who are not currently lactating won't have this superpower.

It is also possible to practice Kangaroo Care continuously or intermittently. Continuous skin-to-skin care might be best with two people sharing the work, switching off between partners. Continuous or nearly continuous skin-to-skin care may be in order if you have an early full-term baby (born 37-39 weeks) who needs extra care. This baby may not be considered premature, but he did arrive a little early in reality (each day counts). True preemies (born before 37 weeks) *absolutely benefit from skin-to-skin* because they have a much more difficult time with body system regulation. If your baby is premature and goes to the NICU, ask about practicing skin-to-skin care in the NICU. It can be remarkably beneficial for some premature infants.

Intermittent skin-to-skin care is Kangaroo Care that is performed now and then for about 90 minutes-two hours. The goal is to make it through a sleep and feed cycle. This option means that you do not need to practice KC all day. Instead, you can hold your baby in KC a few times per day or perhaps just several times per week. Not only are you and the baby experiencing the stability habitat, but you are also providing the best access to the breast. For a newborn, the stability habitat will help relieve state disorganization, stop the defense program, and allow her to run the feeding program. This stability enables your baby to devote all of her energy to growth and development instead of using energy on body system regulation. What better place for her to be than at the food source?

The skin-to-skin environment is the optimal start to breastfeeding. While this may sound obvious, consider the differences between these two common scenarios:

1. The baby is born and immediately whisked off to be weighed, measured, and bathed. He returns to you swaddled in a blanket, wearing a hat. You will likely hold this baby in a cradle hold and begin to breastfeed. The infant cannot use hands, arms, and legs to run the breast-seeking program because all of his limbs are trapped in a tight swaddle. The baby does not use gravity to stabilize his body weight while breastfeeding. The baby will likely approach the nipple from the front in a face-to-nipple position.

2. The baby is born and is placed immediately on your chest in skin-to-skin care. You are semi-reclined in a laid-back position. The baby is dried while in place on your chest. The newborn is naked except for a blanket covering his back. This baby will seek the breast using hands, arms, legs, cheeks, nose, lips, and tongue. Gravity will keep this infant stable on top of you while he is moving toward the breast. This position allows the baby to approach the nipple over the top (if you recline enough).

There are many differences between these two scenarios. While breastfeeding can undoubtedly happen in the first scenario, that environment does not provide for the other essential variables that KC will facilitate. The baby in scenario 2, held in the KC position, will have advantages with body system stabilization, most notably body temperature stabilization, blood sugar regulation, respiratory rate and heart rate stabilization, and more stable oxygen saturation. In addition, the KC baby will be fully able to use all of the neonatal reflexes that accompany the breast seeking behaviors and make more sense in this position. More on that below.

Why Does the Baby Need Help with Body System Stabilization?

Human infants are immature at birth compared to many of our primate cousins. Therefore, human babies need the continuous presence of the parents, particularly the breastfeeding parent, to ensure the infant survives. This constant presence of the parents helps the infant maintain body system regulation, stay close to his food source, and spend less time in a disorganized state. Energy is precious to the newborn. The more time the infant spends in a disorganized condition, the more energy he is spending on running the defense program and not on growth and digestion.

Second to survival is the baby's goal for thriving and growing. To grow, he must be able to run the feeding program. According to Dr. Nils Bergman, infants cannot simultaneously run the defense and feeding programs. It must be one program at a time. As parents, it is our job to help our babies to thrive, allowing for as much time in an organized, stable state as possible. An organized state allows the baby to run the feeding program. As a result, the baby can use all of his energy for growth unless he spends too much time running the defense program, which uses up valuable energy to achieve physical and emotional stability. When we place the baby in skin-to-skin contact, we are helping him stay calm, stable, and organized. This contact is how we maximize his ability to spend his valuable energy on growth, not constantly trying to achieve body system stabilization.

Kangaroo Care for 72 hours doesn't just benefit the baby. Parents who practice skin-to-skin report:

- increased levels of bonding with their infants (lasting for years)
- increased sensitivity to infant cries and signals
- increased milk supply
- increased skills and confidence in providing care for their newborn
- decreased risk of postpartum hemorrhage
- decreased risk of postpartum anxiety and depression
- for parents with infants in the NICU, KC can offer a unique opportunity to make a valuable contribution to infant care while the infant is hospitalized

How to Perform Kangaroo Care

There are some guidelines for practicing KC. Although the practice of holding your infant is intuitive, there are a few things to be sure to do, and a few things to avoid while holding your newborn in Kangaroo Care. Below are guidelines adapted from the American Academy of Pediatrics for skin-to-skin care in the immediate moments after birth and a general outline of practicing Kangaroo Care anytime.

Prerequisites

Before Kangaroo Care begins, there are a few prerequisites.

1. The baby is free of clothing and fabric except for a diaper. The parent may wear an open-front shirt, an open-front hospital gown, or a bathrobe. The infant wears nothing (directly after birth), or the newborn can wear a diaper/nappy.
2. The parent reclines about 30-40 degrees, comfortably supported in a position that they can maintain for at least 90 minutes.
3. If necessary, the parent receives help with placing the baby (may be necessary for newborns in the NICU, connected to monitors).

Immediately Following Birth

The practice of Kangaroo Care directly after birth is slightly different from practicing KC at other times. Here are the guidelines for post-birth KC adapted from the American Academy of Pediatrics procedures for skin-to-skin care.

- After the baby emerges from the womb, he is dried and assessed.
- If the infant is stable, he is placed skin-to-skin with his parent, cord attached.
- The cord can be clamped after a few minutes or after the delivery of the placenta.
- The infant is assessed after the placenta is delivered.
- Continue to dry the newborn, except for hands. The hands that still smell like amniotic fluid will be useful to the baby. Hand-to-mouth movements (smell and taste) will give sensory cues necessary for rooting and finding the nipple.
- Use of infant hat is optional.
- Cover the newborn with prewarmed blankets, leaving the face exposed.
- Caregivers can complete Apgar assessments with the baby in place on the parent at one and five minutes.
- Allow the pair to remain together practicing Kangaroo Care for 60-90 minutes, at least until the first breastfeeding has occurred.

Once again, the parent holding the newborn should be free of clothing and fabric in front and semi-reclined in a comfortable seat or bed. Use pillows to prop up or support the back if needed. If seated, a footstool can be a useful addition.

For infant positioning, the parent (or caregivers) should place the newborn tummy down, with the arms and legs flexed (bent). The infant's chest should be in direct contact with the parent's chest (be sure no arms, hands, or shoulders are in the way). The infant head should turn to one side, with the neck extended slightly to ensure that the airway is open.

Who Should Not Practice Kangaroo Care After Delivery?

There are a few instances when skin-to-skin care is contraindicated. For example, although general anesthesia during birth is rare, it does happen. When general anesthesia occurs, it is best not to perform KC until after anesthesia has cleared the system. In addition, people who received magnesium sulfate during labor may not be able to provide a secure place for KC because of the action of the magnesium as a muscle relaxer. However, it is possible to hold your baby after receiving magnesium sulfate, but you may need supervision or assistance from your partner or your nurse. It can depend on how much magnesium sulfate you received or for how long. It may vary from one person to the next. Other times when KC could be contraindicated are with overly sleepy parents or sedated parents. Allow sufficient time for recovery after any of these scenarios before placing a newborn skin-to-skin with the breastfeeding parent. If the partner is available, the baby can rest in skin-to-skin care on the partner's chest until you are fully awake and ready to initiate breastfeeding.

Caution: Never practice skin-to-skin care while you are sleeping. The baby can and will likely sleep in the KC position, but parents must remain awake throughout the entire experience. If you feel tired or need to nod off, hand the baby off to a partner. In addition, there are times when newborns may not be stable enough to practice KC. This is unique and sometimes ironic because the research clearly shows that KC can effectively stabilize a newborn. Some hospitals and doctors are not inclined to allow KC until after the newborn is stable. The baby may need treatment or observation before being placed skin-to-skin in some cases. In some instances, it can be beneficial to request that your baby is placed skin-to-skin instead of another intervention like using a radiant warmer to increase infant body temperature or formula supplementation for slightly depressed blood sugar readings. It cannot hurt to ask for skin-to-skin but understand that caregivers are more likely to use the intervention they are most familiar with, regardless of whether that is the most protective for breastfeeding or not.

When Can Kangaroo Care Help Protect Breastfeeding?

There are several scenarios where one can utilize skin-to-skin care to keep the breastfeeding dyad together and protect breastfeeding. Consider the following situations:

A. A newborn has *low blood sugar (also called low blood glucose or hypoglycemia). Caregivers are recommending supplementation with formula. What are the alternatives? According to the Academy of Breastfeeding Medicine Protocol #1 on Hypoglycemia, holding a newborn skin-to-skin reduces the risk of hypoglycemia and provides breastfeeding opportunities (Wight & Marinelli, 2014). Kangaroo Care also helps an infant stabilize body systems, so the infant does not have to spend limited energy on system regulation. This practice protects the infant from further hypoglycemia because he can conserve energy.

B. A newborn is experiencing a transient drop in body temperature. Caregivers recommend that the infant be separated from his parents and placed in a radiant warmer or incubator to raise body temperature. What are the alternatives? Again, holding a newborn with skin-to-skin contact facilitates thermoregulation. This practice can prevent separation of the baby from parents, assist the newborn in stabilizing his body temperature, conserve energy that the baby might have spent on raising body temperature, prevent blood glucose drops for healthy full-term infants, and provide unrestricted access to the breast.

C. After birth, a new baby was given formula supplements at the hospital. Now, the infant is two weeks old, and the mother is experiencing less than optimal milk supply. The baby prefers the flow of the bottle compared to direct breastfeeding. The parents want to transition this baby to full breastfeeding and eliminate the formula supplements. Practicing Kangaroo Care as often as possible will help elicit breast-seeking behaviors, even with a baby who seems to prefer the bottle. KC can help stimulate milk production, provide easy and direct access to the breast, and help keep this baby stable. A happy, stable baby will likely have more success with attempts to feed directly at the breast than one who is disorganized and anxious.

You may need to advocate for yourself in some of these situations. Many practitioners are most likely to go with the intervention they know best. If your doctor is familiar with Kangaroo Care and is comfortable with KC as an intervention for stabilizing a newborn in certain instances, you may be in luck.

On the other hand, if your caregiver is not familiar with KC and lacks confidence in skin-to-skin care, they may not offer this option to you for stabilizing your newborn. Be your own advocate and ask for Kangaroo Care if necessary. Keep in mind that there are times when the situation dictates interventions that go beyond the bounds of what Kangaroo Care can offer.

What Happens if You Don't Get to Practice Immediate KC?

If there is a separation between you and your newborn in the immediate postpartum period, or you have been sedated, received large amounts of magnesium sulfate, or are in any situation that prevents you from holding your baby skin-to-skin immediately after the delivery, all is not lost.

The newborn retains instincts and reflexes for breast seeking and breastfeeding long after the first moments of life. So, you can use Kangaroo Care on day two, or even at two weeks or two months. The baby will still be able to reap all of the benefits of skin-to-skin care, no matter his age.

Suppose you had an epidural pain relief, especially with certain narcotics, like fentanyl. In that case, your newborn could exhibit some initial sleepiness and disorganization, which could cause a delay in seeking the breast and possibly a delay in the timing of the first latch. Be patient. Practice Kangaroo Care for 72 hours, and your baby will respond.

Similarities Between Kangaroo Care and Laid-back Breastfeeding

There is a strong relationship between laid-back (LB) breastfeeding and Kangaroo Care in many ways. Consider these commonalities:

- The parent is semi-reclined in both KC and LB breastfeeding.

- Both KC and LB breastfeeding provide the proper physiological context and location to elicit neonatal reflexes and breast-seeking behaviors.
- Breastfeeding is available in both scenarios.
- Both situations support the baby on top of the parent, using gravity to stabilize the baby.
- Parent and baby are chest to chest.

It may seem to some people that Kangaroo Care is simply laid-back breastfeeding without any clothing or fabric between the parent and the baby. This is an oversimplification and does not consider the goals for each of these techniques.

In the case of Kangaroo Care, the main goal is to help the baby achieve body system regulation in the stability habitat, skin-to-skin with a parent or other caregiver. In the KC position, *feeding can happen*, but it is not the primary goal. While being held in skin-to-skin care, a newborn appears to be doing nothing, but many unseen processes occur within the baby. For example, you will not be able to see the baby's body temperature stabilize, but it does. You will not see the heart rate and blood sugar stabilize, but they do. Also, in this position, your newborn will likely fall asleep. Even while the infant is asleep, each unseen process is still ongoing, still protecting the new baby from getting too cold, having swings in blood sugar, heart rate, and so on.

In the case of laid-back breastfeeding, the main goal is to facilitate breastfeeding. While this baby is in the stability habitat, he is also in the place that best facilitates innate breastfeeding reflexes. While practicing laid-back breastfeeding in the first weeks of life, you can see lots of things happening because the baby will perform numerous innate reflexes as he seeks the breast. Suzanne Colson, author of *Biological Nurturing: Instinctual Breastfeeding*, researches the laid-back breastfeeding position. Her studies have documented about 20 innate newborn reflexes that facilitate breastfeeding. The most common innate reflexes are:

- Mouth movements – opening and closing, lip-smacking
- Hand to mouth movements

- Head bobbing toward one breast or the other
- Rooting
- Suck and swallow reflexes
- Flexing and extending the fingers and hands
- Arm and leg cycling (moving arms and legs to aid in a forward movement)

Colson's research led to some fascinating observations about the utility and meaning of these reflexes. However, Colson's studies show that these are dependent on how one holds the infant. For example, in the cradle position, parents interpreted the arms and leg cycling as interference. Similarly, the hand-to-mouth reflex seemed to get in the way of the real action the parents were trying to achieve: effective latching onto the breast. When placing infants on top of the parent in the laid-back position, the arm and leg cycling were truly beneficial movements that the infant used to position himself at the breast to latch properly. In the same way, the hand-to-mouth movements are instrumental and productive parts of seeking the breast when in the laid-back position but misinterpreted for infants in the cradle position (Colson et al., 2008).

Over the many years that I have provided breastfeeding guidance for parents, I have heard numerous comments about how the baby's hands are always in the way when attempting to latch (in the cradle position) and discussions about strategies to trap the hands while breastfeeding. In all cases, it was helpful to position the baby on top of the parent to illustrate how the hand movements are practical and meaningful. Indeed, the cradle hold can be useful at times. Remember that while breastfeeding in the cradle hold, the baby might still want to use hands. Some older babies are adept at using their hands to help position the breast, and some babies likely use their hands for the tactile input and to feel the closeness to their parent.

The purpose of the innate reflexes is to assist the infant in seeking the breast and self-attaching onto the breast for feeding. All mammals are equipped with the skills and reflexes to seek their food source and attach by themselves. Instead of interpreting these skills as unnecessary body movements or even as a nuisance, recognize that these innate skills are the infant's roadmap to food and survival. The newborn wants to use these skills while seeking the breast, and he is not inclined to turn off the innate reflexes just because he is not in the position where the reflexes make the most sense. You can help your newborn make the best use of innate skills and reflexes by holding him in the laid-back position for breastfeeding in the early weeks. As the baby gets older and more adept at nursing, many positions are feasible for effective breastfeeding.

A Final Thought on Kangaroo for 72

If you and your healthy baby had a difficult delivery or your newborn is not adjusting to life outside the womb as well as you would have liked, there is no harm in recovering from birth while holding your infant skin-to-skin. You can even think of it as therapy after labor and birth. This therapy is a gift to your baby and a gift to yourself. Remember, most people do not have a busy schedule planned for the days following birth. Several years ago, I read an article about a woman who attended a Cincinnati Bengals football game just a day or two after her cesarean delivery. The author of the article seemed to celebrate her dedication to the team. Dedicate yourself to team baby instead. I highly recommend avoiding an urge to do anything other than rest, self-care, breastfeeding, and infant care for the first days and weeks after birth. Kangaroo for 72 is both care for you and your baby.

How Can Kangaroo Care Influence Lactation Outcomes?

Over the last few decades, there has been a great deal of excellent research on skin-to-skin care of newborns and its effects on lactation. In this section, we explore the highlights of this research. Consider the following:

- Infants held in Kangaroo Care longer than 20 minutes after delivery are breastfed longer (in terms of total duration, weeks or months) than infants who do not have intense skin-to-skin contact with their mothers after birth (Mikiel-Kostyra et al., 2007).
- In a study of skin-to-skin care after birth versus new parents holding their infants in swaddling blankets immediately after birth, the Kangaroo Care infants had better sucking capability.

They also achieved effective breastfeeding sooner than the swaddled infants (Moore & Anderson, 2007).

- Infants born by cesarean who experience Kangaroo Care in the operating room after delivery are supplemented with formula less frequently before hospital discharge than infants not held skin-to-skin in the operating room (Hung & Berg, 2011).
- Early skin-to-skin contact appears to have a dose-response effect on the degree of exclusive breastfeeding during the hospital stay after birth. For example, a study of newborns held skin-to-skin used a simple metric for comparison. This study connects the number of minutes babies were held in Kangaroo Care with the likelihood of exclusive breastfeeding during the hospital stay. The study revealed that the infants who received more minutes of skin-to-skin contact after birth were more likely to be fed exclusively human milk before hospital discharge (Bramson et al., 2010). This outcome is significant because the recent data from the CDC reports that 19.2% of breastfed infants received formula supplements before they were two days old (CDC, 2020a). Early formula supplementation increases the likelihood that breastfeeding is abandoned early, even among those with strong intentions to breastfeed (Chantry et al., 2014).
- A study of neonatal hypoglycemia (infant low blood sugar) compared the NICU admission rate before and after introducing skin-to-skin care at a hospital in Texas. After implementing skin-to-skin care at the hospital, the number of infants needing NICU care for hypoglycemia decreased significantly from 8.1% to 3.5% (Chiruvolu et al., 2017). In this same study, the number of infants receiving IV dextrose for low blood sugar also decreased significantly (Chiruvolu et al., 2017). Not surprisingly, the study also revealed that the rate of exclusive breastfeeding at hospital discharge increased from 36.4% to 45.7% (Chiruvolu et al., 2017).

True Stories of Kangaroo Care

For many people, the idea of Kangaroo Care sounds beneficial. At the same time, one might consider it *above and beyond* what is necessary. In other words, in theory, Kangaroo Care for all infants would be nice, but some parents and professionals might not consider KC essential. Breastfeeding itself has had a similar reputation for many years, but people are now recognizing that breastfeeding is not a luxury. It is a true necessity for all parents and infants in the postpartum period. Likewise, we now recognize skin-to-skin care as an essential part of the newborn's transition to the world beyond the womb. As discussed above, infants who receive skin-to-skin care are in their stability habitat. If promoting newborn body system stability and providing access to more effective breastfeeding is optimal, why is it still considered optional?

The following are true stories of skin-to-skin care from several parent-baby dyads. Each of the parents in these following stories felt that skin-to-skin care had a dramatic and positive effect on their baby and on their breastfeeding journey.

Kangaroo Care for Preemies

Christine's baby boy was born at 34 weeks, and like many preemies, he struggled with low body temperature. Christine argued with the staff to let her newborn preemie achieve optimal body temperature skin-to-skin with her rather than under the warmer. The nurses were stunned that the baby had better and more stable body temperatures on her chest, skin-to-skin, than they typically see in the warmer. Despite his preterm birth, her newborn breastfed effectively from the start. KC helped Christine and her baby avoid separation. She considered it a massive win for Kangaroo Care.

Lauren's new baby arrived at 32 weeks. Immediate skin-to-skin was not possible with this preemie, but they could initiate Kangaroo Care on day two. Infants born before 34 weeks often have more feeding challenges because they can have difficulty coordinating the suck, swallow, and breathing sequence. Due to her premature status, Lauren's baby could only latch once during her hospital stay. However, the baby did display multiple innate feeding behaviors while in place skin-to-skin. At first, Lauren misread her newborn's head bobbing behavior (an innate breast-seeking behavior) as discontentment, but she continued to place the baby on her chest. After lots of skin-to-skin time over the first weeks of life, her newborn began latching on her due date. After that, she nursed at the breast effectively and eventually transitioned entirely away from bottle feeding. Lauren credits several weeks of Kangaroo Care as the reason for her daughter's effective transition to direct breastfeeding.

Kira had two separate experiences with skin-to-skin for preterm infants. She delivered her first at 36 weeks and her second at only 35 weeks. Both babies were placed skin-to-skin immediately after birth, and Kira tried to do continuous Kangaroo Care as much as she could while at the hospital. Her second baby had hypoglycemia (low blood sugar), and Kira credits supplementation with expressed colostrum coupled with continuous skin-to-skin as the reason her newborn baby rebounded quickly. With each of her birth experiences, Kira and her babies avoided complications, formula supplements, extra observations, and any time in the NICU. She and her babies left the hospital with lactation intact.

Kangaroo Care After a Complicated Birth

Whitney's baby arrived early at 35 weeks via cesarean delivery after a diagnosis of preeclampsia. Cesarean surgery, prematurity, and preeclampsia raise the risk of infant feeding problems and delay lactogenesis II (the rapid transition to mature milk). Whitney's training as a breastfeeding peer counselor gave her the knowledge and the skills she needed to advocate for skin-to-skin care after delivery. Because Whitney was not physically ready for Kangaroo Care immediately after birth, her partner was able to hold their newborn skin-to-skin until she was able to take over. Whitney says that her instincts and knowledge of breastfeeding told her that her fragile preemie needed continuous skin-to-skin care to avoid NICU admission. She held her newborn skin-to-skin as much as she could over the first 48 hours after delivery. During KC, the baby had been stable, exhibiting good blood sugar levels, breathing rate, and body temperature. However, the baby's blood sugar dropped during the separation of the mom and baby (for Whitney's incision care and bandage change). The doctor ordered supplements, but Whitney suggested that instead of formula (which she preferred not to use), the caregivers provide her baby the colostrum she hand-expressed in the days before birth. The staff helped her deliver the baby 5mL of expressed colostrum by cup feeding. After the colostrum supplement, her newborn displayed feeding cues, and she put him to the breast. Whitney believes that skin-to-skin care in the first days of life helped keep her baby stable, which was the key to avoiding NICU admission. She exclusively breastfed her baby for the first six months of life. Whitney says, "I have no doubt that skin-to-skin care is what kept him out of the NICU and helped his little body thrive five weeks prematurely."

Kangaroo Care and Complicated Feeding Challenges

Alexandra and her newborn son had a tough start. Alexandra's baby struggled to feed at the breast from day one. Although she had to supplement with formula, Alexandra never abandoned the idea of getting her baby to the breast and feeding him her milk. Because he was not latching and feeding at the breast, Alexandra initially struggled with low milk supply issues. She began pumping and continued to investigate the source of the breastfeeding challenges. She took her newborn son to several specialists and tried multiple interventions, but she received no answers and failed to correct his feeding problems. Eventually, Alexandra decided to stop trying to fix the mystery problems, and instead, she began to hold him skin-to-skin as much as she could. He spent lots of time skin-to-skin and took his naps naked on her chest. She expressed milk for him as much as possible to build her milk supply in hopes that he would eventually transition to breast milk, no formula. She finally discovered that her baby had a posterior tongue tie that had been undiagnosed, a small lip tie, and oral motor hypotonia (reduced muscle tone of the oral structures). Alexandra continued her skin-to-skin care and attempted to nurse her son for months. Finally, she went from feeding him half breast milk and half formula to exclusively feeding him her milk. This mother-baby pair did not give up on KC or breastfeeding, and eventually, Alexandra helped her baby nurse directly at the breast beginning at five months old. In her words, she says, "Skin-to-skin is magic!" Her son continued to nurse until he was two and a half.

Kangaroo Care for an Adopted Baby

Skin-to-skin care is the infant's natural habitat, whether the skin is the baby's biological mother, father, or adoptive parents. Erika and her husband were ready to adopt. They brought home their newborn baby, who had been in the NICU, exclusively bottle-fed every three hours. When they picked up their baby daughter, one of the nurses told Erika not to hold her too much because the baby needed rest. Erika knew that she would, in fact, do just the opposite to help their fragile four-pound daughter thrive. The baby was only 18 days old when they brought her home. Erika started skin-to-skin care with her immediately and was surprised to see that her new daughter knew what to do, despite having never been skin-to-skin with anyone, even after her birth. Once in place on her mom's chest, the baby threw herself over to the breast and latched on as if she had practiced this hundreds of times. Since it was summertime, Erika got several stretchy tank tops to wear and tucked her newborn inside her shirt, skin-to-skin, dressed only in a diaper. This mother-baby pair spent the first several months practicing Kangaroo Care and feeding at the breast using a supplemental nursing system. At the time of the adoption, Erika had no milk, so she pumped her breasts to induce her own milk supply. She spent hours holding her newborn skin-to-skin and continuing to pump milk every day. She eventually had enough supply to feed the baby exclusively with her own milk. Erika nursed her fragile four-pound adopted preemie for four years. (It is entirely possible to bring in your own milk for an adopted baby.)

Kangaroo Care for Hypoglycemia (Low Blood Sugar)

Some infants are more at risk for metabolic complications after birth, including infants born to a parent with diabetes, babies born preterm, small for gestational age (SGA), infants with growth restrictions, and infants born large for gestational age (LGA).

Karla's son was born large for gestational age and subsequently struggled to stabilize blood sugar levels. He was admitted to the NICU and was given IV dextrose to help bring up his blood sugar. Karla and her husband held their baby skin-to-skin during their entire stay in the NICU except for a short stretch at night so they could both get some sleep. His blood sugar levels stabilized but were not considered good enough for discharge from intensive care. One of the nurses suggested to Karla that perhaps all the skin-to-skin holding was taxing for the baby. The nurse advised her to put the baby down in the infant bassinet for a while. The next glucose reading revealed that his blood sugar had dropped. Upon investigation, the nurse discovered that the IV was not working properly. Everyone surmised that Kangaroo Care with his parents was the reason for his early blood sugar stabilization. Karla decided to resume continuous skin-to-skin care with her newborn. She and her partner took turns holding him for the next 12 hours in Kangaroo Care. His blood sugar stabilized, and the hospital discharged them.

Kangaroo Care for Oxygen Saturation

The stability habitat is not just helpful for stabilizing blood sugar levels. It helps infants regulate their breathing rate and oxygen saturation as well. For example, Gabby's grandson was born by cesarean at full term. He was diagnosed with transient tachypnea of the newborn, faster than normal breathing rate. The baby was observed in the nursery while receiving oxygen and skin-to-skin care with his dad. A few hours after the birth, his mother was mobile enough to join them in the nursery. She held the baby in Kangaroo Care, and soon after, the baby's heart rate, breathing rate, and oxygen saturation levels all normalized. Gabby feels strongly that the magic of skin-to-skin care stabilized her grandson.

Sometimes, infants appear stable by all measures, except for parental instinct. Sarah had a healthy baby who seemed stable, but she was suspicious of his demeanor on the first day of life. She held him skin-to-skin while he made unusual grunting noises throughout the day. Her nurse commented that she was a little worried about his breathing but that keeping him in Kangaroo Care provided the stabilization he needed. Sarah's baby never needed any other assistance beyond KC.

Kangaroo Care for Transitioning Off of the Nipple Shield

Skin-to-skin care can help reboot a previously challenging breastfeeding experience. Danae used a nipple shield for the first few months of breastfeeding. Although Danae tried to latch her daughter without the nipple shield, they had only had success a few times in the first ten weeks of life. She tried all the usual techniques and tricks to wean from the nipple shield, with no luck. Finally, Danae decided on continuous skin-to-skin as her last resort. (Some lactation consultants call this a nursing vacation, with the breastfeeding dyad settling in together to do nothing other than Kangaroo Care and breastfeeding for several hours or even a day or two.) Danae and her 10-week-old daughter snuggled skin-to-skin for 12 hours. As a result, her baby tapped into her innate infant instincts for breastfeeding and to essentially relearn to breastfeed, this time without the nipple shield. Danae threw away the nipple shield that same night. She nursed her daughter for three years, including through Danae's second pregnancy and then as a tandem nursling for 15 months.

Kangaroo Care for the Disorganized Infant

Amber's daughter had several feeding issues. Her baby was unsettled, and they found feeding her to be a struggle every time. After trying several things, Amber found that feeding her daughter while also practicing skin-to-skin improved her ability to organize herself. This was most likely a result of the stability habitat. Amber's baby stabilized body systems while in Kangaroo Care, which allowed for smooth breastfeeding. Several years later, Amber discovered that her daughter had multiple sensory processing issues with her from birth, affecting her ability to breastfeed effectively. According to Amber, skin-to-skin was absolutely the necessary element that provided the path for her daughter's stability and breastfeeding success.

CHAPTER 6

Breastfeeding is a Complex, Whole-Body Wellness, & Sensory Experience

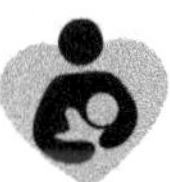

You are not alone if you have always thought of breastfeeding as a food delivery system. Unfortunately, many people tend to think of breastfeeding only as a method of infant feeding, a way to get fuel into a hungry baby. This limited view of breastfeeding only as a food source is likely a hangover from decades of formula feeding, which is an infant food delivery system.

However, research has given human milk a new identity over the last few decades. The old, simplistic view of the "food delivery system" is woefully outdated. To think of breastfeeding only as a food supply is wildly inaccurate and oversimplified, at best. Yes, infants come to the breast for food, nutrition, nourishment, and calories, but that is a limited way to define this type of infant feeding. We need to step away from this old-fashioned view that human milk feeding is just a supply of calories.

An enormous shift would occur if we embraced a much broader understanding of human milk and what it means to feed your baby with human milk. Human milk and breastfeeding are more complex than Western society once thought. Breastfeeding is a *multi-factored health and wellness system.* Breastfeeding is a whole-body sensory experience that has immediate and future impacts on both parent and child, reaching far beyond just delivering calories to a hungry baby.

Consider these outcomes of breastfeeding. Do any of these fit neatly into the idea that breastfeeding is just food?

- Human milk provides antibodies and immune factors to the baby.

- Human milk helps seal the immature infant gut.
- Breastfeeding helps prevent postpartum hemorrhage.
- Lactation can act as reliable birth control under certain conditions.
- Breastfeeding can help people with diabetes lower their need for insulin.

Breastfeeding is, in fact, a complex interaction between parent and child. The underlying messages of this interaction are protection and survival, for both parent and baby. If this were the prevailing view of what it means to feed babies with human milk, our caregivers and families would help new parents protect lactation and this infant-feeding relationship at all costs. For now, our society fails to understand and value human milk and breastfeeding in this way. As a result, many new parents and babies pay the price for this every day.

To broaden our working definition of breastfeeding, let's examine what else besides calorie intake is happening during lactation and through the act of breastfeeding. We will first look at infant feeding in terms of the communication between parent and baby and consider infant feeding part of a whole-body sensory experience. For more information on other wellness and health outcomes of breastfeeding and human milk feeding, see Chapter 2.

Communication Signals

Breastfeeding is an intricate communication experience between parent and child. Some communication signals are obvious, and some are invisible, detectable only at the hormonal level. The communication between a parent and the newborn is a series of ongoing bodily reactions, each one responding to cues from the other. This system is primarily to safeguard the newborn, but it serves both the parent and the baby in many complex and diverse ways.

Scent Signals

Although both partners have been communicating for months in preparation for birth, this interaction changes dramatically after birth, when the new baby is on the parent's chest getting comfortable with her out-of-the-womb environment. Now that she is out in the world, the infant's first goal is to locate her food source, and the parent's body facilitates this by communicating through scent. Once the baby is near the breast, she looks for the nipple. The scent excreted from the Montgomery glands surrounding the nipple guides her. This scent is similar to amniotic fluid, which the baby can taste and smell as she instinctively licks her hands in preparation for latching (assuming there was no immediate infant bathing). That familiar smell given off by the glands surrounding the nipple is the communication from the parent's body that attracts the baby as she looks for her food source.

The newborn also gives off a scent that activates the reward centers in the maternal brain. This smell is why new parents find their newborns irresistible. The smell of a newborn appeals to parents in a delicious way, making it more likely that parents will continue to nurture and care for their new baby. Imagine if babies did not smell so irresistible. Would people be drawn to infants, wanting to hold them and nurture them? Unlikely. It is the design of nature that the smell of infants is so universally appealing.

Olfactory Input

According to studies on information gained from olfactory cues, human body odor contains all kinds of useful information. For example, people can identify others by body odor alone and other characteristics, like family connections, gender, and age (Lundström et al., 2009; Mitro et al., 2012; Weisfeld et al., 2003). Disease conditions within the human body are also detectable by smell (Olsson et al., 2014). Maternal instincts are particularly acute when recognizing changes to infant odors that can signal infant infection, such as foul-smelling urine that could indicate a urinary tract infection. Studies show that when women (especially mothers) smell newborns, it stimulates the reward pathways in the brain, flooding it with dopamine. This effect is equivalent to eating a wonderful meal. In this instance, smelling the baby's pheromones triggers the reward pathway and enhances caretaking and parenting behaviors. Mothers are also better equipped than others to tolerate the scent of their own infant's stool (Case et al., 2006), which helps guarantee that they will keep attending to the baby and his needs.

Hormonal Signals: Oxytocin and Prolactin

The parent takes in sensory information from the newborn while the baby nuzzles and massages the skin around the breast, areola, and nipple. This nuzzling helps facilitate the release of oxytocin, the hormone that prepares the breast for a milk letdown.

Once breastfeeding is underway, the infant suckling sends hormonal signals to the parent. This sucking awakens the innate systems deep within the parent's brain to enhance infant feeding and nurturing behaviors, maximize bonding behaviors, and increase maternal sensitivity to the baby's cues. It also helps to shrink the uterus (helping to prevent postpartum hemorrhage), down-regulate reproduction, and prevent immediate pregnancy. That is an incredible amount of information! Unfortunately, nearly all of these processes diminish without initiating lactation or are absent (especially concerning reproductive status and ovulation).

A fascinating piece of the complex information exchange taking place at this time involves high amounts of specific hormones in the parent's body, bringing essential messages for her own survival and that of her infant.

Oxytocin

Several simultaneous reactions occur when the baby latches onto the breast, communicating complex messages throughout the parent's body. As the newborn latches, the parent responds by increasing maternal oxytocin levels. This hormone is often referred to as the love hormone because it enhances the feelings of love and bonding between people. In effect, by breastfeeding, the baby physically communicates to the parent that the birth has occurred. The parent responds to the baby with nurturing behaviors to ensure the infant's survival. The elevated levels of oxytocin facilitate more nurturing and caring behaviors and help parents respond to the baby's needs. In addition, there are fascinating changes in the human brain brought on by oxytocin. These changes include an increased maternal ability to recognize nonverbal communication and cues from others and increased sensitivity to others' feelings, including her baby's. Aside from enhancing protective behavior, high oxytocin levels help facilitate the milk letdown reflex, bringing breast milk to the baby, obviously influencing the infant's survival.

Oxytocin facilitates letdown and bonding and directs the specific postpartum clamping of the blood vessels in the uterus. In response to the new baby's latch, rising oxytocin levels tell the uterus to begin to shrink back to its pre-pregnancy size. The smooth muscle of the uterus responds to the dramatic rise in oxytocin by contracting and shrinking. As the uterus contracts, the blood vessels clamp down and prevent excessive blood loss, helping to ensure survival by preventing postpartum hemorrhage. In effect, breastfeeding (immediately) after birth tells the body that the pregnancy is over. This signal tells the body that the baby no longer needs a food supply inside the womb. *Instead, the baby receives food and nurturing outside of the womb, at the breast.*

Prolactin

Oxytocin is not the only hormone that makes up the complex communication of breastfeeding. Another essential hormone called prolactin is elevated during breastfeeding. Prolactin's main job is to stimulate milk production, but this also is an important signal for the ovulation cycle. When a baby is at the breast, high prolactin levels inhibit ovulation. In fact, by breastfeeding frequently, the newborn is telling her parent's body not to devote any energy toward reproduction at this time because all the available maternal resources are necessary for sustaining the survival of this new baby.

Interestingly, prolactin levels increase or decrease with the amount of milk needed by the baby, and maternal fertility responds rapidly to this sensitive system. If the baby is exclusively nursing and prolactin levels remain high, this suppresses ovulation and prevents pregnancy. This is Mother Nature's postpartum birth control system, and it can (but not always) last for several months after birth. This also ensures that the parent's physical resources are only devoted to the child who has just been born. As the child gets older and begins eating solid food, she begins gradually shifting the balance of her calories toward solid food. This process is usually a slow one, lowering maternal levels of prolactin over time. As prolactin levels drop, fertility returns and ovulation can begin again. A drop in prolactin can also occur in a person who has just given birth in the absence of breastfeeding. This lack of breastfeeding can cause fertility to return much sooner. For most people, nighttime breastfeeding (or milk removal by pumping or hand expression) appears to be a necessary part of lactation amenorrhea (delayed return of fertility). Sudden shifts in nursing patterns can also cause a sustained decrease in prolactin and a return to regular ovulation.

Demand and Supply Signals

The baby can communicate with the breast regarding how much milk to make through breastfeeding. Although babies have no language skills, they easily communicate their needs concerning milk production. The baby uses her innate sucking reflex to signal precisely how much milk she needs from the breast. Infants are born with an intense need to suck, which is a vital mechanism for their survival. Suppose the baby is meeting all of her sucking needs at the breast. In that case, the parent will likely bring in a healthy milk supply because milk production is stimulated by suckling, and specifically, milk removal. In effect, the more milk a baby removes from the breast, the more milk the body will make. This is a case of demand stimulating the supply. When the baby or pump removes milk, immediate signals go to the milk-making cells in the breast, causing them to produce more milk. The reverse is also true; when there is no demand and little or no milk leaves the breast, communication breaks down, and milk production slows or stops. This delicate communication system can be derailed if a new baby meets her sucking needs with artificial nipples like pacifiers or other feeding methods. Milk production can also break down when the baby is not removing enough milk. This is common for babies with ankyloglossia (tongue-tie), premature babies with weak suck reflex, or sleepy babies who do not wake often enough to nurse. Even missing one feeding per day for many days in a row will effectively down-regulate the maternal milk supply.

Recently, I heard a lactation educator tell an entire class of parents-to-be that the breast is not smart. Her logic was that the breast only knows two functions: increasing milk supply or decreasing it. In my professional opinion, the breast is incredibly "smart," because the supply and demand system of lactation can respond to delicate nuances in the infant feeding pattern. For example, when the baby is ready for a major growth spurt, the baby will come to the breast more often, sometimes in a cluster pattern. The breast immediately responds by increasing supply over the next few hours and days, so the growing baby has more milk. Conversely, when the baby gets additional calories from solid food late in the first year, milk production can gradually decrease but not disappear as it readjusts to lower demand. Milk production can also respond quickly to the lack of milk removal. If the breast is not emptied regularly, a feedback loop rapidly sends signals to the milk-making cells within the breast to slow and even stop milk production. This system is incredibly sensitive and responsive. In many ways, the breast is not only smart; it is brilliant in its ability to regulate supply and demand.

Immunity

Breastfeeding is a way for a parent to communicate with the infant's immune system. Since humans are born with an immature immune system, one fundamental purpose of breastfeeding is to assist the baby with immune function through antibodies delivered through the milk. The parent's body makes antibodies to viruses, bacteria, and pathogens she encounters in her environment. The parent passes them to the baby via the breast milk. For example, suppose the breastfeeding dyad is always close or shares the same environment. In that case, they will encounter the same germs, and the infant will receive added protection from pathogens in her environment from the antibodies in the breast milk.

Given all of this evidence, it is clear that breastfeeding is much more than a food delivery system. Every time the baby comes to the breast, communication occurs between parent and child. The infant's ability to utilize an intricate and delicate communication system enhances maternal nurturing behaviors. It helps to ensure the new baby's survival long before speaking her first words. This complex communication system is an incredible way for each partner to send and receive messages for nurturing, protection, temporarily shutting down fertility and enhancing the baby's immune function.

The Sensory Experience

As we saw in the discussion about communication (above), an incredible amount of information exchanges at the micro-level during breastfeeding. For that to occur, parents and babies use all of their senses to send and receive signals from one another. This connection is what makes breastfeeding a whole-body sensory experience. In addition, at the time of birth, the infant is sensorially primed to make the critical transition to extra-uterine life. In this crucial phase between uterine life and living, breathing in the world, the baby's senses are amplified, ready to take in all the new information.

During the first 60-90 minutes, a healthy infant born without exposure to labor augmentation drugs and pain medications will be able to seek the breast, locate the nipple, latch and begin breastfeeding without the management of caregivers. The baby's senses guide the way.

Breast-Sensing Technology

Breast-sensing technology sounds hilarious, but in a literal sense, your newborn has this tech on board at birth. Immediately after the infant emerges from the womb, the baby comes to the parent's abdomen or straight to the chest. The critical input at this moment is the skin-to-skin contact between parent and baby. This sensory input from the skin is the most significant input for the baby right after birth. This tactile information tells the newborn that the environment has changed. The baby is now ready to let the environment dictate its behavior since it is no longer in the womb. Dr. Nils Bergman, author, researcher, and public health physician states that "place determines behaviours" for the baby (Bergman, 2017). Essentially, this means that the baby's behavior will depend on his location. For example, when a newborn is resting skin-to-skin on the parent's abdomen or chest, sensory input from this environment tells the baby to seek the breast.

The baby's breast-sensing technology also includes visual cues, tactile cues (from the tongue, hands, face, and cheeks), olfactory cues (sense of smell), innate reflexes, hand movements, and tongue movements. In the unmedicated birth scenario, the baby's senses tell him what behaviors to exhibit and when. In fact, there is an eight-step predictable and observable sequence (Ransjo-Arvidson et al., 2001) that the baby will utilize to seek the breast, using only sensory information gathered from his location on the mother's skin and innate reflexes to find the way. Here is how it generally looks. First, the baby is placed on his ventral surface (front side, tummy) on top of a reclined parent. This placement is important because if the baby is on his back, he will not (and cannot) run through the entire breast-seeking program. Newborns held skin-to-skin are routinely placed on their ventral surface (tummy) immediately after delivery, and this is one crucial part of activating the breast-seeking sequence. Infants can exhibit reflexes in many positions, but the laid-back position with a newborn on top of the parent facilitates this particular sequence and makes many movements more salient and useful (more on that in a moment).

Sensing Position and Seeking the Breast

Once in place, the baby might rest there to gather sensory information, adjust to breathing air, and get his bearings. If he is resting on the abdomen, the baby will use an innate stepping reflex to push himself forward, moving toward the breast. If the baby is already in place between the breasts, he will likely bob his head toward one breast and then maybe back toward the other breast. At this time, the baby uses his sense of touch from his hands, face, cheeks, nose, and chin to find the breast. He uses his sense of smell to locate the nipple because the Montgomery glands surrounding the nipple give off a scent that attracts the baby. Studies show the newborn sense of smell is acute. At four days postpartum, newborns who spent at least 50 minutes skin-to-skin right after birth identified their own mother's milk from a group of odors, including human milk from a donor (Mizuno et al., 2007). Visual cues are not as acute as olfactory cues, but babies can use their vision. Even though infants cannot see well at distances greater than about 12 inches or about 30 cm, they can use visual cues to detect the nipple and areola. But most of their breast-sensing tech comes by way of the tactile and olfactory cues he takes in once in place skin-to-skin with his parent.

The baby is now competently running the specific eight-step sequence to seek the breast. The infant uses hands, mouth, tongue, and stepping or crawling reflex to reach the breast. Once there, he can precisely position himself for latching onto the nipple. In the atmosphere of managed birth, these steps and often rushed and even augmented by well-meaning members of the care team because some people assume that all infants need assistance on their way to the breast. We need to shift our assumptions about infants, embracing the idea that they are hardwired for this job and proficient enough to carry out their instinctive mission. One of the main reasons for this is when we are hands-off and allow the infant to run the program, seek the breast, and latch, he is more likely to do it better than he would with over-management. Remember, this is not to suggest that we can never intervene. When an infant needs assistance, I fully support and recommend gently assisting at the breast. However, for healthy newborns, it is more effective to take a hands-off approach. Watch to see if your new baby can self-attach before trying to intervene. Begin by assuming that your baby knows what to do.

Sensing the Latch

The latch process is also a sensory exercise for the newborn. When the baby is facing the nipple at close range, he will use his cheeks, lips, tongue, and chin to determine the exact location of the nipple before attempting the latch. The infant's chin pressed firmly into the breast tissue is a strong signal that he is in the right place. Next, the baby will open his mouth wide for latching. This wide mouth is necessary because the baby must take in more than just the nipple. As we lactation professionals like to say, "It's not called *nipple feeding*!" For a good latch to occur, the baby needs to feel the sturdiness of the nipple in the correct position in his mouth. The sensory input from his tongue and soft palate gives subtle cues to the infant that the nipple is in the correct position. Some people (occasionally) need the assistance of a nipple shield to provide the nipple more structure so that the baby can feel his way to a good latch. Sometimes we see the overuse of nipple shields but if you need one, and it helps your baby transfer milk with a good latch, use it. It does not have to be long-term, but it can help some breastfeeding dyads get lactation off to a good start.

What Does a Baby Need to Achieve Self-Attachment in the First 60-90 Minutes?

People often feel that they must intervene, placing the fully clothed baby with the parent in the cradle position and "assisting" with latch using the rapid arm movement (RAM) method. Years ago, one savvy lactation consultant in Bloomington, Indiana, told me about the inherent problems with the RAM method. She described it as placing the infant in the cradle position, nose to the nipple. Then, when the baby opens his mouth, the parent (or L & D nurse) will use RAM to shove the infant into the breast tissue with hopes of the infant achieving a good latch. I hope this scenario seems ridiculous and unreasonable to you. As I highlight throughout this chapter and elsewhere, you now know that the newborn is competent to seek the breast and latch on his own.

So, as the new parent, what is your role in the first 60-90 minutes while your baby is running the predictable steps of breast seeking and achieving the first latch? The most important things you can provide are:

1. The right environment
2. Time

If your labor was induced or augmented, and/or if you were exposed to pain meds or other interventions, the baby might be groggy, sleepy, and even disorganized. You can do certain things in this instance to help your baby run the breast-seeking program. In this case, the most important things you can provide are:

1. The right environment
2. More time

The right amount of time is usually about 90-120 minutes after delivery. Infants with exposure to pain medications during labor might take more time than infants without. The elements of the right environment are relatively simple but can easily be disturbed. Here is one ideal environment. (Yours may look different based on birth location and/or hospital policies.)

- The newborn is immediately placed skin-to-skin with the parent after delivery. *Skin-to-skin is the newborn environment.*
- The newborn is placed on the abdomen or further up, on the chest in between the breasts.
- The baby can be dried off (except hands) and then covered lightly with a dry infant blanket.
- Avoid hats or clothing and excessive coverings of any kind, if possible, at least for the first hour.

In this scenario, the baby and the parent use their senses to gather and share important information. The parent responds to the newborn through sensory cues that affect hormonal profile and ability to bond with the infant. In fact, the new parent is also using sensory input to become acquainted with the newborn: smelling the newborn activates reward centers in the maternal brain; sensory input from the infant's skin helps release hormones necessary for lactation; tactile input from suckling at the breast helps shrink the uterus; hearing the baby's cries also facilitates hormone release; looking at the newborn's face stimulates the reward center in the maternal brain (Strathearn et al., 2008).

Before your baby is born, watch a few videos of infants performing the breast crawl so you know what to expect. Search YouTube for breast crawl videos. There are several videos available online.

Eight Step Sequence to Seek the Breast and Latch On

When a newborn is in the appropriate habitat (lying tummy down, between the breasts), she will behave in predictable ways as she seeks the breast. These steps are part of the newborn's journey to the breast.

The baby licks and smells her hands and moves her tongue. Then, she will open her mouth. The baby may rest for a while between steps or take steps out of order. When she is ready, the baby will focus on the nipple and begin to move toward the nipple. She may use hands in massage-like movements to stimulate the breast and nipple. When she is in very close range, the baby may lick the nipple before attempting to latch. Finally, the baby will latch onto the breast (Ransjö-Arvidson et al., 2001).

TRUE STORY

After moving into a new neighborhood in Media, PA, many years ago, our family attended a block party. I met lots of new neighbors and their children, all of whom were as old or older than my own. One of my new neighbors, Ellie, asked me what I do for work. Telling people that I am a lactation consultant (LC) almost always sparks the most curious reactions. Some do not know what an LC is or what an LC does, so it often leads to interesting discussions. In this case, Ellie had a serious look on her face, and she said, "Can I ask you a question about breastfeeding?" I was unsure what to expect because I knew that her youngest child (whom I had just met) was 10 years old. She then told me a story that I was familiar with, but apparently, she was not. Here is Ellie's story.

One afternoon, Ellie's neighbor, Silvia, who had just given birth six weeks earlier, asked Ellie if she could watch the baby while Silvia was on a one-hour conference call. Silvia was going back to work the following month but occasionally called in for important meetings during her maternity leave. Ellie agreed to take care of Silvia's new baby during her call. Ellie loved babies, and she was excited to hold a new baby for an hour.

Ellie arrived and got acquainted with Silvia's daughter, who was a bit fussy during the conference call. Ellie, a mother of three, assured Silvia that she could settle the baby, no problem. Ellie tried a few of her infant-settling techniques, and sure enough, the baby calmed down. In the process, Ellie was stunned when she felt the unmistakable tingling sensation that she used to get when her milk let down at the beginning of a feeding session with her own kids. Ellie thought, "How in the world could this be happening?" She was only *holding* her neighbor's baby! There was no feeding or even skin-to-skin! Ellie had not had a milk supply in nearly a decade! So, where was the feeling coming from?

Ellie told me that she was completely surprised by the feeling of the phantom milk letdown. I assured her that she was not alone; many people have had similar experiences. I explained to her that this happened because she was, just for that hour, totally immersed in the sensory input from a newborn. Ellie had a hormonal shift while holding the baby, smelling her head, and hearing her cries. Because Ellie's body had been in this situation hundreds of times before with her three children, her body was responding in the way that it knew how, even if she was not planning to nurse Silvia's baby and even if she had no milk.

The maternal response (in the brain) laid down through parenting and breastfeeding is incredibly strong and is not easily forgotten. After weaning, the body prunes back the milk-making structures in the breast, but the pathways of maternal response in the brain can remain in place. Ellie's body was responding to a shift in her hormones brought on by a newborn, something her body knew how to do well.

CHAPTER 7

Parenting and Breastfeeding Skills

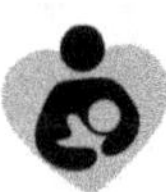

Think of a time in your life when you planned to take on a new project or endeavor. Maybe it was getting a driver's license, writing a term paper, learning a new language, planning a trip or an event, improving your health, writing a blog, painting, cooking, or even reading. Every project you have ever undertaken has likely involved some skill development. You can set an intention to get your driver's license and buy a car, but you won't be getting around until you acquire the skills for driving the vehicle. You may own a bicycle, but you won't be riding until you develop the necessary skills. The same logic applies to parenting and infant feeding. It is necessary to develop parenting and infant feeding skills when you have a baby.

After working with new parents for over a decade, I began to wonder why some people excel at developing the skills of breastfeeding and parenting and some others do not. It might be easy to assume that some of us are more interested in diving into the parenting role more completely than others, but that feels too simplistic as an explanation. After considering many aspects of skill development, I have found four key factors that drive the acquisition of parenting and infant feeding skills: intention, information, instinct, and intuition. The degree to which each person succeeds with developing new skills can be related to the influence of these four factors.

Table 7.1: Factors that influence infant feeding skill development

Intention	Information
Motivation level for breastfeeding Strength of interest in breastfeeding Degree of commitment to producing and/or using human milk	Prior cultural knowledge Books, blogs, webpages about lactation Family experience with breastfeeding Breastfeeding classes and education
Instinct	**Intuition**
Bodily responses to your baby Hormone profile Nurturing behaviors Anatomic structure integrity and capabilities	Tuning in/awareness of your body Observation and awareness of subtleties Tuning into your baby Reading your baby's behavior, body language

Intention

Your intention will be one of the essential factors in developing your breastfeeding skills. Before beginning any endeavor you want to do, you first set an intention to accomplish your task. Regarding breastfeeding, that may simply be deciding to choose human milk as you infant feeding method, or you may combine it with an intention to breastfeed for a certain amount of time. For example, I speak to many people who say, "It is my goal to breastfeed my baby for the first year." However, intention is more than goal setting. Intentions exist in a range of degrees. One person may have a casual intent to breastfeed, while another person can be intent on breastfeeding at all costs, no matter what interference arises on the infant feeding journey. I find that most people's intentions are somewhere in the middle, but there is no right or wrong way to hold your intention. It is what it is, but it does pay to be aware of the strength of your intention. It can factor into your feeding decisions throughout your baby's first year or two.

To set your intention, state to yourself (or to others) your feeding goals and your reasons for choosing those goals. When you decide on your infant feeding goals, consider why you are making the choices you make. What is driving your decisions? What motivates you to choose to breastfeed? Would you consider your intention to be strong, or is it more casual? Be prepared to adjust your intentions as you move along the path of parenting and infant feeding. You may feel differently after your infant feeding experiences. Take some time to reflect.

TRUE STORY

Hayley was interested in feeding her newborn with human milk. During the first few weeks, breastfeeding was going well, but she experienced some mild, ongoing pain during the latch and throughout the feeding. In addition, her baby wanted to nurse quite frequently during the nighttime hours, which left Hayley feeling exhausted. When her daughter was two months old, the baby's grandmother suggested that perhaps using infant formula for some feedings would allow Hayley to have a break and get more sleep during the night. Because Hayley's intention to breastfeed was relatively flexible at that time, she was open to the idea of trying formula. Interestingly, her daughter thoroughly rejected the formula and refused to take a bottle. Instead of trying to force it, Hayley continued to nurse. She sought help and support from volunteer lactation counselors and a lactation consultant. She tried different positions and latch techniques and the painful latch resolved; infant feeding became much easier. After months of breastfeeding, Hayley's motivation to continue breastfeeding was gaining strength. She nursed her first child for a full two years and later nursed her son for three years. Not only had her intention to breastfeed changed over the course of the first year, but it also impacted her feeding experience with her second child as well.

Information

Developing your infant feeding and parenting skills also depends on the information and knowledge you have about feeding babies. Part of this is formal education, like taking a breastfeeding class. Much of the information people have about infant feeding comes from informal channels – your family's infant feeding experiences, how you were fed as a baby, cultural attitudes toward the breast and breastfeeding, and your partner's attitudes toward infant feeding options. Some of this we can control, and some of it, we cannot.

For example, you cannot control how you were fed as a baby; it is part of your past experience. You can, however, control the amount of breastfeeding education and information you encounter now. If you are from a family of formula feeders (your mother used formula, your grandmother used formula, etc.), you may need to read a lot about breastfeeding and take a good breastfeeding class. In addition, you may want to talk to some people who had positive breastfeeding experiences to expand your knowledge about lactation.

On the other hand, if you were breastfed and you observed your aunts and friends feeding their babies at the breast, you may not need quite as much formal education. Based on your current knowledge, you will know how much breastfeeding education you need. Keep in mind that while it does truly pay off to take a breastfeeding class and read about infant feeding before your baby is born, much of what people learn about breastfeeding happens as on-the-job training. Your baby will be your best teacher. Be sure to pay attention in class!

Instinct

Your body has instincts for parenting and infant feeding. While the action of breastfeeding might not be instinctual per se, biology wires humans to care for and to nurture human infants. Interestingly enough, breastfeeding helps enhance parenting and nurturing behaviors by releasing hormones that cause parents to act in more caring, nurturing, and protective ways. You can maximize the chance that innate forces strengthen your parenting skills and infant feeding skills by listening to your instincts. First, hold your baby skin-to-skin in the first days and weeks of your baby's life. This contact will allow you to access instincts by creating the optimal habitat for exchanging bodily signals with your newborn. Second, immerse yourself completely in your baby's cues and signals. Wear your baby in a sling or baby carrier, practice Kangaroo Care, smell your baby's head. Also, be sure to listen closely to your baby breathing, gently massage your baby, make eye contact with your baby while holding her, and provide unrestricted access to the breast. All of these behaviors will provide for the exchange of essential signals between you and your baby that change your hormonal profile, enhancing your natural human parenting and nurturing skill development. While some people are more inclined to be nurturing, every person has this potential. Finally, enhance your parenting instincts by making a point of being physically close to your baby, night and day, in the early days of parenting and breastfeeding.

Intuition

There is no doubt you have heard the term "women's intuition" in the context of a mother's ability to read her child. In the past, intuition may have been more associated with women and mothers because there is a high degree of connection between parent and child (especially when breastfeeding). However, in reality, we should not call this phenomenon "women's intuition." Intuition does not favor any type of person, male, female, or nonbinary; intuition does not care how we identify our gender, sexual orientation, race, ethnicity, or anything else. Every person is intuitive, and anyone can develop these skills by focusing on awareness. Intuitive awareness about your baby comes from careful observation of your baby's habits, behaviors, and tendencies. There is nothing complicated about being intuitively connected to your baby. It is a natural part of human life, and it can factor into your ability to develop parenting and breastfeeding skills. Enhance your intuitive skills by being present when you're with your baby. Observe the baby with all your senses, looking for subtle changes. Be aware of the baby with your inner knowing and trust your gut feelings. If you have ever had a family pet, you have likely used careful observation and intuition to connect with your dog or cat. Our pets cannot speak to us, but we learn to read them and meet their needs by observing their behavioral cues and habits. The same nonverbal information is available from your baby. You will learn to read your baby's subtle cues quickly if you allow yourself to become totally immersed in your baby's physical and emotional signals. Intuition is a *major factor* in developing certain parenting and breastfeeding skills but breastfeeding and parenting classes often neglect these factors. I routinely encourage parents to put down the infant tracking apps and connect physically and emotionally to their babies. You will learn much more about your baby from careful and consistent observation than you might learn from tracking apps.

Ultimately, these four factors are essential parts of skill development for any endeavor but especially for infant feeding and parenting. The degree to which each of the four factors plays into your own skill development will depend on your background and familiarity with breastfeeding and parenting.

Below are some critical breastfeeding and parenting skills that will benefit you on your parenting journey. Assess your intention, information, instinct, and intuition as you learn each skill. These factors are key to learning new skills and will likely change over time as you encounter new knowledge and experiences.

Breastfeeding and Parenting Skills

1. Comprehensive parental evaluation of infant wellness

It is essential that all parents learn to assess infant wellness, regardless of whether the baby is fully breastfed, fully formula fed, or something in between. This discussion focuses on breastfeeding and using human milk but can also apply to partially-breastfed infants. Parents should use these skills without additional apps, charts, or scales. Although these are low-tech skills for assessing infant wellness, they can yield incredible information about it.

It is no secret that many people today favor the use of gadgets, tools, apps, and infant trackers to assess infant wellness. Visual observation gives parents a more informed picture precisely because keen observation can bring together multiple data points and factor in intuition as well. Comprehensive infant wellness evaluation is a skill that uses all your senses. You will observe the baby, listen to the baby's breath, touch your baby's skin, and smell your baby. When you are learning to assess your baby's wellness, consider carefully observing these factors.

Wellness Signs

- Your baby can be comforted by using several simple techniques, including skin-to-skin, gentle bouncing, holding, music, singing, and baby-wearing.
- When your baby is awake, he is aware, alert, and active.

- Your baby's skin color appears normal.
- Your baby displays feeding cues when actively seeking the breast or is ready for feeding.
- Your baby nurses at the breast or is fed 8-12 times in 24 hours and seems happy after feedings. Your baby releases the breast on his own when the feeding is over.
- Your baby produces enough wet and dirty diapers each day. See the chapter on Lactation Promotion Factors for more information.
- Your baby meets developmental milestones.

Warning Signs

- Skin appears blue. This sign indicates that oxygen is low, a condition called cyanosis. Check for a bluish tint around the mucous membranes in babies with darker skin - lips, gums, and around the eyes. You may also see it in the fingernails. Babies with lighter skin may have a bluish tint around the mouth or face.
- The baby does not produce enough wet and dirty diapers. Too few wet and dirty diapers can indicate inadequate intake and dehydration.
- The baby displays lethargy, difficulty waking to feed, excessive sleepiness. These signs indicate that your baby is unwell, has an infection, jaundice, or low blood sugar (hypoglycemia). Babies often sleep more during a growth spurt, so sleeping more can also be normal.
- Infant fever. Although one can assess increases in body temperature by touching your baby's skin, it is not the most accurate or reliable way to determine if your baby has a fever. Use a digital thermometer. Infant body temperature can be assessed rectally, in the ear, mouth, and armpit. Be sure you are using your thermometer correctly. High fevers can be dangerous in infants and indicate infection (bacterial or viral) or other illnesses. A pediatrician should see all infants under two months with an elevated body temperature. In the case of assessing infant body temperature, I highly recommend

using an accurate digital thermometer. (This is one tool every parent must have.)

- Difficulty breathing. This sign could indicate that your baby is struggling to get enough oxygen. Any change in breathing patterns should be assessed carefully by your baby's caregiver immediately.
- Monitor changes in the smell of your baby's breath. This signal can indicate a festering illness, such as a cold or upper respiratory illness.
- Monitor changes in the smell of your baby's urine or stool. Although this sounds somewhat unsophisticated, it is an excellent way to tell if your baby has an infection or an illness. For example, changes in the smell of urine can indicate the presence of urinary tract infections or related infections. Also, expect some changes in the smell of infant stool when the baby begins eating solid food, but if you rule that out, it can also indicate an illness.
- Your baby is not comforted and calmed by soothing techniques. Do not ignore inconsolable crying. Instead, get a full evaluation for your baby. Inconsolable crying can signify ear infection, injury, a stomach bug, colic, hand, foot, and mouth disease, sore throat, or other causes. Seek care if you are unable to calm your baby.
- Mouth breathing. A brilliant lactation consultant in Phoenix, AZ named René Moore, IBCLC, gave an informative talk to a group of lactation professionals a few years ago about the importance of the infant airway and proper breathing. I was lucky enough to attend this talk and I am grateful that I can now recognize some of the warning signs of breathing problems. Mouth breathing is a warning sign that truly needs investigation by a pediatric dentist, by an ENT (ear, nose, and throat specialist), or another airway specialist. Humans are *nose breathers*, night and day. Breathing through the mouth is a significant sign that something is not right. Many parents have connected mouth breathing with a list of oral problems and airway problems. Furthermore, an astute few have connected the dots to associate

mouth breathing with poor childhood sleep quality and childhood behavior problems. If your baby is a mouth breather, seek an immediate evaluation with a specialist. If your older child is a mouth breather and is experiencing snoring, night waking, trouble sleeping, and disruptive daytime behaviors, find a specialist who can evaluate the airway, oral restrictions and conduct a sleep study. You may need more than one specialist. Find more information about obstructive airway from AAPMD Foundation (American Academy of Physiological Medicine & Dentistry). Watch an eye-opening five-minute video on YouTube from AAPMD Foundation called "Finding Connor Deegan" about airway obstruction, disrupted sleep, and behavior problems.

TRUE STORY

My oldest daughter was born with a highly arched palate and tongue and lip ties. It compromised her ability to drain the breast properly, caused painful feeding (for me), and later as a toddler, caused significant airway obstructions, snoring, sleep apnea episodes, and daytime tantrums. Between 12 months and 24 months, she woke from her midmorning nap and cried for about an hour or more every single day. She did not sleep well as an infant or as a toddler. She was 19 months old before she slept through the night one time. At that time, I was not trained in lactation and I didn't have the knowledge to connect the dots between all her earlier problems with breastfeeding and her subsequent sleep problems and general discontentment. In addition, her tonsils were chronically enlarged from mouth breathing, but I did not know the cause. At age 5, she had her enlarged tonsils removed, and somehow, I intuitively knew that tonsillectomy was not the true solution for her problems. Unfortunately, I could not figure out what caused any of the breastfeeding problems, snoring, or sleep problems until she was in the 4th grade. After moving to Phoenix, AZ, we found a new dentist. On our first visit, she casually mentioned that my daughter had a severe tongue tie. Her previous dentist noted the high arched palate but said nothing about the oral restrictions. The pediatricians we had seen over the years had never mentioned anything, even though I questioned them repeatedly about her sleep problems and my previous breastfeeding difficulties. After speaking to the dentist in Phoenix and some local lactation friends, I knew that my daughter had to have some treatment. We opted for laser tongue-tie release (frenotomy) along with a palate expander and later a nighttime retainer. She immediately slept much better, had greatly improved moods and ability to cope with daily routines. Her grades improved as well as her growth.

2. Feeding Cue Recognition

As a breastfeeding parent, it is crucial to recognize your baby's feeding cues because infants fed human milk do not adhere to a predetermined schedule for feeding. Instead, the baby decides when to eat and how much to eat. As you learned in previous chapters, feeding on demand sets the volume of your milk supply. Feeding cues are characterized as *early, active,* or *late*. Try to recognize your baby's early feeding cues because this will facilitate a much more relaxed feeding session. If your baby progresses to late feeding cues, her behavior could become more anxious, upset, and frantic. Babies who are upset (and agitated) cannot latch onto the breast. Feeding is much easier when your baby is calm at the beginning of the feeding. As you learn your baby's cues, you will be relying on information and intuition. Keep in mind that your baby may develop feeding cues that are not on this list. I outline feeding cues in detail in the RELAX chapter. Here is a summary.

- Early Feeding Cues – lip-smacking, tongue movements, opening and closing the mouth, hands to mouth, fist in the mouth.
- Active Feeding Cues – active body movements, rooting at the breast, vocal sounds (happy baby sounds), gentle arms and leg movements.
- Late Feeding Cues – panic, whimpering, larger and more forceful body movements. Behaviors that progress to angry crying, frantic behavior, and screaming.

When you see the early feeding cues, respond to your baby by offering the breast. However, if your baby is already showing signs of irritation, you may need to utilize infant calming techniques before the baby is calm enough to come to the breast.

3. *Assessing Satiation*

How can you tell if your baby has had enough milk? How will you know if your baby is, indeed, satisfied after feeding? There are several indicators of satiation that you can look for to assess whether your baby is content after a feeding (McNally et al., 2016). However, recognizing whether your baby is full and content after feeding is more difficult to accomplish than simply recognizing hunger cues. Research shows that parents can better identify and interpret hunger cues than fullness cues after feeding (Hodges et al., 2013). Because of this, it is essential to learn and recognize your baby's subtle messages and signals that let you know he is full and satisfied after feeding. Carefully observe your baby during and after the feeding to assess your baby's feelings of contentment and fullness.

Observe

- Look for the nutritive sucking pattern while the baby is at the breast. After the initial milk let-down, the baby will take in milk and swallow the milk during active feeding. The pattern might be one-to-one (e.g., suck, swallow, suck, swallow) or perhaps two-to-one (suck, suck, swallow, suck, suck, swallow). Look for this pattern while your baby is actively drinking. You will also see the baby's lower jaw moving while actively feeding, and then he pauses to swallow. This pattern is likely to slow down toward the end of a feeding when your baby feels full.
- Does your baby appear happy and content after feeding? If not, offer more time at the breast.
- Does your baby's body seem more relaxed? Look for a total relation of the body, especially hands. For example, before coming to the breast, the baby may have tightly closed fists. However, the baby will become more relaxed during the feeding, and the hands will open.
- Observe your baby's cues during the entire feeding session. At the outset of feeding, your baby is likely to be focused on you, on the breast, and not much else. As the feeding progresses and the baby becomes full instead of hungry, her behaviors will change (especially for older babies). She may begin to look around, want to touch your clothing instead of

the breast, and could even begin to take breaks from active feeding. You can see that her attention is shifting from being highly focused on feeding to focusing on non-food-related things. As a result, she is more easily distracted.

- Your baby may appear sleepy or fall asleep at the breast. This is perfectly fine except when a baby is not taking in enough milk. For an overly sleepy baby who has trouble staying awake for feedings, you can try to physically stimulate your baby with touch, take off her clothes or even place a cool cloth on the forehead. Use massage and breast compression to push a little more milk toward the nipple. This technique can sometimes help sleepy babies remain interested in nursing. Some babies like to take a short nap before switching sides to the other breast.
- Trust that your baby knows when she feels full and allow your baby to determine the end of a feeding session. Some babies are efficient feeders, while others take a lot of time to transfer all the milk they need. If your baby was born earlier than expected, has low muscle tone, has any oral anatomy restrictions, or has other special needs (e.g., Down syndrome, cleft palate, heart condition, and other special conditions), your baby may need a lot of extra time at the breast. Because some babies tire out more quickly, they may need shorter but more frequent trips to the breast. Trust your baby's signals of hunger and fullness. She knows.

4. Infant Calming Techniques

Some of the best skills you can learn as a parent are infant calming methods. If you recall from the chapter on Kangaroo Care, infants who become "disorganized" lack body system regulation and organization. When they lack organization, babies will signal to you that they need help. Sometimes, those signals look like feeding cues, and sometimes, they do not. For example, when your baby is fussy and irritated, he may be hungry, but to successfully latch onto your breast, he must calm the irritation first. It is difficult to feed a frantic baby. Babies also show irritation at other times, even when they are not hungry. They may be trying to signal that they have other discomforts like feeling too hot or too cold, feeling the lack of security, needing reassurance that you are nearby. Internal body systems may be affected by their lack of organization as well. They could be breathing too fast or exhibiting an elevated heart rate or blood pressure. In these situations, your baby knows that he needs security, calming, comfort, and the physical presence of his parents or caregivers. However, babies need help in achieving body system organization. There are many techniques that people use to calm babies. Here are a few methods for infant calming. Try several until you find what works for you and your baby. Remember, what works for one child may not work at all for another.

- Sucking is an incredibly organizing behavior for infants. It is one of their most essential survival skills, and it helps them feel calm. For tiny babies less than six to eight weeks old, allow for all the sucking to take place at the breast. For older babies, pacifiers/dummies are okay to use in moderation. Perhaps you only use it in the car if your baby screams when you put him in the car seat. Maybe you only use it around 6pm when your baby is particularly irritated. Use the pacifier selectively. Therapeutic use of pacifiers is acceptable for infants who need this kind of treatment. Be sure your baby is not hungry when you offer the pacifier because this can lead to missing feedings.
- Skin-to-skin is another fantastic method for calming your baby. When you hold your baby skin-to-skin, you give your baby calming sensory input from your skin to her skin. This type of human touch is reassuring. It provides warmth, allows eye contact, and helps your baby achieve a full body reset. Read the chapter on Kangaroo care for full details on using this technique.
- Baby-wearing is a handy technique for calming a fussy baby. Find a baby carrier that suits your needs (if you have one that you are not thrilled with, look for other types of infant carriers). Be sure to wear the carrier following the manufacturer's guidelines or in the safest way possible. Once you have the baby in the carrier, you can move around to help calm your baby. Many people say that the carrier provides the feeling of being back in the security of the womb. The movement and closeness to you help to simulate that experience as well.

Many people find that a baby wrap or sling is essential for infancy.Calming noises and sounds, such as soft white noise or gentle music, can help calm your baby. White noise and gentle music can help drown out the other environmental noise. These tools provide comfortable background noise. Be careful not to play white noise or music too loudly for infants. Some babies who get used to a white noise machine while falling asleep may have difficulties falling asleep without it. Use white noise in moderation.

- The classic rocking chair is a bit cliché, but for many babies, it provides comfort. Gently rocking in the chair for a while can offer a slow rhythm that can lull babies into a calmer state or even help put them to sleep.
- Change the scenery. Sometimes taking your baby out of the immediate environment and into a different place can help change her mood. For example, take a walk outside with your baby. Move around your house to a new location. Go for a short drive (if your baby enjoys car rides).
- Combination approach. Try supporting your baby in different positions while you gently sing or shush your baby. Cradle your baby in your arms on his side or on his tummy while rocking him. Wear the baby in a sling while you play calming music.
- Move to a quiet room with low lighting. Babies who are overstimulated often feel disorganized and a little out of control. Reducing stimulation can be as simple as holding your baby skin-to-skin in a quiet room.
- Breastfeeding is effective at helping babies become organized. Sometimes, an older baby will calm down enough to latch right away. Of course, if the baby is highly agitated, latching onto the breast may not be your first step. First, calm your baby using one of the calming methods that work for you. Then, offer the breast. Even if your baby recently ate or is not showing hunger cues, nursing at the breast provides extreme comfort. Babies can latch onto the breast and use a non-nutritive sucking pattern to calm themselves and won't likely lead to active feeding

(unless they decide to change their sucking pattern). Sometimes, people latch babies to the emptier breast if they know the baby truly only needs comfort.

5. Responsive Parenting

Although responsive parenting is different from other practical or hands-on skills on this list, it is equally important, if not more so. Responsive parenting skills and compassion and empathy are the foundation of parent-child relationships that are nurturing and respectful. This topic is much too large for me to address in this book adequately, but it would be negligent to exclude it from a list of necessary parenting skills. In light of that, this will be a brief overview. Please learn more about responsive parenting beyond this short discussion.

What is Responsive Parenting?

No doubt, there are many ways to define responsive parenting. Simply put, responsive parenting is responding to and meeting your child's needs with nurturing and caring behaviors. While that may seem incredibly simple, at times, it can be much harder to practice than it might seem.

Practicing responsive parenting begins the day your baby is born. Many people assume that newborns and young infants cannot understand language, therefore, adult conversations cannot affect them. Truthfully, infants are incredibly astute at picking up signals, even with language. The tone of voice is an important signal. Babies can understand distress or anger in language. Babies quickly learn to associate positive and negative emotions with facial expressions. Use appropriate language and behavior with your newborn. Speak to your child how you would like people to speak to you.

Responsive parenting is also about responding, as the name suggests. The response that you give is totally dependent on your child's needs at any given time. Reading your child's cues and responding as necessary is essential for meeting your child's physical and emotional needs. It pays off to remember that as a nursing parent, you have a unique way of meeting nearly all your baby's needs with one simple action: breastfeeding. One of the main principles of the La Leche League philosophy is that parenting through breastfeeding is a comprehensive way to nurture your baby while meeting all of her needs. For those breastfeeding, this means that throughout your breastfeeding experience, you can meet your baby's needs through breastfeeding, even as your baby gets bigger and her needs change.

Breastfeeding can provide food for your baby, give warmth to a chilly baby, offer a soft place to snuggle, and provide comfort to a toddler after a fall. In addition, breastfeeding allows your baby to practice sucking skills, induces sleep, and breastfeeding can provide emotional reassurance and nurturing for your baby. Breastfeeding is one of many tools you can use to effectively respond to and meet your baby's needs.

Other useful responsive parenting techniques include:

- Use variety in your language; speak directly to your baby.
- Use animated facial expressions to engage your baby.
- Respond to your baby's calls and cues.
- Validate your child's feelings. Acknowledge feelings of hurt or discomfort. Provide reassurance.
- Praise your baby/child for accomplishments.
- Model cooperative behaviors and sharing.
- Provide an older child with choices about her environment, clothing, and food.
- Respond with love and consistency, even when setting boundaries.

Infant, toddlers, and older children all have unique and different needs. You can use responsive parenting techniques at any time with your baby. To learn more about responsive parenting to meet your baby's needs, find books and online resources on attachment parenting.

6. Skin-to-Skin

Skin-to-skin care, also called Kangaroo Care, is vital for anyone caring for an infant. Kangaroo Care is a profoundly effective way to help your baby achieve body system regulation. Your body is your baby's natural stability habitat. When you hold your baby skin-to-skin with no fabric or clothing between you, your body helps regulate and reset your baby's entire system. See the chapter on Kangaroo Care for complete details. Here is a brief summary of how to practice skin-to-skin care.

- Sit comfortably with your body semi-reclined, about 45 degrees.
- Remove clothing, shirts, bras, or any other fabric from your chest.
- Place your naked baby (dressed only in a diaper) tummy down on your chest. Next, position her with chest and abdomen on your chest.
- Turn your baby's head to the side, and make sure to flex her arms and legs. Be sure your baby seems comfortable.
- Cover your baby with a blanket.
- Rest in the skin-to-skin position together, as long as you are comfortable. Try not to wake your baby if she falls asleep.

This position is useful for helping your baby achieve a body system reset. Skin-to-skin can be helpful if your baby is irritable, crying, agitated, too hot, or too cold. Skin-to-skin care can help your baby normalize her blood sugar, blood pressure, breathing rate, heart rate, and oxygen saturation. In addition, it can help babies organize their sleep patterns and help them adjust their emotional state. This tool is an incredible parenting skill and one that your baby will benefit from every time you practice Kangaroo Care.

7. Breast Compression

Under normal circumstances, when your baby comes to the breast, she latches on and begins a rapid suck pattern to stimulate the milk let-down. Once the milk letdown has occurred, the baby will change to a nutritive suck pattern (one-to-one or two-to-one suck swallow pattern). After actively feeding for a while, the milk flow slows down; your baby is likely to pause and take breaks because the milk flow is no longer rapid.

The scenario above works quite well for some babies, but other babies need a little at-breast intervention to get more milk moving. Massaging the breast tissue before your baby nurses can stimulate a let-down. Compression while nursing or pumping can help move more milk toward the nipple. Breast compression and breast massage can increase the number of calories your baby will get during one feeding because you manually move more milk, making more available for her intake. In addition, breast massage and compression can increase the fat content of human milk (Wambach & Riordan, 2016). The true fat content of the milk you make is not increased by breast compression; this technique helps move more fat into the milk delivered to the baby. Here are the basic steps:

- For massage, gently provide pressure with the palms of your hands or knead the breast gently with your knuckles. Roll the breasts between your palms. This massage can help stimulate a let-down. It is also handy when dealing with engorgement or plugged ducts. Use these techniques before trying breast compression.
- For compression, place your thumb on one side of the breast, back slightly from the nipple, and your fingers on the other side. Gently compress the breast and hold for a few seconds. Release and move your thumb and fingers to either side into a new position. Gently compress the tissue again and hold for a few seconds. Release and change hand position again.
- Breast tissue with milk-making structures exists all around the breast and up into the axilla (armpit). So, be sure to massage and compress these areas too.
- Continue with compression until you have moved all around the breast.
- If your baby is nursing, you may see that the suck swallow pattern becomes quicker. If you are pumping milk with a breast pump, you may see an overall increase in your milk output.
- Experiment with different hand positions and see what works best for you.
- Maya Bolman and Ann M. Witt have a fantastic video on YouTube called "The Basics of Breast Massage and Hand Expression." Observe the massage techniques if you are experiencing engorgement. This technique is a brilliant strategy for loosening up the breast and preparing the tissues for milk let-down.

Breast compression and massage can help increase milk output while nursing and pumping, increase the amount of fat the baby gets, help speed up the milk let-down, and move more milk toward the nipple for a baby who has a weak suck or has trouble staying awake at the breast. In addition, compression and massage often help manage low milk supply. These techniques are adaptable, and you can utilize a pattern or method that best suits your breast anatomy and your needs. One size does not fit all. Use the approach that works best for you.

8. Hand Expression

Hand expression of breast milk is just what it seems: using your hands to express milk from the breast. This procedure is a useful technique for relieving breast engorgement, treating plugged ducts, removing milk when separated from your baby, and better emptying the breasts after feeding. There are many techniques for hand expression. Here is one commonly used method:

- Always begin with clean hands.
- Gently massage the breast with both hands. One effective technique is to roll the breast between your hands, one below the breast and one above. Gentle massage, tapping, and kneading can also be effective. Nipple stimulation can also help prepare the breast for hand expression. In addition, the massage, tapping, and rolling helps to prepare and stimulate the breast for milk let-down.
- Place one hand on the breast, holding the breast with thumb over the nipple and fingers under the nipple. Be sure your fingers are a centimeter or two back from the areola.
- Move your whole hand back toward your chest wall as you simultaneously bring the thumb toward your fingers in a squeezing motion. Apply enough gentle pressure to move milk but not to cause any pain.
- While compressing the tissue, milk should start flowing from the nipple. If you get nothing, you may need to massage a bit more. The let-down usually takes about 60-90 seconds. Once the milk starts flowing, collect it in a clean cup or another container.
- If your fingers and thumb are too close to the nipple, you will not be able to compress the structures of the breast that

contain milk. If your fingers are too far away from the nipple, you could move milk, but it will be harder to express milk. Finger and thumb placement should be just beyond the areola but not too far back. Try different positions to see what hand placement is best for you.

- Move your hands around the breast to be sure you drain the tissues evenly.
- Watching videos of hand expression can help if you struggle to express milk. For example, the video mentioned above by Maya Bolman, IBCLC (called "The Basics of Breast Massage and Hand Expression") shows excellent strategies for hand expressing milk.

9. Co-Sleeping

Like Kangaroo Care and responsive parenting, co-sleeping is a parenting skill that deserves a much more extensive explanation than I can give in this book. In fact, entire books are dedicated to the skills necessary for practicing co-sleeping with your baby. This will be a brief discussion of co-sleeping methods and options.

We define co-sleeping as sleeping close to or nearby your baby. There are several ways to achieve co-sleeping. Some options include sleeping in the same room on two different surfaces, sleeping at arm's reach of your baby with the baby in a separate bassinet or small crib, or bedsharing with your baby. Co-sleeping facilitates easy nighttime feeding and increases the amount of sleep for parents and babies compared to non-co-sleeping arrangements. Co-sleeping allows for early feeding cue recognition during the night due to the physical closeness of parent and baby. Parents who sleep with their babies often report that their sleep cycles are in sync with the baby's sleep cycle, and they can wake just moments before the baby wakes to nurse. Co-sleeping (same room or same bed) can reduce the incidence of SIDS (sudden infant death syndrome).

There are seven parameters to safely co-sleeping on the same surface with your baby.

- Breastfed babies can co-sleep. Formula-fed infants should not co-sleep on the same surface as adults. Formula-fed babies can sleep in the adult bedroom in a crib or bassinet.

- Parents must be non-smokers (non-negotiable).
- Parents must be completely sober: no drug use, marijuana use, or alcohol use. Also not negotiable.
- Babies who co-sleep must be full-term infants, not born prematurely.
- Babies who co-sleep must be dressed lightly.
- Babies who co-sleep should always sleep on their backs.
- Co-sleeping surfaces must adhere to safe sleep guidelines for sheets, blankets, and bed types.

If you consider co-sleeping, get the information you need to sleep safely with your baby. Dr. James McKenna, anthropologist and mother-baby sleep researcher at the University of Notre Dame, has two books worth reading for those who want to co-sleep: *Safe Infant Sleep, Expert Answers to Your Cosleeping Questions,* and *Sleeping With Your Baby: A Parent's Guide to Cosleeping*.

Another great source of information for co-sleeping families is a book called *Sweet Sleep: Nighttime and Naptime Strategies for the Breastfeeding Family.* This excellent book, written by Diane Wiessinger, Diana West, Linda J. Smith, and Teresa Pitman, is essential for breastfeeding families. It covers safe sleep and all seven elements of co-sleeping in depth. I highly recommend this book to breastfeeding families.

Even if you do not plan to sleep regularly with your baby, the night may come when you fall asleep in bed with your baby by accident. Please take the time now to learn how to properly prepare an adult bed for co-sleeping situations.

10. Pumping and Storing Human Milk

Many people find that pumping human milk is a regular part of their infant feeding experience. However, while some people pump most days of the week, others pump occasionally, and some parents are exclusively pumping without direct feeding. Each of these situations is a valid approach to using human milk but may dictate differences in the kind of pump used and how milk is stored.

The skills for pumping human milk are not necessarily complex, but everyone should consider a few important guidelines before getting started.

Milk Pumping Guidelines

First, select a pump that will be the right fit for your needs. If you are working full time or planning to pump exclusively, you will need to invest in the highest quality pump that you can afford. In this case, you will be pumping several times per day, and you want a pump that will have the power to last for months. If your pump schedule only includes pumping now and then, you may not need a top-of-the-line model. Some people who do not pump very much could consider a hand pump, wearable pump, or even hand expression (no pump). Evaluate your pumping needs before you invest.

Second, read all the manufacturer's instructions carefully. You will need to thoroughly understand how the pump works, its limitations, and techniques for cleaning and maintaining it.

Third, be sure to understand the proper way to assess flange fit. The flange is the piece of pump equipment that covers the nipple and areola. If this piece does not fit properly, you could experience suboptimal pumping outcomes. Poor flange fit can lead to nipple damage, swelling in the areola, pain, and less than complete milk removal or uneven breast draining. To assess your flange fit, pay attention to how the nipple looks while you are pumping. The nipple should be centered in the tunnel and move freely, not touching the sides of the tunnel. Friction with the side of the tunnel could cause pain and nipple damage. Also, be sure that the areola is not moving up into the tunnel while you are pumping. This movement could cause swelling and pain. If you are unsure about flange fit, speak to a lactation consultant. Another option is to try different size flanges to see what works best for you. In addition, there are inserts available to help improve comfort while pumping.

Additional advice for pumping:

- Wash your hands before pumping.
- Be sure to have everything you will need. This equipment could include the pump kit, a snack, water, something to read, or work to do.

- Find a comfortable spot where you will not be interrupted.
- Connect with your baby through your senses. For example, look at pictures of your baby, watch a happy video, sniff an infant hat or piece of clothing recently worn by your baby.
- Begin pumping. Adjust the speed and suction as needed. Remember that high speed and suction can cause nipple damage. Start slow and low to figure out optimal settings.
- Collect milk and store it according to current safety guidelines.
- Remember that milk production is highest in the morning hours and lowest about 12 hours later (afternoon). You will still have milk in the afternoon, but production/output is higher in the morning.
- Milk output can vary from day to day and certainly from breast to breast. You may notice that your left side produces more than your right (or vice versa).
- Hands-on pumping can increase milk output. Use massage and compression techniques to ensure milk removal.

Milk Storage Guidelines

In general, there are three choices for storing freshly expressed human milk.

1. Room temperature (no hotter than 77 F & 25 C)
2. Refrigerator (40 F & 4 C)
3. Freezer (0 F & -18 C)

If you choose to express milk and leave it at room temperature, it can safely last up to four hours before it must be used or discarded. Milk that is expressed and then put in the back of the refrigerator (do not use the door or the front part of the refrigerator) can safely last up to four days before being used or discarded. In the back of the freezer, human milk can safely last up to 12 months. However, it is best to use the milk by six months. There is additional information about pumping in the RELAX chapter, in the section about pumping using the RELACS technique.

11. Self-Advocacy and Child Advocacy

All of the skills included in this chapter are important, but perhaps no skills are as important as self-advocacy and child advocacy. Simply put, self-advocacy is the ability to identify your needs and seek the resources you need to meet your needs. Child advocacy identifies a child's needs and speaks for them to ensure their needs are met. These are essential parenting skills.

There are many elements involved in the practice of self-advocacy. Self-advocacy is not one skill but a collection of skills that a person can use to bring together various resources and information that can help meet their needs. For this discussion, we will consider self-advocacy through the lens of lactation. Our example here is limited but includes many of the self-advocacy skills as it applies to any area of your life, including 1) identifying your needs, 2) knowing what you are entitled to, 3) communication skills, and 4) decision-making skills.

Identifying Your Needs

While identifying your needs is often a straightforward task, it may not be that easy when it comes to breastfeeding, especially if this is your first experience with babies. Suppose you had not had a baby before or had much personal experience with infant care. In that case, you likely have an incomplete picture of life with a newborn, newborn care, infant feeding, and self-care in the postpartum period. This observation is not a criticism; it is a reality for most of us. This inexperience leaves us in a place where we don't know what we don't know. In other words, many people are unaware of their own incomplete knowledge of infant care and infant feeding before the birth of their first child. This reality makes it difficult to identify and anticipate your needs in advance of birth. Read through the following questions to help you examine existing resources and anticipate possible future needs. There are no right or wrong answers. This guide will help you evaluate your needs, but your answers will differ from the next person.

- Who are your breastfeeding support people?
- Which friends or relatives can you call on for help with breastfeeding?

- Which friends or relatives can you ask for help with daily chores and practical support (e.g., meal making, laundry, picking up an item from the store)?
- Who are your professional support people?
- Have you found a pro-breastfeeding pediatrician? Have you found a local breastfeeding support group?
- What are the items for baby care and infant feeding that you need?
- Can you borrow any of these from a friend or family member?
- What books would you like to read about infant care and breastfeeding?
- Have you considered making several meals ahead of time and freezing them after the baby arrives?
- Would you consider having a friend or sister set up a meal train?
- Have you considered your plans for nighttime sleeping and breastfeeding?
- When will you get rest and sleep?
- When will you have time or make time for self-care?
- Where will you set up your breastfeeding station? Remember, you may need to consider at least two places to breastfeed your baby – one for daytime and one for nighttime.
- Where will the baby sleep?
- Where will you sleep?
- How will other non-baby-related chores get completed?
- How will you divide housework and meal prep with your partner?
- Is it feasible to hire help?
- Would you consider hiring a postpartum doula?

Knowing Your Rights and What You Are Entitled To

Are you aware that most states or local municipalities have laws that protect breastfeeding in public or the rights of parents to breastfeed anywhere they are legally entitled to be? Beyond breastfeeding in public, there are all kinds of situations where breastfeeding has been called into question. Some of those scenarios include:

- Custody disputes
- Pumping milk while working, break time for pumping
- Breastfeeding in restaurants, malls, stores, on airplanes, college classrooms, government buildings
- Carrying pumped milk through airport security
- Pumping milk while serving time in prison
- Breastfeeding in uniform (armed forces)

Knowing your rights can often (but not always) help you in situations where someone calls your breastfeeding rights into question. Be prepared. Know your rights in advance. If you are traveling with pumped milk in a cooler through airport security, read the TSA rules before you go. It may help to print the rules and bring them with you. Each state in the U.S. has different laws regarding breastfeeding and the rights of nursing parents. Familiarize yourself with your local rights. In the U.S., the National Conference of State Legislatures (NCSL) has a well-organized and easy-to-read online resource outlining the breastfeeding laws for each state and territory. Visit ncsl.org and search for Breastfeeding State Laws. Most breastfeeding protection is provided by the "gender equality" clause in the Canadian Charter of Rights and Freedoms in Canada. British Columbia and Ontario also have provincial-level laws protecting breastfeeding rights. Regulations in Australia and the UK also protect rights for breastfeeding.

Communication Skills for Breastfeeding and Parenting

Communication is an important part of any healthcare situation because the stakes are typically high. We usually have limited time to speak with our doctors and sometimes it is hard to discuss everything in a short office visit. In addition, some people are intimidated by speaking to their doctor. Here are some tips to help you optimize communication with your healthcare team.

1. Be prepared. Write down your concerns if you need to in order to remember your priorities and questions.

2. Be honest about who you are and what your needs are. Let your doctor or caregiver know relevant information about you. For example, I always tell my caregivers that I am seeking the most natural solution or remedy first. This is not something they would know about me by reading my health history and it's not something they usually ask. It helps to let your caregiver know "who you are" so they can present the best possible information and advice.
3. Don't be afraid to ask for more information or more time to make decisions. Feeling rushed can often lead to hasty decisions. Ask you caregiver for more information. Ask about resources that you might need: books, websites, local resources, or other education opportunities. Often times, caregivers are a wealth of information but may not readily give you all the details about something unless you ask.
4. If your doctor suggests options that you don't feel comfortable with, be sure to explain your hesitations. Each one of us is unique and that means that what the doctor prescribes to one person may not be right for the next person. It is perfectly okay to reject options that are offered. Gone are the days when people blindly followed all professional medical advice. This can also be a time to consider getting a second (or third) opinion. If you feel pressured or even coerced into choosing between two unappealing options, ask about alternatives. Ask for more time. Consult with your partner or other trusted friend or family member.

Decision-Making for Breastfeeding and Lactation

In the context of healthcare and infant feeding, there are several variables to consider when making decisions. Each person has a unique set of variables to start with so your decisions may be quite different from others you know. Some of the unique factors that may impact your decisions are health history, cultural background, nutrition requirements, current health status, beliefs and attitudes about infant feeding, as well as other factors.

When you are facing an important decision with regard to breastfeeding or lactation, begin by gathering the information you need in order to evaluate all of your options. Once you have learned what your options are, be sure to evaluate how your choices will affect your decision to breastfeed. Assess the positives or benefits of your choices as well as the risks of each choice.

Shared decision-making is a common approach when parents are evaluating health related questions. Be sure to factor in all the necessary participants. For example, you may want to discuss with your partner the risks and benefits of any choice before you make a decision. Sometimes, shared decision-making can involve getting information and discussing pros and cons with professional help, like a lactation consultant or the baby's pediatrician.

Consider any alternatives if you are having a difficult time making an important decision. Seeking out alternatives is an excellent idea and one that is often overlooked. Many times, people see options as only two choices but in reality, there may be several alternative options. For example, imagine that you're deciding whether to get an epidural during labor. At first, it may seem that there are only two options: to get the epidural or to avoid epidural. If you decide that you want to have pain relief during labor but you are concerned about how epidural analgesia may affect breastfeeding, investigate alternatives to epidural pain relief. You might be surprised to find that there are numerous coping techniques and strategies that you can learn before labor that have great potential for providing pain relief.

Check in with your intuition before making significant decisions. What does your gut feeling tell you? Are you leaning toward one option or the other? Are the possible choices aligned with your beliefs and values? Do you need more information? Do you need more time? Listen to your intuition and try to go with your gut.

Sometimes, we overlook the option of "not choosing" to make a choice. In other words, there is sometimes the option to do nothing. This principle does not always apply, especially when you must take action in order to move forward.

These decision-making steps are easy to remember if you use the acronym BRAIN. BRAIN stands for Benefits, Risks, Alternatives, Intuition, Nothing. If you want to be sure you cover all your bases in decision-making, even when you have to come up with a decision quickly, run through the steps by first assessing the benefits and risks of each option. Remember to consider any alternatives and factor in your intuition. Finally, remember that sometimes there is the option to do nothing.

Conclusion

Reflect on the skills listed above. Then, analyze your current skill level for each one and determine if you need more information, new or different intentions, more intuitive awareness, or even more instinctual response to develop your skills. Over time, you will progress from beginner to proficient if you put in the time and effort to learn these skills.

There are many other skills of parenting and breastfeeding that you will encounter. Be open to learning and remember to learn with the beginner's mind. Don't assume that what you already know about breastfeeding and parenting skills is fully informed or accurate. Skill building is a work in progress, and there is always more to learn, even for the experts.

PART II
Lactation Interference Factors

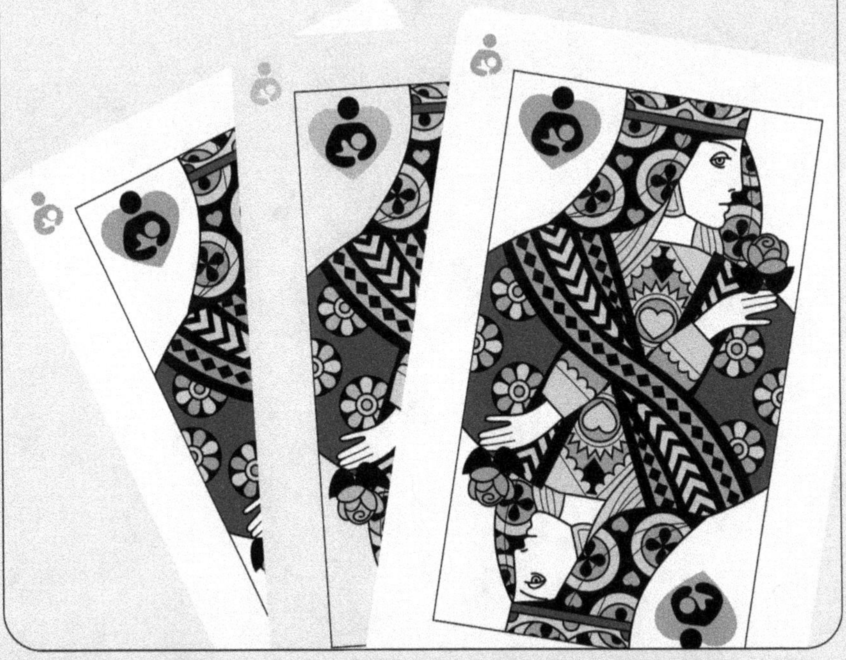

CHAPTER 8

Breastfeeding Interference and Birth-Related Factors

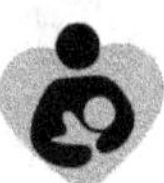

If you think that it makes absolutely no sense, physiologically or evolutionarily, for childbirth to negatively impact lactation, you are exactly right. After all, lactation is the natural progression following the end of pregnancy. Why would the physiology of birth cause negative consequences for lactation? The answer is simple: birth does not cause adverse outcomes for lactation. In fact, childbirth, specifically the expulsion of the placenta, is the trigger for *turning on the mechanisms* that produce human milk. This happens because of a particular hormonal shift.

The hormones of pregnancy, primarily estrogen and progesterone, keep lactation on hold before birth. These hormones inhibit the release of prolactin, the milk production hormone, from the pituitary gland and make mammary tissue less sensitive to prolactin. Once the placenta is expelled from the uterus, the pregnancy is officially over, and a dramatic hormonal shift occurs. The pregnancy hormones give way to a completely different hormonal profile, one that supports lactation. As a result, prolactin levels rise in the days after birth, and milk production transitions from the concentrated, small quantities of colostrum to an abundant milk supply.

If birth does not interfere with lactation, what causes birth-related adverse outcomes for lactation? Birth itself is not the problem. It is our modern and ubiquitous use of intrapartum labor interventions that can have negative impacts on lactation.

Labor interventions vary in terms of their impact on lactation. Some interventions have a low impact on lactation, whereas other interventions have a consistently high impact. Many factors contribute to the overall outcome, including preexisting maternal conditions.

Each person's reaction to labor interventions will be slightly different than another. This explains why some people can experience an intervention or two and not have any lingering or troublesome consequences for breastfeeding. Others can experience the same interventions and have more intense problems. There isn't a "one size fits all" algorithm for predicting lactation outcomes after labor interventions. Still, some excellent studies shed light on the trends. This section of the book will discuss interventions before, during, or after birth that can disrupt milk production and feeding.

Before we dive into interventions, let's discuss why these interventions exist, what purpose they serve, and how and when to agree to or avoid them.

An Overview of Birth Interventions

Have you ever wondered why humans gave birth under trees or in secluded locations for thousands of years, free of today's high-tech interventions, yet today, these birth "routines" seem so necessary? The not-so-surprising answer is that birth interventions are mostly unnecessary. However, we have been led to believe that they are somehow essential.

Birth interventions like labor induction with Pitocin/Syntocin, epidural pain relief, forceps, vacuum, IV fluids, and cesarean birth are intricately associated with hospital birth. These interventions do not exist outside of hospital birth. Generally, hospitals run maternity care on a schedule. There are established guidelines for how long membranes can be ruptured before induction must start. There are time limits on how quickly one must progress through labor before labor might be augmented. There are even limits on how long a typical hospital birth will allow pushing during the second stage of labor. When labor doesn't fit neatly into the predetermined time limits (a rarity), hospitals use interventions to get things back on course. One major flaw with this strategy is that one intervention often does not correct the initial "problem" and another intervention is required for further correction. Sometimes, the full cascade of interventions falls into place. One person may experience induction, Pitocin, epidural, IV fluids, instrumental delivery, or cesarean during a single birth experience. This sounds extreme, but it may surprise you that this is quite common in U.S. hospitals with high rates of interventions.

There are other reasons for the regular use of labor interventions besides heavily scheduled and time-limited maternity care. For example, one reason that interventions are so common is because hospital birth disrupted traditional birth. Long before hospital birth, people would labor in their own environments, choose their own positions and movements during labor, and eat and drink as they pleased. In addition, labor took place in the company of caring, supportive people who could provide massage, counterpressure, hot and cold packs, soothing food and drinks, and other comfort measures considered the first line of relief for the work of labor. Depending on one's preferences, this type of birth may be much more tolerable than the clinical care that often happens in a hospital setting, without the comforts of physical and emotional support, food, and the ability to call the shots.

Today, people often assume that the first line of relief during labor is an epidural. Of course, this requires that birth takes place in a hospital because you cannot get an epidural in the comfort of your bedroom. One ingenious strategy to postpone or avoid using labor interventions is to plan for low-tech comfort measures and person-delivered assistance. For example, you and your partner can learn specific techniques during pregnancy to prepare or hire a labor companion trained to provide this type of support. Studies show that hiring a labor companion/doula will lower the risk of many common labor interventions. Another good way to avoid birth interventions is to avoid the hospital. Consider a free-standing birth center or home birth. Both of these are excellent and safe options for healthy people having low-risk pregnancies.

Another reason that labor interventions are so common in the hospital setting is that birth in the hospital most often occurs in a suboptimal position: lying down or semi-reclined. As you might imagine, giving birth while the pelvis is resting flat on the backside is not optimal. To work with gravity and to optimize the pelvic outlet, opening it to its widest possible point, the pelvis must be upright. Lying down while in labor is often uncomfortable, which increases the need for pain relief. Stay upright and move during labor. Use a squatting position for giving birth. These seem like simple recommendations but staying upright and mobile during birth can make all the difference.

To summarize these ideas, I will quote Lamaze and their Six Healthy Birth Practices because these simple steps are incredibly important (Lamaze, 2021):

1. Let labor begin on its own.
2. Walk, move around and change positions throughout labor.
3. Bring a loved one, friend, or doula for continuous support.
4. Avoid interventions that are not medically necessary.
5. Avoid giving birth on your back and follow your body's urges to push.
6. Keep mother and baby together- it's best for mother, baby, and breastfeeding.

Your Birth Attendant

The vast majority of people giving birth do so with a skilled birth attendant. Usually, birth attendants belong in one of three categories: OB-GYN (obstetrician-gynecologist), midwife, or family doctor. In the U.S., most people are attended by an OB-GYN. Only about 10% of births in the U.S. are attended by midwives. However, midwives attend well over half of the births (up to 2/3) in many European countries.

Does the type of birth attendant you choose impact your breastfeeding experience? According to a recent study from Virginia Commonwealth University, the birth attendant does play a role in your future breastfeeding journey. Consider this:

- People who birth with a midwife or family doctor are twice as likely to breastfeed at least six months than those who birth with an OB-GYN (Wallenborn & Masho, 2018).
- People who choose midwives as birth attendants are six times more likely to breastfeed exclusively for at least six months (Wallenborn & Masho, 2018).

What do these results suggest? Is there something special about midwifery care that teaches people or persuades them to breastfeed and do it longer than if they had selected an OB for their birth? Or is it possible that the people who choose midwifery care were already more inclined to breastfeed their babies? The answer is probably a little bit of both.

Because midwifery has roots in maternity care in the community setting (home birth), midwives have had a long tradition of caring for both the parent and baby after the birth and the parent-baby breastfeeding relationship. Although status as a midwife does not automatically mean that the midwife has any formal lactation training, midwifery care has long been a place where breastfeeding is nurtured and supported.

On the other hand, obstetrical care has roots in the hospital setting, thriving as a model of maternity care at the time when infant formula reached its peak. One criticism of OB care today is that OBs are unlikely to have any training in lactation care at all. This lack of training makes breastfeeding support and education low on the priority list for an OB. Historically, the main focus of obstetrical care is a safe birth, the health and safety of mother and baby, without focusing on breastfeeding. This could be changing, however. In 2016, the ACOG Breastfeeding Expert Work Group issued Committee Opinion, Number 756. In this opinion, there are recommendations for the OB-GYN practice to fully support breastfeeding and even for OB offices to have embedded lactation care available at their offices. Keep in mind, this is an opinion of an expert committee, not necessarily their policy, and certainly not a mandate.

Change is slow to take place in the healthcare setting. It can take about 17-20 years for evidence-based practices to become standard care. Is it likely that a traditionally trained OB will rush out and seek lactation training or hire a lactation consultant for their office after reading Committee Opinion number 756? No, but trends are changing, and in the future, this may be standard care. Until then, be mindful that the prenatal and postpartum support available from midwifery care can be vastly different in the U.S. when compared to prenatal and postpartum care available from an OB. It just might influence your breastfeeding initiation, support, experience, and duration.

Induction of Labor

At first glance, several of the routine childbirth interventions discussed in this book might appear to have no influence on breastfeeding outcomes. Labor induction is undoubtedly in that category. If your caregiver suggests induction of labor, you might be thinking, "Okay, does it really matter if my labor starts today or next Friday?" As you may have guessed, I have included labor induction in this section because it can substantially impact infant health, maternal health, and breastfeeding.

First, some facts: in 2016, the induction of labor rates were different from state to state in the U.S. The national average in 2016 was about one out of four pregnancies ending with induction of labor. According to the CDC National Health Center for Health Statistics, data from 2016 shows that California had the lowest percentage of labor induction (14.3%), and West Virginia had the highest (39.4%) (CRO, 2016). For reference, it is essential to note that the U.S. had an average induction rate of 9.5% in 1990 (Rayburn & Zhang, 2002). Similarly, a 2018 publication in Canada shows that the induction rate was only 12.9% in 1991-1992 and rose steadily through the early 2000s (Public Health Agency of Canada, 2018). Both the U.S. and Canada have had a recent stabilization or modest decrease of induction rates.

It is unclear why induction rates rose steadily for about two decades and remain relatively high. The *Listening to Mothers III* survey shows that at least 14.8% of mothers surveyed said their caregiver pressured them to begin labor by induction (Jou et al., 2015). Like many other aspects of managed childbirth in the hospital culture, induction rates are likely a complex interaction of many factors.

Induction is not risk-free, and although there may not be a direct impact on lactation, induction can cause some downstream problems that affect breastfeeding outcomes. One of the most problematic outcomes of induction of labor is that induction increases the odds for all sorts of other birth interventions, including many that influence lactation. Two of the most important outcomes for labor induction that affect breastfeeding are increased risk of cesarean and iatrogenic prematurity. In this section, we will briefly examine each of these and their potential impacts on breastfeeding. (For more information, see the sections on cesarean and premature infant.)

Induction that Leads to Cesarean Birth

There has been some debate as to whether labor induction raises the risk for cesarean delivery. However, a study done in 2016 analyzing data from 42,950 uncomplicated, singleton births to first-time mothers found that induction of labor leads to a significant increase in delivery by cesarean (Davey & King, 2016). The data showed that people whose labors were induced had a 26.5% cesarean rate. In comparison, those whose labors started on their own experienced a 12.5% cesarean rate (Davey & King, 2016). This study involving thousands of first-time mothers shows a clear relationship between labor induction and cesarean delivery. In short, more inductions equals more cesareans. However, it is not necessarily the induction itself that impacts breastfeeding. Since labor induction appears to raise the risk of cesarean delivery, induction leads to greater risk of cesarean and cesarean birth increases the risk of breastfeeding complications.

Another severe outcome of induction of labor is iatrogenic prematurity. *Iatrogenic* is not a word you hear every day and certainly not one that you're likely to hear from your caregiver. Iatrogenic means that a condition was caused by the caregiver, not by illness or other patient-centered condition. In this case, *iatrogenic prematurity* means an infant who is born prematurely because of doctor's interventions. Without exact information on when the infant was conceived, it is impossible to accurately determine the fetus's gestational age, especially in late pregnancy. This leads to uncertainty in assigning a due date. In addition, there is some controversy about due dates, as the traditional method for calculating the due date was developed using faulty logic and assumptions. In the absence of *known* conception date (e.g., in vitro fertilization or those who were charting their cycles during conception), caregivers are guessing when they assign a due date. Furthermore, they are guessing at a likely gestational age for the fetus. This lack of certainty creates ample opportunity for mistakes to occur when calculating the gestational age and frequently causes an infant born after induction to be less than 40 weeks gestation. In this case, the induction does not create breastfeeding problems;

it intentionally causes the birth to occur before the infant is ready, sometimes much too soon. This premature infant, even one born at 37, 38, or even 39 weeks, is at greater risk of feeding complications. See the section on prematurity for more information.

Other Outcomes of Induction Related to Lactation

Studies show that labor induction can cause separation of the breastfeeding dyad and delay the timing of the first latch and feeding. For example, in a study by Cadwell et al. (2018), results suggested that labor induction decreased the odds that a baby could latch and feed at the breast within 60 minutes of birth time. In this study, 31.3% of infants born after labor was induced could accomplish breastfeeding within one hour. In comparison, 56.6% of infants born without labor induction could accomplish their first feed within 60 minutes (Cadwell et al., 2018). In addition, this study also showed that induction of labor increased the odds that the baby was separated from the parents after birth compared with babies born after non-induced labor (Cadwell et al., 2018). Separation after birth puts into place several risk factors, including increasing the time between birth and first feed, decreasing the number of feedings in the first 24 hours, disturbing the "golden hour," increasing infant stress, and delaying bonding. All of these factors can negatively influence the pathway to breastfeeding.

Another study done by King et al. in 2010 reveals more negative outcomes for lactation when induction of labor is performed. First, elective induction before 39 weeks without valid medical reasons puts the baby at risk for certain conditions affecting breastfeeding. For example, induction before 39 weeks can increase the risk of breathing problems for the baby, increase infection rates and increase the likelihood of admission to the NICU (King et al., 2010). All of these are known to interfere with breastfeeding. In addition, King et al. (2010) confirmed many other studies that have found that induction increases the use of epidural anesthesia, which has several known adverse outcomes for lactation. See the section on Epidural for more details. Finally, similar to factors detailed above, this study found that elective induction before 41 weeks can lead to an increased risk of cesarean delivery (King et al., 2010), impacting milk production and interfering with lactation in the early weeks.

Please know that this is a complex and controversial topic. Many researchers and studies have been performed on labor induction and shown little or no consequences for infant or maternal health. Little information is available that directly connects induction of labor to infant feeding complications. It does not take an expert to connect the dots. Do your own research and make an informed decision before agreeing to induction of labor. Be sure you are an excellent candidate for induction, otherwise, a failed induction leads most often to cesarean. As a quick summary, here are some of the impacts of induction of labor:

Table 8.1: Risks associated with induction of labor

Increased odds of	Lactation Interference
Iatrogenic prematurity	Latch may be difficult, premature babies can tire out easily
Breathing problems	Can increase feeding difficulties
Infant infection	Increases risk of separation
NICU admission	Decreases odds of exclusive breastfeeding
Cesarean delivery	Can delay lactogenesis II

Epidural

I once heard a woman say that her birth plan included walking backward into the delivery room toward the anesthesiologist so that she was 100% ready to receive an epidural. Of course, she was joking, but her comment about facing her back to the anesthesiologist indicated her readiness to opt-in for this pain relief. Many people share this intention because they are highly motivated to avoid any discomfort or pain during labor. However, this intervention does not come without risks, some of which can impact lactation.

Epidural analgesia is pain relief for labor and birth administered into the spinal cord's epidural space. Medications used with this technique are local anesthetics but are sometimes used in conjunction with other medications (opioids, for example). Be sure to ask your OB what medications will likely be used in your situation. Commonly used medications in epidural analgesia include bupivacaine, chloroprocaine, lidocaine, mepivacaine, and ropivacaine. Opioids in epidurals can include morphine, fentanyl, and pethidine.

Epidural anesthesia is used during childbirth, helping to control pain levels during labor. This method is usually adequate for pain relief. However, it has the added side effect of numbing the patient from the waist down, impacting the use of the lower limbs. After receiving an epidural, one is confined to the bed. A urinary catheter is required because it will not be possible to walk to the bathroom. Epidural pain relief is also accompanied by other necessary interventions. In addition, some opioids used in conjunction with epidurals can negatively impact infant feeding, notably fentanyl. Although the infant is not the target of the medication, drugs administered by epidural cross the placenta and reach the baby within minutes.

As mentioned above, an epidural is not used in isolation. This is one specific intervention that has several other co-interventions that are required. For example, use of epidural anesthesia:

- Creates the need for IV fluids
- Is accompanied by a urinary catheter
- Is used in conjunction with continuous electronic fetal monitoring

In addition, there are many potential outcomes from using epidural pain relief that create more prolonged labor and increase the risks for other interventions. Consider these additional risks associated with epidurals:

- Lower Apgar scores (Ravelli et al., 2020), and low Apgar scores are correlated with feeding problems (Thavarajah et al., 2018).
- Vacuum delivery (Hasegawa et al., 2013). Vacuum delivery is associated with lower Apgar scores and birth trauma, both associated with feeding problems.
- Cesarean delivery (Hasegawa et al., 2013). Cesarean is associated with a delay in lactogenesis II.
- Forceps delivery (Newnham et al., 2021). Forceps delivery is associated with trauma that can lead to bruising, jaundice, nerve damage, and feeding problems, all of which can negatively affect breastfeeding.
- Slow labor, longer second stage of labor (Newnham et al., 2021). Longer and more difficult labors are associated with feeding difficulties.

- Increased blood loss (Newnham et al., 2021). Blood loss (maternal hemorrhage) is associated with Sheehan's syndrome, pituitary damage, and higher rates of problems with milk production.
- Exposure to fentanyl. Fentanyl in higher doses has adverse effects on the infant suck reflex and decreases the likelihood of exclusive breastfeeding (Oommen et al., 2021). Authors of this study recommend lower doses of fentanyl (less than 200 micrograms) to have better neonatal feeding outcomes (Oommen et al., 2021).
- NICU admissions (Ravelli et al., 2020). NICU admission is associated with lower rates of breastfeeding (Gertz & DeFranco, 2019).

In addition, some studies find that epidurals during labor:

- Reduce the likelihood of breastfeeding at six weeks, especially among first-time parents (Orbach-Zinger et al., 2019), reducing the likelihood of breastfeeding at three months (Newnham et al., 2021).

Several of the outcomes of epidural pain relief listed above are things that open the door for other interventions or create potential problems for lactation. For example, because one cannot freely stand up, walk, move around, and quickly change positions after administration of an epidural, the infant may not descend through the birth canal as easily. This may increase the risk of instrumental delivery (Antonakou & Papoutsis, 2016). As noted in a later section, vacuum and forceps deliveries can have negative consequences for infant feeding.

Another potential complication (discussed in detail in a later section) is the administration of IV fluids. Fluid can build up in the extremities, including the breasts, and cause swelling and constriction within the breast tissue. This, in effect, slows milk flow and causes painful edema. There are also infant outcomes of extreme overexposure to IV fluid, discussed in the IV Fluid section.

The research literature on the use of epidural analgesia during labor is highly variable. There are studies showing an association with lower breastfeeding rates and studies showing that there is no effect of epidural use on the initiation of breastfeeding and continuation of breastfeeding. Why does the research on epidural use show such variability?

The factors involved in using epidurals are different for each person, and the circumstances differ greatly from one individual to the next. Some people may be surprised to learn that an epidural is not a standard concoction. The anesthesiologist determines the drugs used, based on the individual person who is receiving the medication. Therefore, drug types and amounts in the cocktail will vary from person to person. In addition, the exposure time will vary from one birth to the next. Some people will have slower labors than others, which increases the drug exposure time for parent and baby.

In addition to those variables, the dose makes an impact on outcomes. For example, the amount of analgesia correlates to epidural outcomes; higher drug concentrations are related to worsening effects for neonatal sucking reflexes. Finally, the exposure time is a factor as well. If the epidural is in place for several hours, the parent likely will receive an increased amount of IV fluids. This fluid can affect breast tissue, engorgement, and latch (see section on IV fluids).

One fascinating study on the use of epidurals during labor shows that people who choose to have epidurals prior to labor have decreased success with breastfeeding initiation compared to people who choose no labor medication (Wetzl et al., 2019). On the other hand, women who planned for no medication, but received epidurals as a last resort, did not have decreased breastfeeding initiation success.

Managing or Minimizing the Risks from Epidural Anesthesia

Epidurals are effective at reducing and relieving pain, but this intervention is not risk-free. Many effective alternatives could be considered first-line pain relief, either in place of the epidural or to delay its use until further along in labor. In addition, there are several ways to receive epidural pain relief while also minimizing the maternal and infant risks. Let's consider some of these scenarios.

First, epidural pain relief during labor is certainly not the only way to find comfort during childbirth. Keep in mind that people have been giving birth for literally thousands of years without pain medication. We can tap into the wisdom of our great, great, grandmothers to find an impressive array of techniques that can be comforting during labor.

The most critical factor in finding comfort during labor is likely choosing a labor companion (or companions) who will provide you with authentic emotional and physical support. This cannot be overstated. All people who give birth must be accompanied by companions of their choice – companions capable of providing loving support. These supportive and nurturing companions can be people trained to provide labor support (e.g., hiring labor companions/birth doulas), or they can be partners, family, and friends willing and able to provide emotional and physical support required during labor. If hiring a labor companion is not in the cards, investigate educational options for your partner or friend who will provide support. This is an important job that requires some amount of preparation. Providing high-quality labor support is not something that will come naturally to everyone. Certainly, some people are nurturing and caring by nature but providing labor support is not always straightforward. It does require skills and knowledge about childbirth. If your partner, sister, or friend will serve as your labor companion, be sure that they are prepared. Training options include actual doula training (something for the ambitious person who might want to dive into the birth world), online birth classes to learn the basics of childbirth, and a good guide to providing labor support. Penny Simkin's book *The Birth Partner* is a great guide to help anyone acquire the basic skills to support the parent during labor in both physical and emotional ways. If your partner will provide this support, I highly recommend taking a childbirth class together that will focus on coping measures and comfort techniques. In a comprehensive birth preparation class, you will learn about all the stages of labor. Together, you will practice comfort measures for labor like massage techniques, hot or cold packs, counter pressure, acupressure, walking, supportive standing and kneeling positions, tub and shower options, and many others.

If you are interested in having a labor companion and you're worried about the cost, investigate whether your city has a doula program that offers services for free. One example of this in Austin, TX (and there are many throughout the U.S.) is GALS (Giving Austin Labor Support). Through this program, volunteers who have trained as labor companions provide this service free of charge. Check to see if your area has an organization like this one. Other options include partner support, friends, or family members.

A word of caution: be sure that your labor companion can provide you with the support you will need during labor without getting too stressed or even perhaps needing support of their own. For example, you might think your own mother will be comforting support for you, but in reality, it could be tough for your mom to calmly support you if she perceives you are in any pain. Sometimes, this is why it pays to hire someone who is not emotionally involved in your life. That said, many partners and family members have provided excellent support for people during childbirth; just be honest with yourself about your friends and family, and their potential limitations.

Another crucial step for managing labor without an epidural is to familiarize yourself with and practice the skills you will likely use during labor before it begins. As mentioned above, I highly recommend taking a comprehensive childbirth class. Be sure your birth class is taught by an unbiased person, covers the comfort measures and coping skills you will need, and gives you a firm working knowledge of birthing basics. Look for an independent birth class (not affiliated with the hospital) that focuses on skills for your labor companion. This type of preparation will pay off greatly because you will develop the techniques to move through labor feeling supported and encouraged by your partner. If you cannot find an excellent local option for a face-to-face childbirth class in your area, take an online birth class, learn about comfort measures, read *The Birth Partner*, and do some online research about comfort measures during labor. One good place to start is Childbirth Connection. Find them at childbirthconnection.org.

What if Coping Techniques Are Not Enough for Me?

Despite what you might be thinking, I do not recommend that everyone choose a drug-free birth. This is a personal choice, and while I believe that there are many benefits to a drug-free birth, it is certainly not for everyone. If you want to have an epidural, get one. Know that you may need extra support to get breastfeeding off to a good start. Also, if you are concerned about lactation interference, be aware that there are ways to minimize your exposure to the epidural and thus, minimize the consequences for lactation and infant feeding.

First, delay the use of epidural as long as you can. This can be accomplished by staying home for as long as possible. In your own home, you can rest in the comfort of your own bed. You can take a long, hot bath. You can choose any sitting or standing position you like. You will be free of monitors, cords, IVs, or other attachments. You can eat and drink anything you want at any point. You can watch your favorite movie or listen to music. Once you leave home, you leave your own turf. When you enter the hospital, you enter the arena of managed birth. Now, you are on their clock and their rules. Decision-making at the hospital is not always straightforward. Occasionally, people face scenarios they don't want or procedures they don't need. A good rule of thumb for labor is to stay home for as long as possible.

Other strategies you can use may possibly lessen the effects of epidural anesthesia. For example:

- Request the lowest dose of medication possible to give pain relief
- Turn down the epidural or turn it off when the birth is getting close or is imminent

These strategies are no guarantee that you will be free from lactation interference. In addition to the risks discussed here for breastfeeding, epidurals have other risks for both maternal and infant outcomes. Take the time to educate yourself thoroughly before choosing epidural pain relief.

Infant Bathing

Some birth routines seem harmless when it comes to potential impacts for breastfeeding. Newborn bathing *seems* to fall into this category. I mean, it's a bath! So, how could that affect breastfeeding?

Surprisingly, the timing of the infant's first bath can impact several factors associated with breastfeeding initiation and success. Some of these impacts are directly related to breastfeeding initiation, and some are indirect. All of them can be avoided by delaying the first bath.

1. Separating the parents and baby for the purposes of bathing disturbs the golden hour and immediate skin-to-skin time. This can directly affect the opportunities for breastfeeding within the first hour.
2. Bathing can lower the infant's body temperature. Body temperature regulation outside of the womb is difficult for newborns, especially preemies. Newborn bathing can lower

body temperature, leading to hypothermia. Hypothermic state (body temperature is too low) is a great risk for babies. In this state, infants must use up limited energy reserves to bring their body temperature up to normal. Energy is precious to the newborn; he needs it all for growth. The WHO recommends delaying the bath for 24 hours (WHO, 2018).

3. Blood sugar levels are affected by the timing of the infant's first bath. In a recent study, McInerny (2015) showed that infants whose first bath was delayed had better blood sugar levels, even those at higher risk (e.g., post-mature, small for gestational age, and babies whose mothers were diabetic) for potential blood sugar issues had better outcomes when the bath was delayed. Lower blood sugar levels can sometimes lead to early supplementation, lab testing, and other interventions interfering with breastfeeding initiation (McInerney & Gupta, 2015).

Prevention Strategies:

Delay first bath. WHO recommends 24 hours. If this is not possible due to religious beliefs or local or family traditions, delay for a shorter period, but not less than six hours.

Vacuum-Assisted Delivery

Occasionally, birth is assisted by vacuum extraction, sometimes because of a prolonged second stage of labor, when the parent is exhausted, or to avoid cesarean delivery. A vacuum, also called ventouse, might also be used when non-reassuring fetal heart tones are detected. In theory, the vacuum helps speed the delivery process. The vacuum has a soft cup that uses suction to attach to the infant's head. Then, the infant is born by a combination of pushing and traction from the vacuum. Recent data from the National Center of Health Statistics (Martin et al., 2017) suggests that about 3% of all births in the U. S. are vacuum-assisted.

Vacuum-assisted delivery has various outcomes and risks:

- Soft tissue swelling on the top of the baby's head (caput succedaneum)

- Bruising, blood leaking out of the blood vessels in distinct layers under the skin at the top of the head, blood pooling under the scalp (cephalohematoma and subgaleal hematoma)
- Bleeding within the skull (a rare but severe condition called intracranial hemorrhage)
- Bleeding in the eye (neonatal retinal hemorrhage)
- Break or fracture in the skull bone (skull fracture)
- Broken or abraded skin on the top of the baby's head (superficial scalp injury)

Complications from these outcomes that could affect breastfeeding include caput succedaneum, cephalohematoma, subgaleal hematoma, and intracranial hemorrhage, all of which are associated with bleeding and bruising with varying degrees of severity. Any bruising and bleeding caused by birth injury should be taken seriously, whether from spontaneous vaginal delivery or instrument-assisted delivery. Newborns with bruising are at greater risk for jaundice, directly affecting breastfeeding in the early weeks. See the section on Jaundice for information on how jaundice can impact infant feeding. Preventing jaundice, if possible, can help maximize breastfeeding ease and success in the early weeks. Some of these outcomes, including caput succedaneum and retinal hemorrhage, are quite common in spontaneous vaginal birth but appear more often due to instrument-assisted delivery.

Other studies have found:

- Infants born by vacuum-assisted delivery are sleepy, exhibit less willingness to suckle, and are supplemented more often with formula, and are less likely to feed at night (Vestermark et al., 1991).
- After vacuum-assisted delivery, there may be a delay in the appearance of mature milk (Vestermark et al., 1991).
- Vacuum-assisted delivery is associated with early cessation of breastfeeding and lower scores on a breastfeeding assessment tool (Hall et al., 2002).

Prevention Strategies:

- Avoid an epidural to maximize your ability to move around during labor. This can help prevent the need for instrument-assisted delivery and has other benefits as well.
- If an epidural is placed, adjust the medication downward during pushing to allow yourself to feel more and to potentially move more effectively.
- Change positions often and keep moving during labor. Avoid lying down during labor. Use gravity to your advantage. Maintain upright positions if possible.
- Avoid multiple attempts at using instrument-assisted delivery. Rates of complications are higher if several attempts are made to use the vacuum during delivery.
- Avoid sequential use of vacuum and forceps during your birth. Studies show that when these instruments are used sequentially during birth, vacuum and forceps complication rates are higher (Gardella et al., 2001).

Forceps

Like the vacuum, forceps delivery is an assisted vaginal birth. A physician uses an obstetrical tool to guide the baby's head out of the birth canal during pushing. Forceps look like large salad tongs and are placed inside the vagina on either side of the baby's head. The doctor supports the baby's head in the forceps and guides the head out during a contraction. Forceps delivery rate in the U.S. is estimated to be under 1% of all births. Interestingly, vacuum and forceps deliveries have declined quite a bit in the last two or three decades while the cesarean delivery rate has increased dramatically (Stock et al., 2013). Some researchers have pointed to the high rates of litigation with instrument-assisted delivery to explain why many doctors have largely abandoned instrumental delivery and moved decidedly toward cesarean delivery.

There may be times when opting for forceps delivery is a wise strategy. For example, vacuum-assisted delivery is not an option if the baby presents face first (rare, but it does happen) and is already engaged lower in the birth canal. In this instance, forceps may be useful. It is also important to remember that if you are presented with the opportunity to use forceps or have a cesarean, choosing forceps might not seem appealing but could prevent you from delivering by cesarean (which has consequences for this birth and future births).

The use of forceps during vaginal delivery is indicated by many of the same factors as vacuum-assisted delivery, including maternal exhaustion, pushing is ineffective (i.e., the baby is not progressing), a long second stage of labor, non-reassuring fetal heart rate, or other need to expedite the birth process.

The risks for infants born by forceps are similar to those of vacuum delivery. The risks include:

- Cephalohematoma – blood pooling under the infant scalp
- Nerve damage to facial nerves
- Brachial plexus nerve damage resulting in numbness and loss of control in the arm, hand, wrist
- Intracranial hemorrhage – rare but severe bleeding inside the skull
- Eye trauma
- Skull fractures
- Seizures

Breastfeeding complications can arise from a forceps-assisted vaginal delivery, especially in the presence of facial nerve damage, bleeding, bruising, and head trauma. One of the major concerns with bleeding and bruising is that it can lead to complications with infant jaundice, which can have major impacts on infant feeding. See the section on Jaundice for further information.

Another complication of forceps that has consequences for infant feeding is nerve damage. Infant nerve damage can directly affect the baby's motor skills, coordination, tongue movements, sensation in the mouth, lips, tongue, and cheeks. These problems are usually temporary but can dramatically impact the newborn's ability to organize innate breast seeking and feeding skills in the critical first hours and days.

Can You Prevent the Need for Assisted Vaginal Delivery?

As noted in the section on vacuum delivery, you can use several strategies to minimize the chance of needing an instrument-assisted delivery. This list echoes several recommendations throughout the book, not because I totally reject birth interventions but because these strategies work. Here are some tips to avoid the need for instrument assisted birth:

- Hire a labor companion. Having physical and emotional support during your birth truly improves maternal and fetal outcomes. Read more about how labor support can positively impact your birth in Penny Simkin's book called *The Birth Partner.*
- Stay home as long as you can. In your own environment, you can move around as you please, eat and drink what you want, and feel far less institutional than you would in the hospital environment.
- Stay active and upright during your labor *and during the birth*. Avoid giving birth while you are lying down, especially avoid lying on your back. Instead, keep moving throughout your labor, taking breaks to rest as needed.
- Deliver your baby in a squatting position or on your hands and knees. Use a birth ball, peanut ball, birth stool, squat bar over the hospital bed, or any other position that allows you to use gravity to help your baby descend efficiently through the birth canal without getting wedged in a less than optimal position. (Many people are unaware that hospital beds have the option to use a squat bar. Ask about this if you are giving birth at a hospital.)Birth is highly managed and calculated at a hospital, especially in terms of time. During the second stage of labor, caregivers begin to explore alternatives if pushing lasts more than two hours. If you are faced with an ultimatum or interventions that do not appeal to you during labor, ask for more time. Studies show that arbitrarily terminating the second stage after two hours may be premature (Cheng et al., 2014).
- Avoid epidural anesthesia so that you can maintain mobility. Using your legs means you can walk, go to the bathroom, get in the tub, move around, change positions, and be

upright, supporting yourself during labor and birth. Being mobile helps the baby achieve better positioning for birth.

- Avoid induction. This one single intervention is often the gateway to many other interventions, including Pitocin and epidural.
- If you do have an epidural, turn it down or off when it appears that the end of labor is near. This could enable you to regain a little more mobility, even if it's slight position changes while still in bed.

Dyad Separation

In the long view of human history, parents and babies have almost always been kept together as a single unit following birth. This togetherness facilitates early breastfeeding initiation and enables the infant to maintain homeostasis within body systems and feel safe and calm. When incubators and infant formula became commercially available, parent-baby separation following delivery *became standard practice in the obstetric unit*. Unfortunately, this occurred before the study of such a practice could be subject to randomized controlled trials. Therefore, it was not questioned as a part of routine care for a newborn (Bergman, 2019).

Over the last few decades, mounting research has shown that separation of the breastfeeding dyad following delivery has significant negative consequences. Some of the outcomes are directly related to breastfeeding, and some are indirectly related. Even if parents do not choose to initiate breastfeeding, separation has health implications for both parent and infant. Here are some of the consequences and outcomes of separation after birth:

- The distinct predictable sequence of infant behaviors to facilitate the first latch and breastfeeding that occurs directly after birth (Widström et al., 2011) is disrupted by separation of parent and infant. This can affect the infant's ability to suckle (Crenshaw et al., 2012).
- Studies show that tasks and procedures performed immediately postpartum when the infant is separated from its parent can disturb the baby's sucking ability (Righard & Alade, 1990).

- Dyad separation causes stress for both the parent and the infant (Bergman et al., 2004). Stress increases cortisol for both parent and baby.
- Infants cry more when separated from their mother. Crying is a risk factor for brain bleeds. Crying is also a late stage feeding cue. It is much more challenging to attempt to feed a baby who is highly agitated and crying intensely.
- Separation also increases the risk of postpartum hemorrhage for the parent (Saxton et al., 2015).
- Separation and the use of incubators (or radiant warmers) are not as effective at thermoregulation as skin-to-skin (Bergman et al., 2004). Risk of hypothermia increases if the dyad is separated. See the discussion on hypothermia for more on this.
- Separation *does not facilitate early initiation of breastfeeding.*

One interesting study examined the complex outcomes of separation after labor. The study participants received Demerol, which is a narcotic used for pain relief. The study then tracked people who had received Demerol (pethidine, meperidine) *and* were subsequently separated from their infants. These same infants were unable to latch onto the breast and nurse successfully within two hours after birth (Righard & Alade, 1990).

Another study examined the effects of an immediate separation of the breastfeeding dyad compared to early skin-to-skin contact and feeding initiation. Parents who spent time (25-120 minutes) holding their newborns skin-to-skin directly after birth displayed more maternal responsiveness and sensitivity to their babies one year later compared to those who were separated for two hours after delivery (Bystrova et al., 2009). Even the practice of rooming-in did not compensate for the immediate postpartum separation of the breastfeeding dyad (Bystrova et al., 2009).

Strategies to Avoid Separation Complications:

Keep your baby with you after delivery. Request that the baby room-in with you for the duration of your stay. Keep your baby skin-to-skin (Kangaroo Care) for 90 minutes to two hours after birth. Request that all tasks and procedures be done while the baby is with you or be postponed. If your baby needs medical attention and you must be separated, place the baby skin-to-skin immediately after you are reunited and reboot the process of breastfeeding initiation.

Oral Nasal Suctioning

Before birth, infants swallow amniotic fluid. Although the fluid is squeezed out of the baby during vaginal birth, it can sometimes remain in the mouth and nose in small quantities after birth. It was once thought that routine suctioning of the newborn's mouth and nose was optimal, but research has shown otherwise. According to Wambach and Riordan, authors of *Breastfeeding and Human Lactation*, suctioning can cause nasal swelling that partially obstructs the airway (2016). Without a clear nasal passage, breastfeeding may be suboptimal or even have to wait until nasal swelling diminishes.

Suctioning is another procedure that may appear at first glance to be completely harmless to the infant. Still, problems can arise from the overuse of suctioning techniques when the procedure is not indicated and from heavy, forceful suctioning. Oral aversion, or hypersensitivity of the oral cavity, can result from heavy suctioning of an infant in the neonatal period. This can occasionally cause breast refusal. In its Guidelines for Perinatal Care, the American Academy of Pediatrics states that suctioning is not necessary when the infant is "vigorous." In other words, healthy, active, and alert.

More recent research suggests no benefits to routine suctioning of the mouth and nose at birth for healthy babies born at or near term (Kelleher et al., 2013).

IV Fluids

Perhaps this is one of the most insidious interventions to interfere with lactation. Who would think that fluid could wreak havoc on lactation? To be clear, like so many other factors of managed birth, it can.

Fluid that is administered during labor through the IV is usually done so in conjunction with an epidural. Because the medication in an epidural can lower blood pressure, IV fluids are administered to combat this effect. In addition, it bypasses the need for fluids by mouth and assures adequate hydration. Placement of the IV also allows for easy administration of other medications if that becomes necessary.

But what if there is too much exposure to IV fluids? Is there such a thing? Does overhydration affect the parent? Or the baby? Spoiler: Overhydration can affect lactation for both.

Problems Caused by Overhydration:

People who take on too much fluid through the IV during labor can experience breast edema. This edema, or swelling of tissues, creates constriction within the breast. Constriction around the milk ducts makes it difficult for the milk to flow. The edema puts so much pressure on the milk ducts that it may prevent the ducts from fully dilating. This can slow or stop the flow of milk. Some women experience breasts so swollen with edema that the tissues become hard, with no pliability. Normally, breast tissue is soft and pliable. This allows the baby to easily latch. If breast tissue is too hard, the latch can be difficult or impossible. It is also quite painful and can take time to resolve.

If the IV fluids during labor are excessive for the mother, they are also excessive for the newborn. For example, imagine extended labor that exposed parent and baby to IV fluids for many hours. This fluid immediately reaches the mother and because the infant is still receiving oxygen, fluid, and nutrition from the placenta, he receives a portion of the IV fluid as well. This condition seems innocent enough, but it can create issues that relate to breastfeeding for this baby.

The overhydration caused by maternal IV fluid in the baby's case artificially inflates the newborn birth weight (Chantry et al., 2011). As a result, the birth weight is slightly higher than without all the extra fluid on board. This is easily resolved by urination over the first 24 hours of life (Noel-Weiss et al., 2011). For the pediatrician closely monitoring infant weight loss over the first few days, the weight loss can sometimes seem dramatic. If there appears to be a weight loss of greater than 7-10% of newborn birth weight, breastfeeding is called into question. Is the baby getting enough breast milk? Does this baby need to be supplemented with formula? Supplements are frequently recommended when new babies drop too much weight after birth. Because greater fluid loss is common for babies exposed to excessive fluids, some of these supplements could be unnecessary if the excessive weight loss is related to overhydration and fluid administration during labor.

Prevention Strategies

To avoid IV fluids:

- Choose a caregiver who supports your choice to avoid IV fluids. Choose a birthplace with low induction rates and low cesarean rates.
- Stay at home for most of your labor. At home, you can eat and drink as you please.
- Hire a labor companion. Labor support is associated with lowered rates of many interventions.
- Avoid induction. Induction frequently leads to augmenting labor with Pitocin (synthetic oxytocin), which leads to greater use of epidural analgesia. IV fluid is a co-intervention with epidural.
- Consider home birth. It is increasing in popularity, and it is as safe as hospital birth for low-risk people.

If IV fluid becomes necessary, minimize the impact of IV fluid while it is in place:

- The timing and flow rate of the IV appear to be significant factors, especially during the last two hours of labor (Noel-Weiss et al., 2011). Therefore, try to slow the flow of IV fluid while it is in place and discontinue it during the final stage of labor.
- If the IV is in place for other medications (like antibiotics), remove the tube after administering the meds. This will allow you to walk away from the IV pole and be far less restrictive in terms of movement.
- If you were overexposed to IV fluids, consider using the newborn's 24-hour weight as the "baseline birth weight" as recommended by Noel-Weiss and colleagues (Noel-Weiss et al., 2011). This allows the infant to off-load the excessive weight through urination during the first 24 hours.
- IV fluid is not guaranteed to cause breast edema. It is the overexposure to IV fluid that can do the most damage. If you

are planning a birth without induction and Pitocin, you can forgo the IV fluid altogether. Drink water by mouth and stay sufficiently hydrated.

To relieve breast edema:

- Try reverse pressure softening (Cotterman, 2004)which includes subareolar tissue. Subareolar tissue resistance increases during engorgement, when expanded circulation and excess interstitial fluid compete for space with increasing milk volumes. Physiologic and iatrogenic events often combine to produce distortion of breast anatomy. Resulting latch difficulty, delayed milk ejection reflex, poor milk transfer, pain, and nipple damage discourage many mothers. The rationale and technique for a simple intervention developed in practice are described: reverse pressure softening (RPS. This technique involves using your fingers to push back on the breast toward the chest, which helps move some fluid out of the breast tissue. Techniques can be found online (e.g., YouTube). Reverse pressure softening can help relieve engorgement, as well as edema.
- Do not pump breasts that appear to have edema. This can exacerbate issues of tissue distention.
- Do not use heat. You can apply a cold pack for 15-20 minutes in conjunction with reverse pressure softening.

Pitocin

Pitocin, a synthetic form of oxytocin, is a ubiquitous drug used for induction or augmentation of labor. However, it's related to several lactation issues through downstream effects. In other words, it may not be the primary cause of breastfeeding problems, but it can make things more difficult by indirectly causing other problems that do affect lactation. Here is a brief look at some of the downstream effects of Pitocin and the potential breastfeeding outcomes.

- Pitocin is always used in conjunction with IV fluids. It is well established that the overhydration common with excessive fluid causes breast edema and painful engorgement that can create rock-hard breast tissue, making the latch difficult or impossible. In addition, edema can cause milk stasis (restricted flow of milk) and lead to decreasing supply if not remedied immediately. Review the section on IV Fluids for more information.

- Using Pitocin increases the likelihood of epidural pain relief. In short, Pitocin increases contractions unnaturally, causing higher degrees of pain than labor without Pitocin. In addition, epidural analgesia is associated with greater instrumental delivery (use of vacuum or forceps), maternal fever, and other outcomes, each of which may impact lactogenesis or the opportunity for immediate breastfeeding in the first hour of life. See the section on Epidural use for more detailed information.
- Over exposure to Pitocin may lead to more cases of postpartum hemorrhage (Grotegut et al., 2011). Too much synthetic oxytocin coming from a source external to the body (as opposed to oxytocin that is made and released internally) can cause desensitization of the oxytocin receptors and result in uterine atony (i.e., failure to contract). This disrupts an intricate system designed to stop blood loss after the uterus releases the placenta. The continued contractions are necessary to help the blood vessels clamp down and stop bleeding in the area where the placenta separated from the uterine wall. Postpartum hemorrhage can impact lactation. For more information, see the section on Postpartum Hemorrhage.
- Pitocin is often used to induce labor. Induction of labor can and does frequently cause a baby to be born prematurely. This can negatively impact breastfeeding because preemies sometimes exhibit a weaker suck reflex, have uncoordinated suck-swallow-breathe patterns, and are more likely to lack full capabilities displaying feeding cues. As a result, breastfeeding is more complex for preemies. Do what you can to avoid this situation. See the section on Induction of Labor for more information.
- Be aware that using Pitocin generally does not come on its own. It comes with a host of other interventions, often called the cascade of interventions. Pitocin is the first of a long line of factors that contribute to difficulties in breastfeeding. It is incredibly challenging to tease out the exact outcomes

(i.e., which intervention caused a specific lactation problem), but in general, more interventions results in more risk for lactation issues. Pitocin is usually one of the first steps on that road.

Prevention Strategies

Pitocin is used for labor induction and augmentation (speeding up labor). If your caregiver recommends induction or augmentation, it can be advantageous to do your own research into the reasons why induction is being recommenced in your case. There are some valid reasons (medically indicated reasons) for induction of labor. These include placental abruption, blood pressure disorders including preeclampsia, fetal growth restriction, low amniotic fluid, uterine infection, other severe or life-threatening maternal medical conditions, or your pregnancy is past term (two weeks beyond due date).

While some of those constitute emergency situations, the list of medical reasons to induce (above) has a little wiggle room. Suppose your due date is not 100% certain. In that case, there is an opportunity to argue for more time, especially if the baby is in good shape. Also, the diagnosis of low amniotic fluid (oligohydramnios) is not an exact science. Do some research while you're hydrating yourself. See if you can buy more time on this one. (I was told that I had low amniotic fluid with my first, but that was not the case at all). Ultrasound to diagnose the baby's age, weight and the amount of fluid at the end of pregnancy are often inaccurate. This is a wildly overused justification for the "need" for induction.

Avoiding Pitocin

Usually, the first rule of thumb for avoiding Pitocin is to avoid induction of labor. Your body and your baby know exactly when the time is right to start labor. Be patient and let it happen. Work with caregivers who support the same approach, allowing labor to start on its own. Be positive and confident that your labor will begin at the right time. Use guided meditation if needed to relax and release fears. Remember that recommendations for induction of labor because the caregiver thinks your baby is too big or your amniotic fluid is too low are often completely bogus. Stay hydrated and wait for labor to start.

If your water breaks and contractions do not start right away, talk to your caregiver about stimulating labor without Pitocin. Use guided meditation, stay upright and active, take a walk, maybe consider acupuncture.

If your caregiver wants to speed up labor that has stopped or slowed down, try an hour or two of position changes and continuous movement. Sometimes, if labor has stopped or slowed, it makes sense to go home and come back to the hospital when labor is more established. (This may be an opportunity for you if you have avoided breaking the water and avoided other initial interventions.) Otherwise, if you are in the hospital and labor is not progressing, caregivers will attempt to get things moving. On the other hand, if you are in your own home, you can simply wait without the arbitrary pressure of immediately starting labor.

Cesarean Delivery

For birth and breastfeeding, no intervention is likely more complex than cesarean delivery. In 2018, 31.9% of all infants in the U.S. were delivered by cesarean (Martin et al., 2019). According to the World Health Organization's Global Health Observatory data, Canada, the UK, Australia, Germany, and Switzerland have similar cesarean rates right around 30%, giving or taking a few points (World Health Organization, 2018a). In some other parts of the world, rates are near or above 50%, including Brazil, Chile, Ecuador, Turkey, Lebanon, and Egypt (World Health Organization, 2018a). Considering that cesarean birth is widespread, parents and healthcare providers should learn about the downstream lactation outcomes associated with cesarean delivery and how to mitigate them.

Cesarean delivery has several known negative effects on breastfeeding. This issue is quite complex and discussing every angle of the cascading effects of cesarean delivery on lactation is beyond the scope of this book. This section will look at some general outcomes of cesarean birth and how these outcomes relate to lactation. Keep in mind that cesarean surgery may not *directly* affect lactation for many of the following factors. However, it gives rise to conditions that do affect lactation. For example, cesarean birth is associated with more risk of infant hypothermia. Suboptimal body temperatures for newborns can cause dyad separation while the baby is moved to an incubator or radiant warmer. Separation is often a factor in disrupted or delayed breastfeeding initiation. In this case, cesarean does not cause lactation issues. However, it does increase the risk for infant hypothermia, which can create breastfeeding problems.

Cesarean surgery is associated with many risks, some major and some minor. First, and most importantly, cesarean surgery raises the risk of maternal mortality. Compared with vaginal delivery, the risk of maternal death after a cesarean birth is 3.6 times higher (Deneux-Tharaux et al., 2006). Maternal mortality is a grim subject, but it is a reality that we simply cannot ignore because it is a distressing discussion. Obviously, maternal death from any cause reduces the chance that the infant will receive his mother's own milk to zero. Fortunately, human milk can be acquired through formal and informal channels, but it can be difficult to obtain. Cesarean birth also increases the risk of infant mortality (MacDorman et al., 2006; Signore & Klebanoff, 2008).

Other significant cesarean outcomes that may affect lactation:

- One of the major concerns for cesarean delivery and its impact on lactation is that this intervention is associated with a delay in lactogenesis II, the transition to mature milk. This raises the risk of using formula supplements, which is associated with early breastfeeding termination. Infants born by cesarean benefit greatly from skin-to-skin care and from having unlimited opportunities to come to the breast in the early days after birth. If you deliver by cesarean, keep your baby close and nurse as often as you can. If your transition to mature milk is delayed beyond day four, seek help immediately. If you need to supplement, consider human donor milk first if it's available.
- Infants experience greater weight loss after cesarean delivery (Preer et al., 2012). Greater weight loss is associated with more use of supplements, which can decrease breastfeeding duration. If you must supplement, do everything you can to preserve and protect your milk supply. Express milk and/or put the baby to the breast about ten times in 24 hours. Consider human donor milk if necessary.

- Cesarean birth increases the risk of delivering preterm (Bettegowda et al., 2008). Premature infants have an increased risk of breastfeeding difficulties. The more breastfeeding difficulties that one person encounters, the more likely they are to abandon breastfeeding. See the section on breastfeeding premature infants. Seek help from skilled lactation care.
- Cesarean delivery also increases the risk for preterm birth in subsequent pregnancies (Zhang et al., 2019), potentially setting up lactation obstacles for infants born from future pregnancies.
- Compared to vaginal birth, cesarean delivery increases breastfeeding difficulties, especially when the surgery is unplanned (Hobbs et al., 2016). People who encounter many breastfeeding problems are more likely to abandon breastfeeding early on.
- Cesarean birth is associated with a shorter duration of breastfeeding (Hobbs et al., 2016). Compared to vaginal birth, planned cesarean delivery increases the likelihood that breastfeeding stops by 12 weeks postpartum (Hobbs et al., 2016).
- Infants born by cesarean are at greater risk of hypothermia, which creates potential problems for breastfeeding because of the probability of mother-baby separation. Practice skin-to-skin care after cesarean. This can help stabilize body temperature for your baby and provide the opportunity for feeding.
- Cesarean delivery is associated with increased neonatal respiratory problems, potentially causing dyad separation and breastfeeding difficulties.

Cesarean Accompanied by Multiple Interventions

Sometimes the road to delivering by cesarean is planned and straightforward. This can often result in birth without any labor (which has its own consequences). Other times, cesarean surgery happens after a host of different interventions, and the surgery is a last resort. This can lead to a compounding effect of interventions that can cause a delay in the transition to mature milk and full milk volume, which usually occurs between days 3-4 postpartum. Consider this: Nicole's labor is induced with Pitocin, and she needs an epidural for pain relief. Unfortunately, the induction does not go smoothly. It takes many hours for labor contractions to become organized and strong enough to make progress. After another 18 hours of labor, Nicole is exhausted but is still working. She also has the routine IV fluids that accompany epidural, now in place for several hours. After several hours of active labor with little progress, Nicole's doctor recommends a cesarean delivery. During and after the surgery, Nicole loses an excessive amount of blood and requires a blood transfusion shortly after birth. On day six postpartum, she is only able to express a few drops of colostrum. What was the cause of the delay in transition to mature milk with increased volume?

There are many variables to Nicole's story. The delay in full volume milk production could be affected by any of these factors: induction, IV fluids, extended labor, cesarean, and blood loss. It is probably impossible to tease out the exact cause of the delay in full milk production, but the compounding effect cannot be ignored.

Although cesarean delivery can be lifesaving for both parent and baby, it can also raise the risk for poor feeding and health outcomes. One way to avoid cesarean is by avoiding unnecessary induction of labor. If your caregiver recommends induction of labor or cesarean, do some research before agreeing to either of these interventions. If cesarean is necessary for you, breastfeeding is possible. Remember that cesarean can raise the risk for specific situations (see above) that can impact breastfeeding. Be prepared for these potential scenarios and be ready to seek help from an IBCLC.

Retained Placenta

The hormones of pregnancy, especially those delivered and maintained by the placenta, inhibit the production of a copious milk supply during pregnancy. After the placenta is delivered, there is a rapid drop in progesterone, and this removes the inhibitors that were previously in place, allowing the onset of abundant milk production to occur. Typically, there is a rapid increase in milk volume from 38 to 98 hours after birth if all goes well (Wambach & Riordan, 2016).

Suppose the placenta is not completely removed from the uterus. In that case, milk production can be inhibited, and the rapid increase in milk volume will be delayed. This can lead to delay in lactogenesis II, deficient supply, and sometimes postpartum hemorrhage. Most sources say there is not much one can do to prevent a retained placenta but digging into the scientific literature reveals many risk factors for retained placenta, some of which can be avoided.

Risk factors associated with retained placenta:

- Previous cesarean delivery (Ashwal et al., 2014)
- Previous abortions (Ashwal et al., 2014)
- Induction of labor (Ashwal et al., 2014)
- Vacuum-assisted delivery (Ashwal et al., 2014)
- Birth between 24 and 28 weeks gestation (Coviello et al., 2016)
- Birth in a teaching hospital (Coviello et al., 2016)
- Use of epidural analgesia (Ashwal et al., 2014; Zmora et al., 2019)
- Preterm delivery (Zmora et al., 2019)
- Previous history of multiple miscarriages (Zmora et al., 2019)
- Prior history of retained placenta

It is not always possible to prevent these risk factors. Sometimes, retained placenta is related to the anatomical structure of the placenta itself or how it is embedded into the uterine wall. A quick glance over the risk factors above reveals that some can be avoided, especially induction of labor and use of epidural medicines. If you know that you have one or more of the risk factors above, be aware that your risk for retained placenta may be higher than average. If you experience delayed onset of copious milk production, if you don't see a rapid increase in milk volume by day three or four postpartum, consider retained placenta as a cause and speak to your physician immediately. Some signs of retained placenta are persistent bleeding more than normally expected, continued cramping and contractions, fever, delayed onset of copious milk production, passing pieces of tissue fragments, and foul-smelling discharge.

Strategies for Prevention

Avoid the use of synthetic oxytocin (Pitocin) because synthetic oxytocin can cause your uterus to tire and lose tone, commonly called uterine atony. Uterine atony (i.e., failure of the uterus to contract) is associated with the use of Pitocin, and it can lead to postpartum hemorrhage. Avoid induction of labor. Try natural comfort techniques and /or hire a labor companion instead of planning for epidural pain relief. Do what you can to avoid cesarean and instrumental delivery.

Postpartum Hemorrhage and Sheehan's Syndrome

Postpartum hemorrhage is best described as losing a greater than normal amount of blood following childbirth. This type of hemorrhage can negatively impact lactation. The average blood loss following a normal vaginal delivery of a singleton is about 500 ml (a little over 2 cups of blood). For cesarean birth, the average blood loss is about 1000 ml (about 4¼ cups of blood). When blood loss is excessive, greater than 1000 ml, there can be potential negative downstream effects on the pituitary gland, which plays a significant role in lactation.

Hemorrhage after childbirth can directly affect the pituitary gland, also known as the master gland. The pituitary gland produces prolactin, which is an essential hormone for milk production. When the pituitary gland suffers significant blood loss, as in the case of postpartum hemorrhage, substantial damage to the gland is possible. Without a fully functional pituitary gland to produce prolactin, lactation can fail. This phenomenon is called Sheehan's syndrome. In short, the lack of blood flow to the pituitary gland can cause cell death within the gland. It can reduce or stop the production of prolactin and other important reproductive hormones, such as thyroid-stimulating hormones and adrenal hormones.

What Causes Postpartum Hemorrhage (PPH)?

Uterine atony is the most common cause of postpartum hemorrhage. Uterine atony is the failure of the uterus to strongly contract after the delivery of the placenta. The contractions are necessary to cause the uterus to clamp down the blood vessels in the uterine wall, where the placenta was previously attached. Unless the uterus contracts strongly and provides the pressure to close the blood vessels, the placental attachment site could continue to bleed freely, causing excessive blood loss.

Other causes of postpartum hemorrhage include delivering multiples, placental abruption, placenta previa, and other abnormal attachment of the placenta, vacuum or forceps delivery, high blood pressure, infection, obesity, and injury to vaginal tissues during labor.

Can PPH be Prevented?

Preventing PPH is not always possible, but there are ways to manage the risk factors. First, there are several causes and risk factors for uterine atony. Several common risk factors include induction of labor, the use of synthetic oxytocin during labor (Pitocin), distention of the uterus, long labor or short labor, and magnesium sulfate infusions during labor. While controlling the length of labor (especially quick labors) is not always within our control, other factors like induction of labor and use of Pitocin are sometimes optional (remember that it is best to let labor begin on its own). Prevention is not likely for other causes of hemorrhage like placenta previa, placental abruption, and multiple pregnancy. The use of birth interventions like vacuum and forceps, on the other hand, can be preventable. Again, planning a low intervention birth without the routine use of labor induction and Pitocin can reduce PPH risks.

Is Breastfeeding Possible After PPH?

It is possible to breastfeed your baby, even if you experience PPH. An interesting study examined the breastfeeding outcomes of 206 people who experienced hemorrhage with blood loss greater than 1500 ml in the 24 hours following delivery. Not surprisingly, the people who lost the most blood (greater than 3000 ml) had the greatest difficulty with breastfeeding (Thompson et al., 2010). However, overall results showed that 58% of people who suffered PPH were fully breastfeeding at two months (Thompson et al., 2010).

Tips for Breastfeeding After PPH

In the case of PPH, there could be some separation of the breastfeeding dyad after birth because, obviously, excessive bleeding is an obstetric emergency and needs immediate treatment. Separation should be minimized as much as possible. Begin skin-to-skin care as soon as possible and bring the baby to the breast at least ten times each day. If you experience a low milk supply, follow all the tips for low supply, and work with qualified lactation care to develop a plan for feeding your baby. You may need to supplement with donor milk or formula. Consider using an at-breast nursing supplementation device to provide nipple stimulation while your baby receives the supplement. In the case of PPH, it may take much more time for the onset of mature milk to appear. Building a full milk supply can take a lot of extra time and effort. Work with a skilled lactation consultant to develop a plan for your infant feeding goals.

CHAPTER 9

Lactation Interference and Infant Factors

Babies bring their own unique factors to the nursing relationship. There is no doubt that babies are born with incredible instincts for feeding, but sometimes, other elements at work can prevent an infant from having an uncomplicated feeding experience. This section will highlight several factors that can present challenges for the infant.

Baby Struggles to Latch

Breastfeeding can be frustrating and challenging with an infant who cannot latch. There are various reasons why a baby would be unwilling or unable to latch in the first hours, days, or weeks. Some of the reasons include:

- Oral anatomy issues (tongue-tie, recessed chin, cleft palate, low muscle tone, weak suck)
- Premature infants, babies born small for gestational age (SGA)
- Baby is born with special needs (heart condition, Down syndrome, other congenital conditions)
- Infant is disorganized and groggy after an epidural with narcotics
- Infant struggles with nipple shape or size (flat nipples)
- Introduction of bottle-feeding first

Infants who were never introduced to feeding at the breast (e.g., adopted baby, NICU baby) or even a baby who was previously weaned from the breast can learn to latch and breastfeed. Dr. Christina Smillie has studied innate infant feeding behaviors, and her research shows that in the right conditions, babies can access their feeding reflexes for months after birth, with many older babies learning to nurse at the breast well beyond the newborn period (Smillie, 2017).

The key to helping a baby latch is facilitating the right conditions. Several elements make up the right environment for better latching. In general, the best environment will allow babies to access innate feeding behaviors. Remember, the baby's environment will dictate her behavior. As a result, it is essential that parents must create the right environment for latching and feeding. As I said at the beginning of this book, there are many right ways to nurse your baby. Since we are all individuals with unique anatomy and needs, we will all approach infant feeding differently. One can adapt these elements of the right environment to suit your baby's ability to latch and your own needs.

Conditions for the Right Environment for Latching

- If you are trying to persuade a baby to latch, especially one who has not latched previously or one who is fussy when put to the breast, be sure your baby is *not overly hungry* when you try to latch. This strategy may sound counter-intuitive, but trust me, a baby who has already taken the edge off her hunger will be easier to latch. Feed your baby expressed milk or formula first. *Try to persuade your baby to latch when she is calm.* If she is frustrated, she may associate feelings of discontent with the breast. Strive for happy or at least neutral experiences at the breast.
- In the right environment, fully support the infant's body, ensuring no gaps between your body and hers. The baby will respond better to feeding if her body is well supported and completely touching you. If semi-reclined, you can position the baby tummy down, fully supported by gravity, on your torso/chest. If you are seated, gently hold the baby as close to you as possible, providing proper support so that she is not stretching to reach the breast. It can help to have a pillow on your lap in this case. Also, in the seated position, you can slide yourself forward in the chair to achieve a little recline. This position can help mimic the laid-back posture.
- Help your baby access innate feeding behaviors by using the laid-back feeding position whenever possible. When a baby is tummy down on your torso/chest, all of her senses are engaged, and the sensory information tells your baby to

run her feeding program. The skills she can access in this position require the free use of her arms, hands, cheeks, lips, and tongue. In addition, she will use visual and olfactory cues to move into a good position close to the nipple. Finally, she will use hands and face to determine where and when to latch. Babies are totally capable of latching onto the breast by themselves when they can access these inborn skills. Given the right environment and the right amount of time, most infants will demonstrate innate feeding behaviors and use them to latch onto the breast in this position. (Be sure to search for images online if you have trouble visualizing how to position your baby for laid-back breastfeeding.)

- Try skin-to-skin. If your baby is refusing the breast, feed your baby so that she is content. Then, after she is calm and fed, plan a long stretch of skin-to-skin care with your baby in a relaxed environment. The key to this technique is that you are not presenting the breast with the intention of latching. It will be more of a "take it or leave it" attitude. Your main goal is just to relax skin-to-skin with your baby. She may or may not latch this time but keep practicing Kangaroo Care without expectations for feeding her. She will likely access her innate feeding behaviors on her tummy when she is ready.
- Try co-bathing. In this situation, you and your baby relax in a warm bath. You should get in first and have another adult hand the baby to you after you are safely sitting in the tub. Support the baby in the bathwater on her back. Ensure her body is submerged and her face is totally out of the water. The back of her head may be in the water but be sure to provide total support behind her head. She can lie there for a while, relaxing in the warm water. This is a calming sensory experience that mimics the womb environment for many babies. Some people even call this technique "rebirthing." Once you are ready to lie back and try nursing, bring your baby to your chest and relax into a reclined position. Place a wet hand towel over the baby's back to keep her warm. (Continue to drip warm water over her back while she is between the breasts to keep her warm.) Be sure your upper body and breasts are out of

the water. Hold your baby between the breasts and allow her time to explore. She will likely access her innate feeding behaviors in this environment. She may move toward the nipple and use hands and face to determine how to get her best latch. Allow her to discover her skills and the latch process without much management. Keep her supported so that she does not slip into the water. Be mindful of the room temperature. Do not allow your baby to become too cool. After relaxing in the bath with your baby, hand her to another adult to dry her in a warm towel. Never try to get up while holding your baby in the tub. Wet babies are slippery.If your baby will not latch and you feel you have tried everything, work with a lactation consultant to determine why there are latch difficulties. The LC can help you develop a strategy to coax your baby to the breast.

- As always, while you are moving toward your goal for latching, do everything you can to protect your milk supply. Express your milk about eight to ten times per day, around the clock.

You can read more about co-bathing and other valuable techniques in *Complementary and Alternative Medicine in Breastfeeding Therapy* by Nikki Lee, RN, IBCLC. This book is packed full of valuable techniques and strategies that can be therapeutic for the breastfeeding dyad.

Circumcision

Many people have anecdotally observed that circumcision affects early attempts at breastfeeding. However, little published research is available on the subject. In 2000, Nikki Lee, RN, IBCLC, and author of *Complementary and Alternative Medicine in Breastfeeding Therapy,* posed a question to the lactation community via a letter to the *Journal of Human Lactation* editor concerning breastfeeding and circumcision. She wrote, "I have noticed that boys who are circumcised before breastfeeding has been established have more problems with breastfeeding. Conversely, boys who are recovering from a traumatic birth but are left intact have fewer breastfeeding difficulties. Could we recommend that circumcision be delayed in cases of traumatic birth until the boy is feeding well? What do readers think?"

Although this is anecdotal, it is one perspective on circumcision causing interference with breastfeeding. It is one perspective that many lactation consultants and nurses share because they see first-hand evidence of this every day. In online forums for LCs, discussions about circumcision do not question *if* the procedure has negative consequences for early attempts at breastfeeding but rather *if parents receive education about potential feeding problems.* LCs and nurses often observe the scenario that Nikki Lee referenced in her question above; more specifically, baby boys often experience a shut down after circumcision that interferes with subsequent attempts to latch onto the breast and feed effectively.

What Do We Know About Circumcision That Could Lead to Breastfeeding Interference?

- There is often an observable period of withdrawal or shut down after the procedure. The infant will sleep (or appear to sleep) in response to being overwhelmed by the procedure and pain. Some LCs report that infants who were feeding well previously sometimes refuse the breast in the post-op hours following circumcision.
- Some hospitals do not treat for pain after the procedure.
- Some baby-friendly hospitals do not perform the procedure if breastfeeding is not already going well. If the dyad is struggling to establish effective breastfeeding, some hospitals will recommend delaying circumcision.
- COVID related: Newer "early discharge' of the family after birth may impact the timing of circumcision. For example, if a family opts for circumcision and wants early discharge, the infant might be circumcised in the first 24 hours of life. This certainly seems too early because the infant has only had a few attempts to come to the breast before the circumcision.
- Many hospitals and practitioners do not educate families about the lactation interference that sometimes follows circumcision.
- Delaying circumcision has benefits; breastfeeding dyads can establish effective feeding for several days (or even a

week or two) before circumcision, lowering the risk of lactation interference.

- Foregoing circumcision is an excellent option for breastfeeding outcomes and other measures of infant health. Consider this: circumcision raises the risk of infant bleeding and hemorrhage; circumcision is only a cosmetic procedure with zero hygienic benefits; intact foreskin has a protective function for the penis.

Are you Considering Circumcision?

Before deciding about circumcision, please watch the short ten-minute video on YouTube called "Circumcision, the Elephant in the Hospital Excerpts." Consider that not only does circumcision cause breastfeeding interference, but it is also a decision that you are making for someone else who may not want to give up his foreskin.

Premature Infant

A premature infant is a baby born before 37 weeks gestation. Preemies arrive early for various reasons and can present certain challenges for breastfeeding. Ironically, babies born preterm are the most in need of human milk and are less likely than full-term babies to get it. As a result, breastfeeding rates are lower for preemies because the infants and their parents face significantly more challenges than healthy, full-term dyads.

Breastfeeding a preterm baby of any age is less than optimal, but generally, the younger the gestational age, the more challenges are likely when it comes to infant feeding. Prematurity is a complex topic, and there are entire books dedicated to this issue. As a result, it is not possible to cover everything here. Here is some general information you may need if your baby arrives earlier than 40 weeks.

- Many babies born early can still feed directly at the breast. However, feeding may take longer and require more perseverance and support than feeding a full-term infant.
- Human milk is the perfect food for most preemies. If your baby cannot feed directly at the breast, you can pump your milk, so the baby gets the benefits of specific nutrition and antibodies for preemies. Remember, your body knows that

the baby arrived early and changes the milk composition to make up for the lost days of pregnancy. (Milk for preemies has a different and preemie-optimized composition of protein, minerals, and fats that are perfect for preterm infants.)

- Some preemies with low birth weight (under 2000 gm or 4.4 pounds) may need Human Milk Fortifiers (HMF). HMFs are derived from cow's milk or human milk.
- Colostrum is highly beneficial for premature infants.
- If you need to supplement, ask about the availability of human donor milk before using infant formula.
- Skin-to-skin care (or Kangaroo Care) is an excellent technique for stabilizing a preterm baby and providing access to the breast.
- Some preemies who cannot manage latching onto the breast can still benefit from spending time at the breast. Nuzzling and licking the nipple are ways the baby can learn about feeding at the breast even before he is ready for direct feeding. He can also come to the breast for non-nutritive sucking (i.e., practice at the breast after pumping). In addition, he gets sensory input from the feel and the smell of the breast. With the baby at the breast, the parent also gains sensory information that is highly beneficial for making milk.
- Preterm infants ready to feed at the breast should come to the breast in a quiet alert state. Babies who are too sleepy during breastfeeding are less coordinated and may have a disorganized sucking pattern. Babies who are actively crying need help calming down before attempting to feed. Try skin-to-skin.
- For infants who are not ready for direct breastfeeding, the progression of preterm feeding may consist of:
    1. pumping your milk and tube feeding the baby (your milk or your milk with HMF, donor milk, or special formula for preemies)
    2. lots of skin-to-skin care and non-nutritive sucking at the breast
    3. nutritive sucking and complementary feeding
    4. fully breastfeeding

One of the main goals for anyone with a preemie is establishing a good milk supply. Because dyad separation can sometimes accompany premature birth, the parent must begin pumping immediately after birth. In the past, caregivers recommended that pumping begin within the first six hours, but research shows that earlier pumping is more beneficial to establishing a healthy milk supply. When one establishes pumping earlier, the transition to mature milk may come sooner than if the initial pumping session is delayed several hours (Wambach & Riordan, 2016). Try to begin pumping within 60 minutes to two hours after birth. If not possible, begin as soon as you can. To bring in a full milk supply:

- Begin pumping your milk right away within the first hour after birth. You will likely only get drops of colostrum first. This output is normal, and you can feed it to the baby. Sometimes, hand expression of colostrum is easier.
- Use a hospital-grade double electric pump.
- Plan to pump at least eight times in 24 hours, including overnight. Milk production is enhanced during the early morning hours, so you may notice you pump more milk at that time. Take advantage of this and pump several times during the morning hours. Conversely, milk supply is lowest in the afternoons. Pump around the clock but don't fret if you notice you do not get as much in the afternoon hours.
- Practice Kangaroo Care with your baby to enhance your milk supply. Touch the baby, sniff the baby's head, kiss the baby. Remember, sensory input from your newborn drives the production of oxytocin, milk-making, and bonding.
- Keep a pumping log – pumping time, duration, and milk output.
- Get support! Exclusive pumping for a preemie can be isolating, tiring, and difficult. Contact local groups by phone, email, or text for support and information. National groups also offer hotlines. In addition, many local groups have social media accounts online.

Low Birth Weight

The average newborn weighs about 8 pounds (3628 grams). However, some babies, classified as low birth weight (LBW), are born well under the average weight. Low birth weight is defined as a newborn weight less than 5 pounds, 8 ounces (2500 grams). The incidence of low birth weight is increasing in the United States. Due to the growing use of fertility treatments, multiple births are helping increase the number of LBW babies. For example, twins, triplets, and higher-order multiples are much more likely to be born with low birth weight than singletons. Low birth weight is associated with preterm birth but can also result from other situations during pregnancy related to maternal or infant health conditions.

Breastfeeding is possible for infants with LBW. There are some complications and concerns to consider. For example, many of the complications of infant feeding for LBW babies are the same as the difficulties experienced by preterm infants. Therefore, many of the recommendations are the same as well.

What to Feed Your LBW Baby

Your milk is the optimal nutrition for your LBW baby (Kumar et al., 2017). Sometimes, human milk fortifiers (HMF) are added to human milk to optimize nutrients and protein content for LBW infants. If your milk is not available, the next best option is human donor milk. If no human milk is available, one could use special infant formula for preterm and LBW infants. If your baby cannot come to the breast after birth, begin pumping your milk as soon as possible (within an hour or two after birth). Bringing in your milk supply and protecting your milk production will be the first step to successful breastfeeding with a preterm or LBW baby. Do not delay with pumping in the hours after birth. Instead, begin an immediate protocol for pumping your breasts within an hour or two of the birth.

Several complications make infant feeding more difficult with an LBW or preterm baby. You may experience some of the following situations while feeding an LBW baby:

- Overly sleepy baby
- The baby is easily overwhelmed and irritated

- Feedings can be difficult, tiring for the baby
- Feedings require lots of extra time
- The baby coughs or gags
- Lack of coordinated feeding and breathing pattern
- Difficulty latching effectively

It may seem overwhelming to breastfeed your LBW baby, but some interventions can help. First, remember your intention to provide human milk to your baby. A baby with LBW has special needs, and your milk provides the best nutrition possible. Only you can provide this for your baby. Next, keep in mind that Kangaroo Care is the stability habitat. Your LBW baby needs help with stability, and skin-to-skin care is an excellent way to provide that stabilization for your baby. Other useful strategies for LBW infants include: 1) frequent small feedings, 2) low lighting and reduced noise in the environment, 3) paced bottle feeding strategies, 4) slow-flow bottles (if bottle feeding), 5) latching to the breast after the letdown has occurred to minimize gagging, 6) using an at-breast supplementation device, 7) cup feeding, and 8) maximizing a stress-free environment as much as possible for the breastfeeding dyad.

Cautionary Advice

It is likely that parents of LBW infants, preemies, and babies with other special needs require more breastfeeding and parenting support than other new parents do. Find the right support for your needs. Begin by connecting to a community breastfeeding support group in your area. Next, work closely with a lactation consultant who can help you develop a viable plan for infant feeding once your baby is stable. Finally, get support for your own mental health and take time for personal self-care. It is impossible to provide the best care for your special needs baby if you lack supportive and empathetic care. Make this a priority. You may need to enlist your partner, a friend, sister, or relative to assist you in finding the right support for your needs.

Infant Weight Loss

Babies are born with a little extra fluid on board. This is from living in an aqueous environment for months, and it helps them while they are transitioning to receiving nutrients by mouth instead of through the placenta. Weight loss is normal for babies during the first few days of life. Typically, babies lose weight because they are off-loading extra-cellular fluids and meconium.

A recent study shows that the average weight loss for healthy breastfed infants is about 5.5% of their birth weight (Grossman et al., 2012). In this study, the authors note significant differences concerning feeding methods. Specifically, breastfed infants lost slightly more weight during the first week than formula-fed babies (Grossman et al., 2012). Keep in mind, it could be easy to assume that this shows some superiority of formula feeding but be cautious with interpretations. Since human milk is the standard for humans and healthy breastfed infants are losing an average of about 5.5% of their birth weight, this should be the standard. Could it be that formula feeding causes an unnatural weight retention in the first days of life?

Further, in this study, nearly 20% of healthy breastfed infants lost more than 7% (but less than 10%) of their birth weight (Grossman et al., 2012). This is still considered normal weight loss for breastfed babies. Like other research on this topic, this study notes that maternal IV fluid administered during labor can ultimately affect the total weight loss in breastfed babies (Grossman et al., 2012).

Another fascinating study on infant weight loss appeared in 2018. In this study, the research team compared infant weight loss at a hospital before and after receiving Baby-Friendly status. (The Baby-Friendly designation is an accreditation a hospital receives after meeting particular breastfeeding support practices.) The results showed that after the hospital received Baby-Friendly accreditation, the infants born at this hospital had a significant decrease in weight loss in the first few days of life (Procaccini et al., 2018). This outcome shows that breastfeeding support and education can minimize infant weight loss for breastfed newborns.

There are risks associated with infant weight loss, including failure to thrive. Another concern for families who exclusively breastfeed and have an infant who experiences weight loss of more than 7% is the recommendation of formula supplements because this can impact lactation.

Important Facts About Infant Weight Loss

Babies born via cesarean generally lose more weight than babies born vaginally (Kellams et al., 2017).

- Babies born to first-time mothers may experience more weight loss than babies whose mothers have breastfed before because milk tends to come in sooner for parents who have already made milk before (Lawrence & Lawrence, 2016).
- Maternal IV fluid during labor can artificially inflate neonatal baseline weight, which makes weight loss appear excessive. This could lead to unnecessary supplementation.
- Pediatricians may assume that infant weight loss of more than 7-10% results from failed breastfeeding, but exposure to excessive IV fluid should be considered before recommending supplements.
- Formula supplements, often recommended when infants lose more than 7% of their birth weight, are associated with suboptimal breastfeeding practices and early weaning (Chantry et al., 2014).

Prevention Strategies

For efforts to prevent infant weight loss of greater than 7-10%, it is best to use effective breastfeeding practices, especially in the first few weeks (and, well, all the time).

- Feed your baby colostrum within the first hour after birth. If the baby has trouble latching, hand express what you can (colostrum is only available in tiny amounts) and feed that to your baby.
- Practice rooming-in at the hospital. Separation decreases infant access to the breast.
- Practice skin-to-skin. This closeness creates ample opportunity for breastfeeding.
- When possible, practice cue-based or responsive feeding with your baby. Feed your baby whenever you see feeding cues or

at least 8-12 times in 24 hours. Wake a baby who is not waking enough to feed adequately, about ten times in 24 hours.

- Watch for adequate urine and stool output.
- If you delivered by cesarean, you are a first-time parent or had lots of IV fluid (or all three), plan to feed your baby a *minimum of ten times* or more in 24 hours.
- If you received an excessive amount of IV fluid, be aware that you may be at risk for breast edema, and the baby may appear to lose too much weight. Alert your caregiver if they are concerned about the baby's weight loss. Use cold packs and reverse pressure softening to relieve breast swelling and edema.
- Use breast compression and massage to more fully drain the breast while the baby is latched and feeding well.
- Use hand expression, if necessary.
- If you and your baby separate for any reason, begin pumping with a hospital-grade double electric pump within 60 minutes of birth. Pump around the clock and feed your baby the expressed milk.
- If caregivers recommend supplements, express your milk (pumping or hand expression) and supplement with your own milk first.

Warning Signs

If your baby is experiencing normal newborn weight loss but is otherwise thriving and feeding well, no intervention is often necessary. Be sure to assess the whole picture, not just the single factor of weight loss. If your baby is experiencing any of these warning signs, intervention may be needed.

- Minimal amounts of urine or urine with crystals that resemble brick dust
- No urine output or stool output
- Baby poop that has not entirely changed to yellow by day six postpartum
- Breastfeeding problems: painful breasts, poor latch, baby not transferring milk effectively, engorgement, breast edema

- A sleepy baby who will not wake easily for feeding
- (Wambach & Riordan, 2016)

Also, please see the section called IV Fluids in Part II, found in the Birth Factors chapter. If you received IV fluids during labor, this could contribute to infant weight loss.

Infant Hypoglycemia

Hypoglycemia, a condition of low blood glucose (low blood sugar), can be potentially problematic for infants. Glucose is the main source of fuel for the infant body and brain. If hypoglycemia is persistent, it can result in specific and troublesome symptoms for babies, including rapid heartbeat, sweating, lethargy, feeding problems, difficulty maintaining body temperature, and oxygen saturation. In extreme cases, it can lead to brain damage.

One puzzling fact about hypoglycemia is that there is no consensus in the medical community on the tolerable lower limit of blood glucose for newborns, nor is there agreement on how long newborns can tolerate low blood sugar. To complicate the hypoglycemia picture even further, it appears that a temporary drop in blood sugar is completely normal after birth, which is usually self-limiting and resolves during the first day of life whether the infant receives food or not (Hoseth, 2000). In other words, most healthy full-term infants experience a temporary drop in blood sugar in the first two hours after birth. This drop is normal for other mammals as well. After the initial drop in blood glucose, most infants experience a rise in blood sugar over the first day of life.

The problems arise when this temporary drop in blood sugar is mistakenly interpreted as a major red flag and leads to unnecessary supplementation with formula, sugar water, or even IV glucose in some cases. Scholars cite concerns about over-screening for low blood sugar in newborns as the main driver behind the trend of unnecessary treatments for hypoglycemia. As the Academy of Breastfeeding Medicine Protocol #1 points out, low-risk infants without symptoms of hypoglycemia do not need routine blood sugar screenings. Over-screening can potentially lead to the overdiagnosis of infant hypoglycemia and can lead to unnecessary treatments, often involving formula, which can impact the normal course of breastfeeding.

Dr. Jack Newman, Canadian pediatrician, and IBCLC, accurately explains the excessive and unnecessary treatment that can result when caregivers regularly utilize screening for hypoglycemia: "There has developed a sort of 'hyper'-concern about low blood sugar that is simply not warranted. As a matter of fact, most of the babies who are tested for low blood sugar do not require testing, and most of those who receive formula do not need formula. By giving the formula, especially as it almost always is given by bottle, we interfere with breastfeeding and give the impression that formula is good medicine" (International Breastfeeding Centre, 2009).

Who is at Greater Risk for Hypoglycemia?

Hypoglycemia can be a severe condition for infants, but routine screening is unnecessary for healthy full-term infants. Infants who are at-risk for hypoglycemia, however, should be carefully monitored. Some babies who are more at-risk for hypoglycemia include preterm infants, small for gestational age (SGA) babies, infants exposed to cold stress, babies born to diabetic mothers, and large for gestational age (LGA) babies born to diabetic mothers. Please know that large babies are not at greater risk unless poorly controlled maternal diabetes is also present. It is also essential to monitor infants who are ill or are experiencing metabolic problems.

Treatment

Treatment options will vary depending on the severity of the hypoglycemic condition. For example, treatment could begin with breastfeeding, supplementation with expressed colostrum and skin-to-skin care. In some cases, infants will require treatment beyond regular breastfeeding or expressed colostrum. If you cannot express colostrum, ask about the option of using donor milk. If formula supplements are necessary, investigate using alternative feeding methods instead of bottles. Alternatives include cup feeding, spoon-feeding, using an eyedropper, syringe feeding, or finger feeding.

Other times, infants need special care for hypoglycemia and are admitted to the NICU. If you have concerns about the recommended treatments because of the potential negative impact on breastfeeding, be sure to read Academy of Breastfeeding Medicine Protocol #1

Guidelines for Blood Glucose Monitoring and Treatment of Hypoglycemia in Term and Late-Preterm Neonates, Revised 2014 (Wight & Marinelli, 2014). In this protocol, the authors astutely point out that parents should protect breastfeeding and the maternal milk supply by breastfeeding or expressing colostrum frequently. In addition, the treatment of hypoglycemia "should not unnecessarily disrupt the mother-infant relationship and breastfeeding" (Wight & Marinelli, 2014)

What if Breastfeeding is Temporarily Interrupted?

If it appears that your baby needs treatment for hypoglycemia, protecting your milk supply is a top priority, especially if caregivers introduce formula supplements. You can protect your milk supply by consistently practicing the following strategies:

- If breastfeeding is interrupted, begin pumping immediately or as soon as you can. Pump whenever your baby receives formula supplements. Be sure to feed your baby at the breast or express your milk at least eight to ten times in 24 hours.
- Practice skin-to-skin care, even if your baby receives an IV for treatment of hypoglycemia.
- Put your baby to the breast as soon as you can and as often as you can.

Prevention Strategies

- If you have diabetes (types I or II) or gestational diabetes, be sure to manage your blood sugar during pregnancy.
- Practice skin-to-skin care immediately after birth to help stabilize your baby's body systems, including blood sugar levels.
- Avoid cold stress or anything that can potentially cause cold stress after birth (for example, infant bathing).
- Plan for a low-stress birth. This is not always within your control but planning for a low intervention birth is an excellent way to start.

Small for Gestational Age

An infant who is born weighing below the 10th percentile is called small for gestational age (SGA) in North America. In other areas of the world, the threshold for determining SGA varies. There are many causes for SGA, all of which can differ in severity. Infants who are SGA face several potential problems during birth and in the early postpartum period, including 1) meconium aspiration (taking meconium into the lungs during birth), 2) low blood sugar (hypoglycemia), 3) low body temperature (hypothermia), 4) lower than normal oxygen levels, and 5) low Apgar scores (the baby's first assessment). These potential problems for the SGA infant can impact feeding in various ways. Consider these potential risks and outcomes for the SGA infant.

- Meconium aspiration, sometimes associated with SGA, can lead to airway suctioning for the upper respiratory airways (mouth, nose, and throat). Heavy or vigorous suctioning can sometimes cause irritation and oral aversion for babies. This outcome can temporarily impact an infant's willingness and ability to feed at the breast effectively.
- Low body temperature (i.e., hypothermia), is a substantial risk for SGA infants. When an infant's body temperature falls too low, caregivers introduce warming interventions to help the baby recover normal body temperature. However, these interventions can cause separation of the breastfeeding dyad and sometimes disrupt feeding. If possible, practice skin-to-skin to prevent hypothermia and ensure that you and the baby are not separated. For more information, see the section on Hypothermia.
- Low blood sugar (i.e., hypoglycemia) is also a substantial concern for SGA infants. Because of their small size, these babies lack appropriate glycogen stores. In the case of low blood sugar, a person with adequate glycogen stores will first utilize stored glycogen to counterbalance the drop in blood sugar. Because SGA infants lack glycogen stores, a drop in blood sugar is a severe condition that they cannot resolve independently. Caregivers remedy neonatal hypoglycemia by feeding the baby. This food may include human milk or formula supplementation, and occasionally IV glucose if the hypoglycemia is severe. The Academy of Breastfeeding Medicine's protocol for hypoglycemia emphasizes the need to protect the maternal milk supply while an infant is receiving

> supplementation. The ABM protocol states: "It is important for the mother to provide stimulation to the breasts by manual or mechanical expression with appropriate frequency (at least eight times in 24 hours) until her baby is latching and suckling well to protect her milk supply. Keeping the infant at the breast or returning the infant to the breast as soon as possible is important" (Wight & Marinelli, 2014).

Studies of SGA infants reveal that human milk feeding and human milk supplementation are as good or better than formula supplements (Morley et al., 2004; Visuthranukul et al., 2019). If caregivers introduce formula, practice skin-to-skin care, bring your baby to the breast at least 8-12 times in 24 hours, or remove milk with a hospital-grade double electric pump every two to three hours.

Kangaroo Care for SGA

An infant who is small for gestational age has a tiny window of bodily regulation and homeostasis. As a result, this infant may tire easily, experience difficulty maintaining appropriate blood sugar levels, and struggle to maintain body temperature. These are all serious conditions for newborns and can lead to major problems and interventions if not appropriately treated.

Kangaroo Care (KC) is beneficial for infants who are SGA. As noted in the chapter on KC, skin-to-skin care provides excellent support for infants who experience low body temperature, low blood sugar, erratic heart rate, and varying oxygen levels. Holding your baby skin-to-skin provides the critical stability habitat that allows your baby to achieve balance in bodily systems. You may need to request the opportunity to practice skin-to-skin care with your newborn, especially if your hospital favors other protocols that do not include Kangaroo Care for SGA infants. Be a vocal advocate for yourself and have your family and support team be active in helping you achieve your goals for infant care and breastfeeding.

Large for Gestational Age

An infant born with excessive weight may be classified as large for gestational age (LGA) if the baby weighs above the 90th percentile.

At first, it might be easy to conclude that if SGA babies are fragile, larger babies must be more robust, but this is not true. Just like SGA infants, LGA babies may have some complications that affect breastfeeding.

First, it is essential to note that the number one cause of LGA is maternal diabetes. In the presence of this condition, especially if maternal blood sugar lacks tight control during pregnancy, the baby will be exposed to higher blood sugar and will respond with higher-than-average insulin production. These factors come together to create excessive growth and more fat deposits. The result is a larger than average baby.

There are several potential outcomes for LGA infants that can interfere with breastfeeding, including problems during delivery with downstream consequences for breastfeeding, hypoglycemia, respiratory distress, and increased risk of cesarean delivery. Consider these potential risks and outcomes for LGA infants:

- LGA babies can present challenges for normal vaginal delivery. For example, research has shown there is a greater risk for a more extended first stage of labor in people delivering LGA infants (Blankenship et al., 2019). Similarly, delivering an LGA infant can also increase the length of the second stage of labor (Rosen et al., 2018). This outcome can impact breastfeeding because longer labor is associated with a delay in lactogenesis II, the onset of copious milk production (Dewey et al., 2003). When there is a delay in the transition to mature milk, infants are at risk of supplementation, leading to problems with full milk production and sometimes early weaning.
- LGA infants are at greater risk for birth injuries. Neonatal birth injuries that lead to any type of blood pooling under the scalp or skin raise the risk for jaundice conditions and increase the potential for dyad separation and other risks. See the section called Jaundice for more information.
- The risk for jaundice is also present for LGA babies, even without any bruising or birth injuries, because the risk of jaundice is elevated for LGA infants born to insulin-dependent diabetic mothers (Peevy et al., 1980)appropriate for gestational

age (AGA. So again, jaundice can lead to various outcomes for breastfeeding. See the section on jaundice for more information.

- Delivering an LGA baby increases the risk for cesarean delivery. Surgical birth has many diverse implications for lactation. Please see the section on cesarean delivery for more information.
- Even though it may seem counter-intuitive at first, LGA babies are at greater risk for low blood sugar (hypoglycemia). After birth and the cutting of the umbilical cord, an LGA baby can experience a sizable drop in blood glucose because of the termination of the maternal glucose supply. Caregivers remedy neonatal hypoglycemia by feeding the baby. These food sources include human milk or formula supplementation and IV glucose (if hypoglycemia is severe). The Academy of Breastfeeding Medicine's protocol for hypoglycemia emphasizes the need to protect the maternal milk supply while an infant receives supplementation as a treatment for hypoglycemia. The ABM protocol states: "It is important for the mother to provide stimulation to the breasts by manual or mechanical expression with appropriate frequency (at least eight times in 24 hours) until her baby is latching and suckling well to protect her milk supply. Keeping the infant at the breast or returning the infant to the breast as soon as possible is important" (Wight & Marinelli, 2014).
- LGA infants are at greater risk of developing respiratory distress syndrome. This can occur because exposure to higher insulin levels while in utero increases the risk of delayed lung maturation. Treatment for respiratory distress syndrome varies according to symptom severity but can include a high degree of monitoring and ventilation. If caregivers treat your baby for respiratory distress that necessitates separation from you and/or NICU admission, begin pumping immediately and continue removing milk about ten times in 24 hours. When you are reunited with your baby, practice skin-to-skin care as a way to stimulate your baby's breast-seeking skills and reflexes. Continue pumping around the clock until your baby can feed directly at the breast.

Prevention of LGA

Sometimes, infants are born weighing more than average because of their genetics. Most often, LGA is the result of maternal diabetes. If you have diabetes, pre-diabetes, or gestational diabetes, it is essential to control your blood sugar during pregnancy. Work with your primary caregiver to help determine a plan for managing diabetes during pregnancy. In addition, be sure to get good prenatal care and eat a nutrition-packed, well-balanced diet, avoiding processed foods and sugar.

Jaundice

Before your baby is born, she needs extra red blood cells to carry oxygen. After birth, the baby no longer needs as many red blood cells, and the infant manages this by breaking them down. During red blood cell destruction in the liver, bilirubin is produced. It is a brownish-yellow substance found in bile and requires that the baby excrete it through bowel movements. Essentially, baby poop moves bilirubin out of the body. If the baby cannot move bilirubin efficiently, it can build up in the infant's skin, blood, other body tissues, and even cause brain damage if levels are excessive. These jaundice conditions can be mild, moderate, or dangerous. Therefore, it is important to monitor bilirubin levels in any infant exhibiting jaundice.

Jaundice typically presents with a yellowing of the skin and whites of the eyes but this condition cannot be diagnosed based solely on appearance. Instead, babies are screened based on appearance in conjunction with a skin test using a transcutaneous bilirubinometer and blood testing for bilirubin levels. If you notice that your baby has a yellowish appearance in the skin or whites of the eyes, see your pediatrician for a physical exam.

This condition occurs in newborns for several reasons. First, as mentioned above, newborns have an increased amount of bilirubin because of the destruction of red blood cells. Second, newborns are still developing liver function at the time of birth. Because they lack mature liver function, their ability to effectively clear the bilirubin from their bodies is somewhat compromised compared to older children and adults. Third, newborns have an increased ability to reabsorb bilirubin in the intestines, and this causes bilirubin levels to increase in the bloodstream.

Jaundice occurs in newborns in several different types and can occur at other times in the newborn period. The timing of the onset of symptoms can signal the cause of jaundice. In the first day or two of life, high bilirubin levels are characterized as *pathological jaundice*, and this condition needs immediate attention and treatment. Jaundice that occurs later in the first week of life with a gradual rise in bilirubin levels is called *physiologic jaundice* (or normal *newborn jaundice*) and is likely to resolve with frequent feedings. Physiologic jaundice should resolve in one to two weeks, but it can linger as long as three months. Finally, jaundice can occur in newborns as a direct result of suboptimal breastfeeding, in which not enough milk is ingested, slowing the rate of bowel movements. Caregivers refer to this outcome as breastfeeding jaundice, but a more accurate term used by the Academy of Breastfeeding Medicine in their protocol on jaundice is *suboptimal intake jaundice* (Flaherman et al., 2017).

There are many risk factors for jaundice. You can prevent some of these, but not others. Risk factors include, 1) prematurity, 2) delay in lactogenesis II (delayed onset of abundant milk supply), 3) blood type incompatibility, 4) East Asian descent, 5) suboptimal breastfeeding, and 6) birth injuries that cause bruising.

Jaundice can impact breastfeeding. Further, depending on the cause, the severity and the treatment approach for jaundice can vary. Treating jaundice can include:

- Ensuring adequate, frequent, and effective feeding at the breast or by cup, bottle, or other supplementation methods. Regular milk intake encourages bowel movements and helps eliminate bilirubin.
- Supplementing the baby with additional expressed milk or donor milk.
- Treatment may include phototherapy using bili-lights to help the baby break down bilirubin. The baby can be placed in a phototherapy unit or under a fiberoptic blanket covering the skin. Light therapy is usually intense and continuous to be effective. Taking some breaks from the light therapy to put the baby to the breast can be safe for some babies, while others need to stay under the lights without interruption.

- Formula supplementation. There is rarely a need to supplement with infant formula, but this was a standard recommendation in the past. Be aware that if your caregiver recommends that you supplement with formula or interrupt breastfeeding temporarily to use formula, there could be a better solution (e.g., expressing your own milk and supplementing or using donor milk to supplement) to increase your baby's intake. If one must use formula, be sure to begin pumping immediately to protect your milk supply.

Is There a Way to Prevent Jaundice?

The chance of developing jaundice can be minimized for your baby, especially if any known risk factors can be effectively remedied or promptly treated. Consider these ideas:

- Prevent prematurity. Avoid smoking, secondhand smoke, avoid alcohol. Eat well and get good prenatal care. Avoid elective or unnecessary induction at all costs.
- Do everything you can to ensure early, effective, and frequent feedings. Bring the baby to the breast 8-12 times in 24 hours. Nurse your baby around the clock. Respond to all feeding cues. Adjust the positioning if first attempts at nursing are not successful. Try laid-back breastfeeding.
- If you have any risk factors for delayed lactogenesis II (diabetes, metabolic impairment often associated with overweight conditions, long or stressful labor, cesarean delivery), begin immediately after birth with strategies to maximize your baby's opportunities to come to the breast. Practice skin-to-skin to promote milk production and provide more feeding opportunities. Diabetics with well-controlled blood sugars during pregnancy have better outcomes for lactation and neonatal health than those whose blood sugar is not well controlled.
- Avoid birth interventions that are known to raise the risk of birth injuries (vacuum, forceps, cesarean).

Tongue Tie, Lip Tie, Ankyloglossia, and TOTS

Tongue tie, also called ankyloglossia, and other oral restrictions are conditions that limit the movements of the tongue, create problems for speech, and can cause a multitude of problems for breastfeeding.

The tongue tie condition generally refers to the piece of skin (called the frenulum) under the tongue that tethers the tongue to the tissues in the bottom of the mouth. A normal, healthy frenulum is long enough to allow the tongue to move all around the mouth. In infants, a normal, healthy frenulum also allows the tongue to stick out over the lower gum ridge, and it is a key part of achieving a good latch during breastfeeding. However, in the case of tongue tie, the frenulum is too short or too tight, and the movement of the tongue is restricted. In addition, tongue tie is often accompanied by a high arched palate, which contributes to breastfeeding problems.

Lip ties are also possible. The lip is tethered to the upper gum by the labial frenulum, just above the center of the upper gum. You can find the labial frenulum in your own mouth above your two front teeth. Sometimes this frenulum is too tight, and it restricts the upper lip. This can create problems when the baby is trying to seal the lips during the latch process. Restrictions can also be present in the buccal tissue along the inner cheeks. Together these conditions are called TOTs (tethered oral tissues).

TOTs can interfere with breastfeeding in several ways. Many people notice that feeding a tongue-tied infant at the breast is ineffective and painful, but these are not the only issues. The baby and the parent each experience the effects of TOTs differently. Here is a brief overview of potential difficulties for both partners.

Table 9.1: Potential feeding problems and difficulties from TOTs conditions.

Infants	Parents
Shallow latch	Painful latch
Clicking sound	Misshapen nipple after feeding
Poor latch	Breasts not drained properly
Ineffective feeding	Nipple trauma, damage
Feeding constantly	Plugged ducts or even mastitis
Poor weight gain	Engorged breasts could lead to low supply
Unhappy baby	Unhappy parent

When infants have oral restrictions, it leads to ineffective feeding. Sometimes, if the restrictions are mild, the baby may achieve a better latch with changes to positioning at the breast or some extra management of the breast by the parent. For example, I had a friend whose baby clicked while nursing at the left breast and could not make a tight seal on that side. However, the latch seemed fine on the right side. Position change was the solution for this dyad. Instead of using cradle position for both sides, the baby nursed in cradle position on the right side and then in football (or clutch) position on the left. This strategy enabled the baby to achieve a good latch on both sides without clicking or sliding off the nipple. Sometimes, position change is not enough to overcome the complications of tongue tie and other oral restrictions. Many infants with TOTs need treatment to release the restrictions. This treatment allows for better tongue and lip movements, improving the ability to feed at the breast.

Treatment for Tongue Tie

Releasing the restrictions by a minor surgical procedure called a frenotomy can dramatically improve breastfeeding effectiveness. The frenotomy allows for a more normal range of tongue movements, eliminates painful breastfeeding, eliminates nipple compression, help infants overcome potential speech problems, improves infant weight gain, promotes better infant oral health, and reduces the odds of tooth decay.

Who Provides Diagnosis and Treatment for TOTs?

A wise lactation consultant told me that tongue tie and other oral restrictions should only be diagnosed by someone who can also treat the condition. In other words, if one is not qualified to treat the condition, they are not likely qualified to diagnose it either (although, this is not always the case). Over the last decade, I have talked with numerous parents who have had concerns about tongue tie, wondering where to seek diagnosis and treatment. Most of the time, parents get an evaluation from their pediatrician, who may recognize the tongue tie, but more often, they do not. Since most pediatricians are not qualified to perform frenotomy (tongue tie release), they are also not experts at recognizing the sometimes-subtle nuances of this condition. The solution is to seek an evaluation from a qualified doctor to diagnose and treat the condition. In many cases, the best option is a pediatric dentist. Pediatric dentists are, in fact, highly trained experts in oral anatomy and function for babies, toddlers, and children. If you have concerns about tongue tie, lip tie, or other oral restrictions, seek an evaluation from a pediatric dentist in your area who is known for working with TOTs. In addition, pediatric ENTs (ear, nose, and throat specialists) are often an excellent resource for TOTs. They can diagnose and provide treatment.

Alternatively, there are many pediatricians across the U.S. who are tongue tie experts. These practitioners have been highly trained to diagnose and treat tongue tie issues. Some of the pediatric doctors I have encountered over the past few years make treating tongue tie the sole focus of their business. Many pediatricians are well known for TOTs treatments, and families travel from neighboring counties and states to receive treatment from these experts. If you cannot find local help for TOTs, join online groups and look outside of your immediate area for an expert. It is worth the extra effort to find skilled care for resolving the present and future complications from tongue tie restrictions.

The key to resolving infant feeding issues concerning TOTs is getting a prompt evaluation as soon as you have any suspicions about oral restrictions or ineffective feeding. Get another expert opinion if you have received conflicting information (for example, an LC notes some oral restrictions, but the pediatrician sees no tongue tie). Do not delay with evaluation or treatment. Sometimes, undiagnosed tongue tie can lead to early weaning. It may also be necessary to follow the tongue tie release with bodywork or oral exercises for the infant. Consider pediatric chiropractic care, cranial sacral work, or other gentle bodywork designed for infants (or toddlers).

Special Needs Babies

Many families wonder if breastfeeding is a practical choice for special needs infants. Generally, special needs infants benefit from human milk like other infants do, but the benefits are dramatic for some special needs babies.

Many special needs infants may need extra support for feeding. For example, babies with heart conditions, Down syndrome, cleft lip or palate, preemies, small for gestational age, babies with jaundice, low muscle tone, sensory processing issues, or conditions of the mouth and throat are just a few examples of the special needs infants who need extra care and support to establish lactation.

Supplementing

Suppose your baby is born premature or small for gestational age. In that case, human milk provides superior nutrition but be aware that there may be recommendations to supplement your baby if he is not gaining weight well. Ask about supplementing with your own expressed milk or donor milk. Also, investigate the possibility of supplementing with an at-breast supplementation device. This device allows the baby to receive supplemental milk or formula while nursing at the breast. Syringe feeding, spoon feeding, and cup feeding are good alternatives if you decide to avoid bottle feeding.

What Will Help Me Feed My Special Needs Baby?

The short answer to that question is 1) patience, 2) time, 3) trial and error with positioning, 4) experimenting with various hand positions to hold the breast, 5) additional tools and feeding devices (e.g., supplementer device, feeding cups, other tools), 6) supportive pediatrician and healthcare team, 7) peer-to-peer breastfeeding support groups, 8) supportive family and friends, 9) lactation consultants, and 10) mental health support team for parents.

For many special needs infants, feeding can be tiring, and it may take a lot of extra time to get one feeding session accomplished. This effort can require a great deal of patience on your part. Remember to build your support team.

Taking Care of Your Own Needs

Many parents with special needs infants feel isolated and overwhelmed with feeding and infant care. Find a local or online group that you can rely on for support and advice. Do not neglect your own feelings of overwhelm or frustration. Seek support for your mental health if you feel even the slightest bit of anxiety or depression, anger or disappointment. Infant care can be incredibly difficult even without physical or emotional challenges, and special needs can compound that. Seek the support you need promptly. You and your baby will benefit from having the right team in place.

Illness in the Infant

Some people wonder if they should continue breastfeeding when babies get sick. The quick and simple answer is "yes."

Infants and toddlers who develop short-term illnesses (e.g., colds, pneumonia, respiratory infections, bronchitis, ear infections, diarrhea, constipation, vomiting) should continue consuming their regular human milk diet. There are several reasons for this, including the fact that babies are comforted by nursing. In addition, your milk provides antibodies to fight illness. Finally, nursing will provide all the nutrition and hydration your baby needs while recovering from illness.

Even though the medicinal action of human milk is widely recognized, many people still receive outdated advice when it comes to breastfeeding a sick child. For example, you might hear that it is best to stop (temporarily) breastfeeding while your baby is sick. Some people even claim that milk can contribute to mucous production, and therefore, it is best to suspend breastfeeding for a time. The only problem with this logic is that human milk does not contain the same proteins as bovine milk, which may increase mucous production in some individuals.

Other people suggest that it is simply too difficult to nurse a baby with nasal congestion. On the advice of her doctor, my mother "temporarily" suspended breastfeeding when my sister was six weeks old and was stuffed up with a head cold. He claimed that bottle-feeding during a cold would be easier. Unfortunately, my sister never re-established breastfeeding. (It is important to note that this also happened during an era when there was little breastfeeding support. Sadly, because infant formula was so widely used and my parents had become familiar with bottle feeding, my mom did not breastfeed her next two children. One of them was me.)

Temporarily weaning can cause more difficulties than it might solve. For example, assuming you want to resume nursing after the illness, you would have to initiate an around-the-clock pumping routine in addition to taking care of a sick baby. Also, temporary weaning deprives babies of necessary antibodies and other immune factors in human milk when they need it most. Most importantly, abrupt withholding of nursing at the breast will be highly distressing for an infant who has already established breastfeeding. Finally, remember that breastfeeding is extraordinarily comforting for infants and toddlers. Withholding that comfort during an illness seems cruel and can cause distress for the dyad.

Challenges of Feeding a Sick Baby

One of the greatest challenges during an illness is that a sick baby may not be as eager to nurse as he is normally. Fewer feedings can lead to engorgement and slowed milk production. This can have immediate implications for the milk supply. In addition, if your baby loses his usual appetite and is taking less than the typical amount of milk, he may also have dangerous setbacks for weight gain. One can remedy both of these situations by offering more nursing opportunities. If your baby is sleepy and takes less milk for a day or two, your milk will not immediately dry up. It is better to express milk than to take a risk that things will just work themselves out. Try hand expression if you are uncomfortable (or inexperienced) with pumping.

Hydration is another concern. Many acute illnesses are associated with the increased risk of dehydration, especially diarrhea and vomiting. Be sure that your baby gets enough of your milk to be sufficiently hydrated. Watch for signs of dehydration and remember that because infants and toddlers have small bodies, they can become dehydrated much more quickly than adults.

Signs of Dehydration in Infants

- Decreased urine output, fewer than six wet diapers in 24 hours
- Sunken soft spot (fontanelle) on the baby's head
- Sunken eyes
- No tears or cry is weak
- Fever
- Lethargy
- Rapid breathing

If your baby becomes dehydrated, take steps immediately to encourage milk intake. For example, you can feed directly at the breast or express milk and feed by cup, spoon, or syringe. Do not give your baby any other beverages or medications unless you have specific medical recommendations to do so. Seek care immediately if your baby is vomiting and consistently unable to keep down any milk you are feeding.

Other Cautions

Be aware that cold remedies and OTC cold/cough products are never suitable for infants and toddlers. Do not use essential oils on infants or toddlers. Also, do not give your baby fruit juices or any soda (e.g., Coca Cola). Never give aspirin to infants, toddlers, or bigger children. Seek medical care if your baby has a fever, refuses to nurse effectively, or becomes overly dehydrated.

Tips for Breastfeeding a Sick Baby

- Continue nursing your baby.Prevent dehydration by offering ample opportunities to nurse.
- Use a suction bulb and saline solution to help gently clear congested nasal passages.
- Wake your baby if he is sleeping instead of nursing.
- Monitor your baby's urine output.
- Practice lots of skin-to-skin care.

Infant Hypothermia

All newborn babies are at risk of losing too much body heat just after birth. Hypothermia is a serious condition that occurs when the core body temperature drops dangerously low. In infants, this is a substantial risk because babies lack the mechanisms adults have for robust body temperature maintenance. For example, infants lack generous body fat stores, making it even more difficult to adjust to the surrounding environmental temperatures. As you might imagine, preemies, babies born with low birth weight, and babies who are born small for gestational age (SGA) are at even greater risk for hypothermia.

Infant hypothermia and breastfeeding have an interesting relationship. Early breastfeeding can protect infant body temperature (World Health Organization, 1997). In contrast, if a baby's body temperature drops too low, the baby will need treatment to rewarm the core temperature. This treatment can take place in a radiant warmer or an incubator. Both of these options will require the baby to spend time warming up in the device, which may interrupt early attempts at breastfeeding. In addition, infants who experience hypothermia can subsequently exhibit hypoglycemia (low blood sugar). As stated in the section on infant hypoglycemia, infants with low blood sugar are at greater risk for formula supplementation, which can be disruptive of breastfeeding.

In well-resourced settings (e.g., hospitals and birth centers in the developed world), caregivers account for infant thermoregulation during post-birth procedures. Of course, that does not eliminate risk, but infant hypothermia is lower in well-resourced settings than in low-resource communities (e.g., developing nations).

The World Health Organization recognizes that hypothermia is a dangerous risk for any infant regardless of birth setting and has guidelines for the "warm-chain" of thermoregulation for newborns (WHO, 1997). The warm-chain consists of interlinked elements of protection that help newborns with thermoregulation in the immediate postpartum period and minimize the risk for hypothermia.

The WHO warm-chain includes several elements that are not only protective of infant thermoregulation but are also protective of early breastfeeding. The WHO warm-chain is summarized below:

- Be sure all people who attend the birth are trained in infant care.
- Be sure the delivery room is sufficiently warm.
- Dry the baby immediately after birth.
- Place the baby skin-to-skin with the parent.
- Initiate early breastfeeding.
- Delay bathing of the baby.
- Keep the baby warm with appropriate clothing.
- Be sure the baby is warm during transport if that becomes necessary.

The elements of skin-to-skin contact, breastfeeding, and delay of the infant bath support breastfeeding, and each of these factors protects against hypothermia *and hypoglycemia*.

As I mentioned, most birth settings in well-resourced settings will take all of these factors into account but be sure to incorporate these if you are planning a home birth or if birth unexpectedly takes place in an unplanned location.

CHAPTER 10

Lactation Interference: Maternal Factors

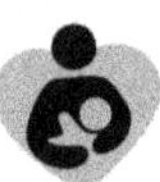

Like babies, each parent brings their own unique primary factors into lactation. Sometimes, there are factors that were present before pregnancy and breastfeeding that can interfere with lactation. In addition, there are maternal complications that arise only once lactation is established. This section will highlight several maternal factors that can present challenges for the breastfeeding.

Breast Pain and Nipple Pain

Which of the following statements is true?

A. Breastfeeding should not hurt.

B. Breast and nipple pain are common reasons for early weaning.

Yes, this is a trick question. Both statements are true. Let's examine each of these ideas.

Breastfeeding should not hurt. This claim is valid. You can imagine that if breastfeeding is supposed to hurt, humans would not have such a long history of infant feeding at the breast. However, breast pain and nipple pain are relatively common and can lead to early weaning if the first days of lactation are not managed well (Kent et al., 2015; McClellan et al., 2012). There are many diverse causes of breast and nipple pain, including 1) poor positioning, 2) shallow latch technique, 3) infant's palatal abnormalities, 4) tongue tie and or lip tie, 5) various infections, and 6) vasospasm. According to Wambach and Riordan (2016), pain falls into two main categories: *early-onset* and *late-onset*. The early-onset pain is usually present during weeks one through three of breastfeeding and is mainly attributable to position and latch techniques (or other mechanical factors). Late-onset pain arrives after a period of smooth sailing for the breastfeeding dyad, in which latch and feeding were pain-free. Late-onset pain is more often associated with breast or nipple infections. Because nipple pain is a primary cause of early abandonment of breastfeeding (McClellan et al., 2012), it is imperative to prevent pain or to get an accurate diagnosis and effective treatment strategy as soon as possible.

Prevention and Treatment Strategies

- If pain presents during the first month of breastfeeding, look for mechanical causes. Investigate different and better positions and latch techniques. Get a full oral evaluation for your baby.
- Look for misshapen nipples (creased or flat on one side after feeding). This can indicate that the nipple is too far forward in the baby's mouth during feeding. Try to achieve a deeper latch with the nipple aimed up toward the roof of the baby's mouth at the juncture of the hard and soft palate.
- Try laid-back breastfeeding with the baby managing the latch. (Don't overmanage: remove your hand from the back of the head; bring the baby to the nipple, not nipple to the baby; wait for wide-open mouth; unlatch if you cannot achieve a deep latch).
- Clicking sounds could indicate that the baby fails to maintain secure contact with the breast. Change positions and/or evaluate the baby for tongue and lip ties or other oral structure anomalies.
- If pain presents only after several weeks of pain-free nursing, first be sure the latch is deep and the position is good. If that does not resolve the pain, consider infection as the source of pain. Infections include mastitis, yeast, Staphylococcus aureus (staph), or other bacterial infections.
- If infection is suspected, seek care from your primary care physician in conjunction with skilled lactation care. Keep in mind that, although the pediatrician can diagnose and treat the baby, they cannot diagnose or treat your infection. In addition, some conditions, like yeast, require treatment of both the parent and the baby.

- If engorgement is causing painful breasts, use cold packs and reverse pressure softening to relieve swelling and edema. Only after treating the swelling/edema should one start milk removal.
- If breasts are not drained after each feeding and cause painful plugged ducts or engorgement, investigate poor latch and/or tongue tie. Also, consider breast massage and compression in conjunction with feeding and pumping.
- If the nipple looks blanched (loses most of its color, looks white) after breastfeeding, vasospasm might be the cause. Investigate vasospasm and Reynaud's phenomenon. Remember that Reynaud's could be more likely in people who experience vasospasm of other body parts like fingers and those with thyroid issues and other autoimmune conditions.

The best thing to do to resolve breast and nipple pain is to find the direct cause of the pain and eliminate it. Using "Band-Aid" strategies (e.g., nipple shields, pumping instead of direct feeding) can help for a time, especially if you have nipple trauma and need to heal. Be cautious about relying on these methods without also finding the cause and making the necessary changes to eliminate the problem.

Dysphoric Milk Ejection Reflex (D-MER)

As far as lactation interference factors go, this one is mysterious and quite disturbing for the people who experience it. Dysphoric Milk Ejection Reflex (D-MER) is a frustrating condition in which the physiology of the milk letdown also triggers sudden feelings of anxiety, depression, melancholy, sadness, misery, anger, and other negative emotions. Usually, the feelings appear abruptly, just before the milk letdown, and last for a few minutes. Although this sounds somewhat innocuous, it can be highly unnerving for some people and even lead to weaning.

D-MER is a physiologic response to the hormonal change that brings milk letdown. The negative feelings that are associated with D-MER are not in any way related to postpartum mood disorders. These feelings are not negative reactions to the baby, infant feeding, or breastfeeding, or pumping. The negativity is not an emotional response but a physical response. D-MER ranges from mild to severe, and for some, the extremely negative experience decreases the overall quality of life.

There are treatments available for D-MER. Alia Macrina Heise, IBCLC, founder of D-MER.org, states that mild cases of D-MER can often be treated (or tolerated) with education about the condition. This education includes helping people understand that the condition is physical, not psychological. For moderate symptoms of D-MER, Heise recommends education and becoming aware of lifestyle cofactors that could aggravate the negativity (such as dehydration or stress). For severe cases, prescriptions have been effective.

Other research has connected D-MER with an inappropriate fight-or-flight response that connects to the rising levels of oxytocin that must occur to facilitate the milk letdown. Because the fight-or-flight response is a protective measure, it can play a positive role during motherhood. Anytime a mammal mother feels threatened, she can easily become aggressive and highly protective. While these hormones are protective, they go haywire in this case, which researchers believe manifests as the negative emotions of D-MER (Uvnas-Moberg & Kendall-Tackett, 2018).

A fascinating article called "The Mystery of D-MER: What Can Hormonal Research Tell Us About Dysphoric Milk-Ejection Reflex?" appeared in *Clinical Lactation* in 2018. This article is free and available on the *Clinical Lactation* website. I highly recommend reading it if you are dealing with D-MER. In the case of D-MER, the authors suggest a connection between a fight-or-flight reaction to hyperactivation of our stress response. Because of the possible link to stress, the authors recommend taking measures that help encourage feelings of safety. Likewise, avoiding situations that feel stressful can also be advantageous. Other recommendations include skin-to-skin care, self-care, and nutrition (Uvnas-Moberg & Kendall-Tackett, 2018). Above all, if you are experiencing D-MER, get help from a knowledgeable care provider. You do not need to suffer through this experience. There is more information about this condition at D-MER.org.

Low Milk Supply

While low milk supply can be a genuine problem for some, it is a perception problem for many others. In other words, sometimes low supply is suspected, but it is not a reality. So, oddly enough, one of the main complications with low supply issues is determining if insufficient milk supply conditions exist or not.

Several situations seem to indicate low supply but are not indicators of low supply (unless these indicators appear in conjunction with other true red flags). One of the most significant false indicators that can raise the suspicion of low supply is pumping volume. Over the years, I have had several clients complain that they must have a low supply because they cannot pump much milk. This assumption is wrong. It is well known in the lactation field that the volume of milk a person can pump is not an accurate indicator of true milk production. Some other examples of false red flags are 1) lacking a physical feeling of milk letdown, 2) your baby wants to feed all the time, 3) the breasts do not feel full anymore, 4) the breasts don't leak, 5) your baby wants holding all the time, 6) your baby is too needy, 6) your baby is fussy in the later afternoon and evening, 7) your baby lingers at the breast (slow feeder), 8) your baby appears hungry after nursing, and 9) your baby wakes too much at night for feeding.

None of these situations (mentioned above) indicates inadequate milk volume unless accompanied by genuine indicators of low milk supply. Often, unrealistic expectations pave the way for parents to assume low supply exists when it does not. In addition, decades of formula feeding and unethical formula marketing to new mothers have had a tremendous negative impact on our collective beliefs about how infant feeding works. Some professionals, even today, are still operating under a particular set of infant feeding rules that apply only to formula. Remember that human milk feeding and formula feeding principles, logic, and wisdom are different. These different feeding systems do not follow the same rules.

When Should I Worry About Low Milk Supply?

Some signs can indicate a truly low milk supply. For example, if your baby is not gaining weight well, does not produce enough wet and dirty diapers, or becomes dehydrated, a full evaluation of your baby and breastfeeding is necessary. Be aware that weight gain for an exclusively breastfed infant should always be charted on the WHO growth chart normed for breastfed infants, not formula-fed infants. See the section on Growth Charts for more information. Further, poor weight gain, not enough wet and dirty diapers, or dehydration are indicators of something wrong, and low supply may exist. Other milk transfer issues could complicate the whole picture. A full evaluation with an IBCLC is essential.

What Are the Causes of Low Supply?

When it does happen, low supply can connect to many factors. Here are some factors that can cause low milk production (this list is not exhaustive; there could be other factors):

- Maternal endocrine, hormonal, and metabolic problems: PCOS, thyroid imbalance, diabetes, or other conditions associated with insulin resistance or metabolic impairment
- Insufficient glandular tissue
- Postpartum hemorrhage greater than 1.5 liters of blood with damage to the pituitary
- Heavy consumption of parsley, sage, or peppermint
- Cold medicines like Pseudoephedrine (also called Sudafed), other cold or allergy meds
- Sleep training
- Lack of sufficient nighttime feeding or expressing milk
- The infant has tethered oral tissues (TOTs), also called tongue-tie/ankyloglossia
- Too much pacifier use
- Scheduled feeding times, lack of cue-based feeding
- Baby is too sleepy, sleeps through feeding times (can happen with preemies, jaundice, high tech sleep bassinets, routine swaddling, anything that causes/promotes too much sleep)
- Supplementation with formula (without also fully expressing your milk *every time*)
- Poor latch, poor milk transfer
- Not enough feeding every day (eight times, the often-cited minimum number of feedings, may not be enough for some babies to bring in and maintain a full milk supply)
- Limiting the feeding duration, the baby does not get enough high-fat milk Heavy use of nipple shields (sometimes inhibits excellent milk transfer)
- Maternal smoking

- Weak infant suck or oral motor dysfunction (preemie, cleft lip or palate, low muscle tone, Down syndrome, special needs)
- Retained placenta
- Low maternal prolactin levels
- Insufficient pumping time (if pumping exclusively)
- Wrong pump settings, old or worn-out pump parts, wrong flange size
- Introduction of hormonal birth control pills, IUD, injectables, implants, rings
- Milk stasis due to heavy engorgement
- Anemia
- Previous breast surgery or trauma (including any childhood trauma to the chest)

Remedies for Low Milk Supply

Once you have determined that you have an insufficient milk supply, you can work to find the best ways to boost your milk production but proceed with caution. The remedy for low supply must be a good match for the cause of the insufficiency. For example, if poor latch and poor milk transfer cause the problem, increasing the number of feedings is unlikely to make much difference unless you also correct the poor latch and milk transfer issues.

In general, the best way to make more milk is to remove more milk from your breasts. Removing more milk can mean bringing the baby to the breast more often. Allow the baby to nurse for a longer duration at each session, using hands-on pumping and feeding techniques (breast compression and massage). This may also include nursing more during the nighttime, adding a pumping session in the morning, or hand expressing after each feeding. It is imperative to remove milk from the breast to signal your body to increase milk production.

Other Ways to Increase Milk Supply

- Improve the latch
- Improve milk transfer (compression and massage can help)

- Practice skin-to-skin as much as possible (plan two days for nearly continuous skin-to-skin and lots of feeding)
- Decrease the length of time between overnight feedings (increase nighttime feedings, wake the baby if needed)
- Eliminate pacifiers
- Wean your baby off supplements gradually while increasing milk removal
- Give only breast milk to infants under six months
- Stay hydrated, eat well
- Consult with an IBCLC
- Read *Making More Milk: The Breastfeeding Guide to Increasing Your Milk Production* by Lisa Marasco, IBCLC and Diana West, IBCLC.

Controversial Impact of Placenta Pills

Over the past two decades, placenta encapsulation has become popular, based on anecdotal promises of preventing postpartum depression and increasing milk supply. Unfortunately, there is a considerable amount of myth and controversy involved in the lore surrounding the consumption of the placenta. For example, some people claim that consuming the dried placenta helps lactation, and others find it hurts lactation. However, many IBCLCs over the past ten years have begun to connect the dots among their clients experiencing low supply, recognizing that consuming placenta pills may be a strong contributor to low milk supply issues.

Recall that the hormones of pregnancy, specifically progesterone and estrogen, are responsible for putting the transition to mature milk *on hold*. These two pregnancy hormones obstruct lactation during pregnancy because they keep prolactin in check. Prolactin can only experience its dramatic rise after the placenta is delivered, allowing lactation hormones to bring on lactogenesis II, the full transition to mature milk. Retained placenta fragments can prevent the increase in prolactin, thus preventing the onset of the abundant mature milk supply. In light of this, does it make sense to consume the placenta and re-introduce pregnancy hormones back into your body?

For some people, this appears to have a dramatic effect on lactation, but consumption of the placenta may not affect everyone to the same degree. This outcome mimics what we see with birth control. Some people can tolerate certain forms of birth control and maintain their milk supply and others notice a measurable drop in supply immediately after starting hormonal birth control. There is enough anecdotal evidence from IBCLCs to recommend using extreme caution with placenta consumption. Even the Academy of Breastfeeding Medicine Protocol #9 lists consuming placenta as a potential cause of low supply (Brodribb & the Academy of Breastfeeding Medicine, 2018). Use extreme caution. Remember that what could be medicine for one person can be toxic to another. We are all individuals, and consuming placenta may not work well for you, even if it worked well for your friend or cousin.

Words of Caution for Those Experiencing Low Supply

If you are experiencing low supply and your baby is not thriving, you may receive the recommendation to use formula or possibly a prescription galactagogue to increase milk production. This recommendation may indicate that the doctor you are working with could not accurately identify the cause of low supply and suggested these other remedies instead of investigating the root of the problem. Be sure to explore the cause of low supply before beginning any treatments. Seek an evaluation with a skilled lactation professional. Using formula is sometimes necessary. Using prescription meds can sometimes help but many other solutions are available to you. Work with a lactation consultant to develop a plan to increase your milk production. Remember that breastfeeding problems have *breastfeeding* solutions.

If you seek to increase milk production, choose a caregiver who will most likely help you with that goal. IBCLCs, board-certified lactation consultants, are highly trained in the anatomy and physiology of the breast and the principles of breastfeeding. Work with an IBCLC rather than your primary care doctor or the baby's pediatrician if you need help boosting your milk supply and creating a plan for effective breastfeeding. Other professionals without lactation training simply do not have the depth of knowledge to effectively support complex cases.

Cold and Allergy Medicines and Herbs

Sometimes, using over-the-counter cold and allergy medications and herbal-based products can affect milk supply by causing a drop in milk production. Cold medicines are effective at helping to dry up a runny nose, but that same action affects milk production. The cold and allergy remedies that are most often to blame for this are decongestants with pseudoephedrine. For most other medications, the reason for caution while breastfeeding is because of the potential for the drug to pass into your breast milk. For cold, allergy, and flu remedies, the worry is not about infant exposure to the medication but the effect on milk production. Read labels thoroughly and use caution when ingesting any cold, flu, or allergy remedy while breastfeeding. Any cold or allergy remedy that inhibits mucous flow could potentially impact milk production.

In addition to pseudoephedrine, some herbal products are available for use as cold remedies. Some of these contain herbs known to reduce milk supply. Any product or preparation using peppermint or sage can influence milk production. Avoid cold lozenges with menthol or peppermint. Avoid peppermint tea.

Prevention Strategies

Some people find that pregnancy and breastfeeding are a time of discovery when it comes to natural remedies. Because one should avoid many medications during pregnancy and breastfeeding, people must look for alternatives. This can be an entry into the world of natural remedies that are great for pregnancy, breastfeeding, and home remedies that are useful with small children. Consider the following (short) list of natural remedies and approaches for the common cold while breastfeeding.

- Prevent a cold by taking good care of yourself. For example, limit your sugar intake (it lowers your immune response), get lots of good quality sleep, or as much as possible with a tiny baby, and eat well.
- Rest. Practice breastfeeding lying down. Remember that your baby is getting antibodies through your breast milk. Keep nursing while you're sick with a cold. It's safe.

- Fluids. Your granny was right! Stay hydrated. (Using a humidifier can help overnight.)
- Sleep when the baby sleeps.
- Garlic supplements (or fresh garlic) has antiviral properties.
- Homeopathic cold remedies may be compatible with milk production.
- Use a saline nasal rinse or neti pot for sinus congestion.
- Gargle salt water. This remedy temporarily helps relieve sore throat.
- Ask for help and support when you're not well. For example, having a friend make you a meal can be a huge relief.

Birth Control

Fertility is not only a hot topic for new parents; it is a crucial element of maternal healthcare. Maternal (and infant) outcomes are better off with optimal child spacing. When pregnancies are close, maternal morbidity and maternal mortality risks increase. Similarly, pregnancy following closely after the birth of a child raises the risk for a baby to be born preterm, with low birth weight and low Apgar scores. Short birth intervals also increase the risks for stillbirth, miscarriage, and neonatal mortality (death in the first 28 days of life). While there is no agreement on defining the most optimal child spacing, the World Health Organization suggests that two to three years is good and three to five years may be better (WHO, 2007). Of course, it depends on your health and personal circumstances.

Controlling fertility during lactation is essential, and some types of birth control are more compatible with breastfeeding. Hormonal birth control pills, the patch, four times yearly injectable birth control, and the vaginal ring are all methods of contraception that contain estrogen. Any birth control that contains estrogen has the potential to decrease milk supply. Therefore, it may be best to avoid estrogen-containing birth control options if breastfeeding. Other options don't contain estrogen and will be less likely to impact your milk supply.

Birth Control Options

LAM

Lactational Amenorrhea Method (LAM) is temporary birth control available to people who are breastfeeding exclusively. This method has three essential criteria. First, after the lochia (initial postpartum bleeding) has stopped, no other menstrual bleeding or spotting has started. In other words, you have not had any periods. Second, the baby receives only breast milk and is fed on demand, day and night. Third, the infant is less than six months old.

If you meet these three criteria, LAM provides a reliable way to prevent pregnancy. Conversely, if you fail to meet all three of these criteria, this method is no longer a reliable source of birth control.

Barrier Options

Barrier options include condoms, sponges, cervical caps, and diaphragms. These methods block the sperm from reaching the egg and do not contain estrogen. These are all excellent options for anyone who is lactating.

Progestin-Only Options

The standard birth control pill, called a combination pill, contains both estrogen and progestin, and is not a good option while breastfeeding because it can reduce milk production. The "mini" pill is a progestin-only option that can prevent pregnancy but does not contain estrogen. This pill works best when it is taken at the same time each day and is less likely to impact milk supply. Wait until your baby is six to eight weeks old before starting the mini pill for best results. For some individuals, the progestin-only pill may impact milk production. The positive feature of these pills is that you can stop taking them instantly if you notice a drop in your milk production. Anecdotally, I have heard from many LCs who say that, although research claims that the mini pill does not impact lactation, LCs are seeing a decrease in supply with many individuals who take the mini pill. Use cautiously.

The Depo-Provera shot is a longer-lasting progestin-only option. This injection option provides a progestin-only birth control option with effects lasting 12 weeks. Caregivers administer this shot four times per year. If you are interested in this option, it may be best to try the mini pill first to observe any potential effects on your milk supply. Otherwise, you may have to deal with the long-lasting effects of the injection and possible low milk supply while the shot is still in your system. On the other hand, if you take the mini pill first and you discover that it decreases your supply, you *can* stop taking the pills. There is no way to reverse the effects of the injection after you get it. It may be best to avoid this type of birth control during lactation.

Internal Devices for Birth Control

An IUD (intrauterine device) is a small T-shaped device placed inside the uterus to prevent pregnancy. IUDs offer long-term birth control and are available in hormonal and non-hormonal options. The hormonal IUDs contain progestin. The non-hormonal option is a copper device that does not contain any hormones. There are several brands of hormonal IUDs available with varying lengths of contraceptive effectiveness. Although these contain no estrogen, there is still a chance that you could experience a drop in milk supply. As recommended above for the injection, consider trying the mini pill first to see if progestin agrees with you before placing an IUD. Also, there are several class-action lawsuits in progress against multiple IUD manufacturers. It may be worth investigating the safety of these devices before considering one. Do your own research. As a word of caution, if you do notice a condition of low milk supply after having an IUD placed, consider having it removed and following a plan to boost milk production.

The birth control implant, a small device implanted under the skin on the upper arm, is a long-lasting contraceptive option, providing birth control for up to four years. This device is also hormonal, delivering progestin only. Although many people are unaffected by progestin-only methods, there is evidence that it may negatively impact some breastfeeding mothers. Stuebe et al. (2016) published a report of one infant with suboptimal weight gain whose mother had received the Nexplanon implant. The mother received the implant when her baby was four weeks old, and one month later, the infant had fallen from the 44th percentile down to the 6th percentile for growth (Stuebe et al., 2016).

Be cautious with all forms of hormonal birth control and long-lasting birth control options. Be aware that if you choose a long-lasting method and experience low supply in connection with that birth control method, it may be difficult or impossible to reverse the effects immediately.

Postpartum Mood Disorders

There is a large body of research on the complex relationship between breastfeeding and postpartum mood disorders (PMDs). Many studies have shown evidence with highly contrasting conclusions and outcomes about postpartum mood disorders and breastfeeding. Nevertheless, there is some evidence that parents with postpartum mood disorders are at a greater risk of early weaning and that people who do not breastfeed are at greater risk of PMD.

One study of 594 parents investigated the relationship between postpartum mood disorders and breastfeeding. The study found a clear relationship between higher scores (greater than 12) on the Edinburgh Postnatal Depression scale and early abandonment of breastfeeding (Dennis & McQueen, 2007).

Maternal endocrine response could also be a factor in postpartum mood disorders. A recent study found that lower oxytocin levels during feedings can be associated with higher levels of anxiety and depression. At eight weeks postpartum, this study found that people who report more feelings of stress, depression, less happiness, and more overwhelm had lower levels of oxytocin while they were feeding their infants. These lower levels of oxytocin were also corelated to higher scores on the Edinburgh Postnatal Depression scale (Stuebe et al., 2013).

Fascinating research on the root causes of PMD reveals an interesting array of factors at work, including 1) history of depression and depression in pregnancy, 2) poor sleep quality, 3) stress, 4) pain, 5) past trauma, and 6) inflammatory responses in the body. a closer investigation by Kathleen Kendall-Tackett)shows that one should not view inflammation as an equal c-factor with others that increase the risk for postpartum mood disorders. Instead, Kendall-Tackett's research shows that inflammation is the umbrella that all the other factors fall under and are influenced by (Kendall-Tackett, 2007). In other words, inflammation can cause other factors that exacerbate postpartum moon disorders. In addition, pro-inflammatory factors increase during the third trimester of pregnancy, making people giving birth at a higher risk for depression and mood disorders than the average person.

Prevention and PMD Coping Strategies

If you have had a history of depression, trauma, pain, and stress, you may be at greater risk of PMD. Breastfeeding can help mitigate PMD because of the action of oxytocin. Oxytocin has a calming effect on mother and baby, and can help calm the stress response within the brain (Donaldson-Myles, 2012). In addition, because breastfeeding increases oxytocin every time the baby comes to the breast, breastfeeding may offer a protective effect on postpartum mood disorders. Other preventative or treatment strategies include:

- Reduce maternal stress during pregnancy and in the postpartum period.
- Enlist help from supportive friends and family.
- Increase your high-quality sleep.
- Exercise. This option may seem impossible for some because baby care consumes life for new families. But it is possible. After the lochia (initial bleeding after childbirth) has stopped, aim for gentle exercises like walking or yoga a few times a week. One can walk (and stroll) with the baby, so there is no requirement for a babysitter. Some yoga instructors are offering free content oneYouTube. You can try these activities in your own home, on your own time.
- Expose yourself to sunlight- especially in the morning hours. This exposure is a mood enhancer and one good way to help regulate sleep. If you live at higher latitudes or have your baby during the cold winter months without much sunshine, consider bright light therapy.
- Acupuncture.
- Massage or other bodywork.

- Remove inflammatory foods from your diet. This change can help reduce the bodily inflammation that exacerbates all the other factors for PMDs. Be sure to include healthy fats in your diet. (That may sound counter-intuitive for the postnatal period, when most people are interested in"getting back in shape" the advice to avoid dietary fat is not only outdated bus dangerous. Humans need high-quality fats to thrive.) Inflammatory foods to avoid: junk food, highly processed foods, poor quality oils and fats, sugar, sodas of every kind, fried foods, fast food of every kind. Sugar is highly inflammatory and is the main pathway for encouraging your body to store body fat. Avoid sugar and sugar substitutes.
- Therapy, herbs, vitamins, and pharmaceuticals are useful options for many people. Most anti-anxiety and depression medications are compatible with breastfeeding but be sure your prescriptions are safe for lactation
- Work with a caregiver that has experience with PMDs and breastfeeding.
- Caution: get help with supplements or herbal remedies if you choose this route. Over-the-counter supplements, herbs, and vitamins can be beneficial. However, only use them under the direction of a qualified caregiver.
- Before starting any treatment for depression or anxiety, check your vitamin and mineral status with complete blood work. Check the status of vitamin D, B12, B9 (also called folate). Request a full iron panel. Check magnesium, zinc, selenium. Always test before supplementing, especially with iron, zinc, and selenium, because too much of these can create toxicity. Be aware that the lab ranges for B12 in the U.S. are considerably lower than in many other nations. Our "normal" ranges for B12 may be too low. In general, it can be best to get your vitamins and minerals from food sources, but sometimes, supplementation is necessary.
- Increase your intake of omega-3 fatty acids, which are known to reduce inflammation.

Trauma Survivors

In 2014, author and psychiatrist Bessel van der Kolk published a brilliant book called *The Body Keeps the Score*. In this book, van der Kolk outlines how trauma affects people and how our bodies hold onto the lasting impact of trauma, whether we know it or not.

Once physically lodged inside our bodies, trauma can exist as memories that we can recall, or it can live under the radar of our conscious awareness. For example, if a person experienced trauma or abuse as a child, they may not remember the trauma, but their body will hold the memory and its effects. These memories are trapped inside our bodies and can be triggered by events that activate those memories or feelings of frustration, discomfort, anger, rage, sadness, loneliness, helplessness, and even dissociation.

If you recall from Part I in the chapter called Whole Body Sensory Experience, breastfeeding is a total body experience- acting as an exchange of sensory information between bodies. Sometimes, the physical experience and sensory intensity of breastfeeding can trigger the memory or feelings of trauma. Occasionally, this is unexpected and can cause quite a startling and devastating surprise.

Some trauma survivors may choose to opt for formula. Honestly, there is no reason to choose breastfeeding if the experience will be a source of re-traumatization. In this case, breastfeeding may not be the best path because feeding your baby should be a happy experience and, if not, at least a neutral experience. Feeding your baby should not detract from your mental health, and it should certainly not be a source of trauma for any parent. If you are struggling with the idea of breastfeeding because you have an experience with trauma, childhood mistreatment, sexual abuse, intimate partner violence, perinatal trauma, or other traumatic experience, please know that choosing to feed your baby in a way that supports your mental health and past experiences is perfectly acceptable. For you, that may mean choosing infant formula. No one can know what is best for you as a parent *except you*. Give yourself the power to make this decision based on your instincts, self-awareness, and trauma history.

However, many trauma survivors do choose to produce milk and feed it to their babies, either by direct feeding at the breast or by pumping milk and feeding by bottle. There is some evidence that survivors of childhood sexual abuse have similar breastfeeding rates to people who did not experience that trauma (Elfgen et al., 2017). Research shows that for trauma survivors, breastfeeding may be more challenging. Some studies show that those with a history of previous childhood trauma report more breastfeeding complications like pain or mastitis (Elfgin et al., 2017), while other studies report that previous childhood trauma may lead to a shorter duration of breastfeeding (Channell Doig et al., 2020).

Occasionally, people find that minimizing the sensory experience of breastfeeding can mitigate some of the triggering aspects of the feeding sessions. For example, if you are affected by the intensity of skin-to-skin contact, try placing a small infant blanket between you and the baby. Others have suggested that using distraction may be a way to keep thoughts or memories from dominating the feeding sessions. For example, you could try watching short videos or listening to music. Pay attention to what causes you the most discomfort or distress and test out ways to lessen the stress. Find what works best for you.

There is no guarantee of a poor breastfeeding or lactation experience for someone with a history of trauma. On the contrary, many people with a history of trauma find that breastfeeding can be a healing experience. People even report that breastfeeding after trauma can be empowering (Channell Doig et al., 2020). this is ay individual path, and what works for one may not work for others. Therefore, if you are keen to try breastfeeding, even if you feel reluctant and unsure of the potential outcomes because of past trauma, I urge you to find support for yourself as you begin breastfeeding.

Look for an IBCLC who is familiar with breastfeeding after trauma. Trauma-informed care is still in its infancy, but many knowledgeable people in the lactation field are educating themselves about working with trauma survivors. In addition to lactation care, you may find working with a therapist or counselor helpful. Online communities and local peer support groups are also excellent resources.

Again, breastfeeding is entirely possible for people with a trauma history. keep in mind, as with all breastfeeding scenarios, you are the person who creates your breastfeeding story. You can choose whatever path works for you, your mental health, and your family.

If you are currently pregnant, you may want to check out Penny Simkin's book, *When Survivors Give Birth*. This book is specific to the subject of childbirth. However, it offers great information for those who have a history of trauma and for those who work with clients who have had past trauma. In addition, I highly recommend reading Bessel van der Kolk's book, *The Body Keeps the Score*. This book explores the impacts of trauma on individuals and how we store that trauma in our bodies. The author also details new paths for treatment beyond traditional therapy.

Previous Breast Surgery

Surgery of the breast, for any reason, including augmentation or breast reduction, can potentially impact lactation outcomes. Unfortunately, there is no way to prevent possible negative outcomes if the surgery has already occurred. However, there are several important things to know if you have had breast surgery in the past and are now planning to breastfeed your baby.

First, it's important to note that breastfeeding can be successful after breast surgery, even after reduction. This is because several surgical techniques are now available to preserve a column of tissue from under the areola to the chest wall. When surgeons use this preservation technique, the anatomy of lactation can remain intact. Without these preservation techniques, you may still make some milk, but supplementation may be necessary.

There are several other important considerations for breastfeeding after breast surgery:

- If you are currently pregnant, consider how best to minimize your risk of experiencing other factors that contribute to low supply and early breastfeeding issues.
- Risk of nipple trauma after breast surgery is higher because breast surgery can compromise the sensation of the nipple. If you have lost sensation in the nipple, detecting poor latch and nipple damage may be challenging. Observe any nipple trauma, abrasions, or nipples that appear misshapen after feeding. These are all signs of a poor latch.

- Be aware that if your breasts were widely spaced prior to augmentation, tubular-shaped, underdeveloped, or asymmetrical, these are all signs that milk production could be compromised (not by surgery but by lack of tissue growth and development).
- Pay close attention to positioning, latch, and suck-swallow patterns. Look for signs of effective milk transfer.
- Closely monitor how your breasts feel before and after feeding. Does the breast feel fuller and heavier before feeding? Does the tissue feel softer and emptier after feeding? Use your hands to assess the fullness of the breast tissue manually.
- Breast compression and massage can help drain the breast but be aware that if you have implants, it may be necessary to use a light massage or avoid compression and massage in the area closest to the implant.
- If you need to supplement, you can consider using a supplemental nursing system that allows the baby to feed at the breast and get milk or formula via a small feeding tube attached to the nipple. The tube is attached to a reservoir that contains the supplemental milk or formula. This tool allows the baby to continue to receive your milk, preserves the bonding of breastfeeding, and delivers supplemental milk simultaneously.
- Be diligent about counting dirty diapers. This is a good indicator of milk intake. In addition, watch the baby closely for other signs that indicate that she is growing and thriving.
- Visit your lactation consultant or pediatrician's office for frequent weight checks in the early days of breastfeeding.
- Before and after feeding, test weights can be useful to check milk intake but be aware that one test weight does not reflect the average amount of milk that the baby gets in other sessions during the day. The volume of milk intake varies from one feeding session to another, and people produce more milk during the morning hours than later in the afternoon or evening. Therefore, be cautious with reading too much into test weight as a general reflection of total milk intake.
- Work with skilled lactation care (likely someone other than your baby's pediatrician) who can help you get breastfeeding

established and manage the risk factors associated with breastfeeding after breast surgery. Find an IBCLC or other qualified lactation specialist.

There can be considerable confusion and misinformation about lactation after breast surgery. This misinformation may come straight from your surgeon. Be aware that plastic surgeons have limited or no specific training in lactation. While they may know a great deal about the anatomy of the breast, they do not see patients for managing clinical care of lactation. Consequently, many surgeons may think they know about lactation, but breast anatomy is only one small part of the puzzle regarding applied lactation knowledge and management. while you may have done your due diligence in gathering information about augmentation, you may have been misled by a well-meaning doctor who lacks training in this domain.

Be aware of the following complications:

- There are four commonly used incision sites for breast surgery to place implants: transaxillary, inframammary, periareolar, and transumbilical. The incision near the areola (periareolar incision) is most likely to compromise nipple sensation and damage necessary nerves that serve the nipple. This incision site can hide the scar but puts the nipple nerve supply at greater risk.
- Larger-sized implants can cause increased chest pressure and put added pressure on the surrounding milk ducts. This pressure may cause slow flow of milk or even milk stasis, which can slow milk production.
- Milk production may be possible after implant placement, but some individuals may not bring in a full milk supply and may need to supplement.

Helpful Resources

Some excellent resources are available for people who have had breast surgery and plan to breastfeed their babies. Look here for more information: www.bfar.org, and the books by Diana West and Lisa Marasco.

Delayed Lactogenesis II - Where is My Milk Supply?

The ability to make human milk develops over time through a process called lactogenesis. The first stage, lactogenesis I, occurs from about mid-way through pregnancy until about day two postpartum. During lactogenesis I, specific cells within the mammary gland develop into secretory cells to secrete milk. From the middle of pregnancy onward, your breasts increase in size to accommodate these changes. At this time, your breasts are ready to make colostrum, and many people notice that colostrum can be expressed or may leak from the breasts during the last weeks of pregnancy. The breasts are now ready for the onset of lactogenesis II, the transition to an abundant supply of mature milk. that transition, however, cannot happen without a significant hormonal trigger. The hormones of pregnancy strongly inhibit lactation, and until the shift occurs, the breasts will not produce an abundant supply of milk.

Lactogenesis II, the Onset of Mature Milk

Some people mistakenly believe that childbirth is the trigger for the onset of lactogenesis II, but that is not entirely accurate. The trigger is a rapid drop in progesterone levels after the placenta is delivered. After the placenta emerges, the pregnancy is over, and maternal hormones make a rapid shift away from the hormonal profile of pregnancy to the hormonal profile of lactation. This shift essentially removes the lactation inhibitors and allows the breasts to move into lactogenesis II, called secretory activation. This process results in the abundant secretion of milk. Lactogenesis II lasts from about day three postpartum to about day eight. During these six days, the amount of milk you make will increase dramatically day by day before abruptly leveling off. As a result, you may feel that your breasts are larger in size, you may notice milk leaking while you are nursing or in between feedings, and your breasts may feel warmer and heavier. By day eight, your milk supply will begin to shift from being controlled by hormonal signals to being controlled by the "demand and supply" rules that govern lactation. For example, suppose continuous milk removal from the breasts is not consistent and timely. In that case, milk production will slow down, and eventually, the breasts will prune back the milk-making structures in a process called involution.

During lactogenesis II, certain hormone signals are essential to facilitate the transition to abundant mature milk. These signals include prolactin release from the pituitary gland, a dramatic drop in progesterone levels (after the placenta is delivered), and an increase in oxytocin. These hormonal changes must be accompanied by consistent milk removal from the breast to enable the onset of mature milk. If one or more of these hormonal processes does not occur, there could be a major delay in lactogenesisIII, and your abundant supply of milk will be delayed or will not appear at all.

What Are Other Causes of Delayed Lactogenesis II?

There are many variables in lactogenesis. First, let's look at some obvious factors that could cause delay. The essential hormones could cause a delay if they are inhibited for some reason. For example, if the pituitary gland suffered damage following postpartum hemorrhage, it may fail to release prolactin. This failure can cause delays (or lactation failure in extreme cases). If progesterone remains high, as in the case of retained placenta, there may be a delay in lactogenesis. There may also be delays in lactation If oxytocin levels do not rise sufficiently.

Other Known Factors That Can Delay Lactogenesis II

Besides the obvious hormonal signals mentioned above, other factors are also at work in the lactation puzzle. These factors operate in conjunction with the dysfunctional hormonal situations mentioned above.

Some of the more well-recognized factors that can delay the onset of mature milk include:

- Cesarean birth
- Maternal diabetes (including gestational diabetes)
- A long second stage of labor, stressful labor and delivery
- Pain medication used during labor
- Maternal metabolic impairment (often associated with obesity)
- Retained placenta fragments
- Postpartum hemorrhage leading to Sheehan's syndrome
- Previous breast surgery

- First time giving birth
- PCOS
- Low thyroid levels
- Ovarian theca lutein cysts
- Hormonal birth control beginning during the immediate postpartum period

Less well-known factors that can delay the onset of mature milk

- Poor sleep in the third trimester of pregnancy (Casey et al., 2019)
- Alcohol use during pregnancy (Rocha et al., 2020)
- Smoking
- High levels of cortisol (Caparros-Gonzalez et al., 2019)

If you know that you have any of these risk factors, it is good to alert your caregivers and have a plan in place if you encounter a delay in lactogenesis II. Also, be aware that there are no guarantees of a delay in your transition to mature milk just because you have a risk factor on the list above. Not everyone who has the risk factors will encounter a significant delay.

What to do if Your Mature Milk is a Little Late to the Party

First, do what you can to promote healthy lactation: Practice skin-to-skin care with your baby, put the baby to the breast (or pump breasts) at least 8-12 times every 24 hours, avoid birth control of any kind at this time, rest and try to maintain a low-stress level, and investigate the possibility retained placenta fragments if abundant milk does not appear by day four or five postpartum. If you are experiencing a delay in the onset of mature milk, work with an LC to determine the cause and develop a plan for feeding your baby.

Research shows that people who experience a delay in lactogenesis II have higher odds of abandoning breastfeeding (or exclusive breastfeeding) by four weeks postpartum (Brownell et al., 2012). Delayed onset of lactogenesis II can create significant issues for lactation, but working with skilled lactation care can help you preserve your lactation potential. Work quickly to find a lactation consultant if you notice that your transition to mature milk is slow. Expressing milk as frequently as needed (about 8-12 times in 24 hours) in the first few days postpartum will go a long way to prevent delayed lactogenesis II.

Postpartum Hemorrhage and Sheehan's Syndrome

Postpartum hemorrhage (PPH) leading to Sheehan's syndrome is a complex maternal condition that can present major lactation interference. Please read about PPH and Sheehan's Syndrome in Chapter 8: Breastfeeding Interference and Birth Related Factors.

Breast Abnormalities and Insufficient Glandular Tissue

Breasts come in all sizes and many different shapes. There are countless variations of what is normal and functional. Even many of the"abnormalitie" of the breast still render them fully functional, but some conditions interfere with the ability to make milk. Some deviations from the normal breast include:

- Additional nipples occurring on the milk line
- Accessory breast tissue, sometimes located in the axilla (armpit)
- Absence of nipples
- Insufficient mammary tissue (also calle: insufficient glandular tissue, IGT, hypoplasia)

In the case of additional or accessory breast tissue or additional (supernumerary) nipples, likely, the primary breasts (and even the additional ones) can adequately produce milk. However, some people have found that the additional tissue, especially when it is located in the axilla, can experience unwanted swelling. Occasionally, the extra breast tissue present in the axilla is missing a nipple or may have an underdeveloped nipple. One may not even recognize this as breast tissue until sometime during pregnancy, when the tissue begins to swell. After pregnancy and breastfeeding, this tissue can be removed without compromising the milk production structure in the two primary breasts. Other nipples that can occur on the milk line may be mistaken for moles until late pregnancy or postpartum when they can produce milk. These areas may be quite sensitive. Apply cold packs, as needed, for comfort. After a week or two, the swelling and discomfort should alleviate when the glandular tissue begins to shut down milk production (because milk is not leaving the breast). Sometimes, this process is slow, and it can be frustrating. Seek care with a skilled lactation consultant if problems arise or speak to your primary caregiver.

One significant breast abnormality that can interfere with lactation is insufficient glandular tissue (IGT). This condition is when the breast does not develop enough glandular tissue, the milk-making structure, during breast development in adolescence. It can result from endocrine disorders and can occur in conjunction with other hormonal imbalances. This condition is not to be confused with small breasts. The normal breast consists of adipose tissue (fat tissue) and glandular tissue. The breast that lacks glandular tissue can be a regular size because of fatty tissue deposits, but it could lack regular function. On the other hand, the small breast that lacks abundant adipose tissue but does have adequate glandular tissue can function quite well.

People who have IGT may not be aware that they lack adequate glandular mammary structures until after birth. There are some signs, however, that can give clues that IGT may be present.

These factors are sometimes associated with IGT:

- Asymmetry of breast development (noticeably different-sized breasts)
- Wide spacing of the breasts
- Breasts appear tubular, lacking a round shape
- Lack of sizable breast development during puberty in conjunction with stretch marks on the breasts
- Lack of breast changes during pregnancy and in the early postpartum period

Notice that these factors are sometimes associated with IGT. If you have had asymmetrical breast development and none of these other factors, you likely do not have IGT. Sometimes, breasts appear normal but lack function. On the other hand, some people report that they have several of the IGT associated factors but cad bring in a full milk supply. Do not rely on these factors alone to determine your IGT status.

IGT Can Interfere With Lactation

If IGT is present, the lactation outcomes may vary. Some people find that they can produce milk and provide some percentage of their baby's needs at the breast. Some others report that IGT makes it challenging to provide any milk for their baby. It can be frustrating and stressful to realize that your potential for making milk is lower than you expected. If breastfeeding is the preferred choice and IGT is preventing full breastfeeding because of low supply, some options are available for feeding your baby with human milk. First, it can help to adjust your definition of successful breastfeeding. You can succeed with breastfeeding in ways outside of the typical norm. Consider some of these alternative solutions:

- Supplement your supply with donor milk. There are multiple strategies for obtaining donor milk. Check around in your area and online groups for possible options. For example, Eats on Feets is an organization that facilitates milk sharing in local communities. There are chapters all around the world. Check them out online.
- Use an at-breast supplementation device with donor milk or with formula. This option allows you to nurse your baby directly without the need for bottles and provide the supplement simultaneously.
- Investigate the possibility of using herbs or medication to boost supply.
- Read about IGT. I recommend Diana Cassar-Uhl's *Finding Sufficiency: Breastfeeding with Insufficient Glandular Tissue*.
- Find others who are also experiencing IGT using online or in-person groups. Sharing experiences and relating your own insights can be cathartic.
- Remember that IGT is a complex issue, and it is likely that everyone will approach their solutions in a unique way. Therefore, one size does not fit all.
- Polycystic Ovary Syndrome (PCOS), diabetes, and hypothyroid are three conditions with hormonal and metabolic dysfunctions that can affect producing human milk. Although many people with known hormonal and metabolic disorders can

produce a sufficient milk supply, some struggle with exclusive breastfeeding. Below is a discussion of three of these conditions that can interfere with the process of lactation.

Hormone and Insulin-Related Conditions:

Polycystic Ovary Syndrome (PCOS), diabetes, and hypothyroid are three conditions with hormonal and metabolic dysfunctions that can affect producing human milk. Although many people with known hormonal and metabolic disorders can produce a sufficient milk supply, some struggle with exclusive breastfeeding. Below is a discussion of three of these conditions that can interfere with the process of lactation.

PCOS

Polycystic Ovary Syndrome (PCOS) is a complex condition involving several distinct dysfunctions of the ovaries, hormones, and metabolism. PCOS is associated with infertility, excessive body hair growth, overweight and obesity, cystic ovaries, ovulatory disturbances, menstrual irregularities, acne, insulin resistance, excessive androgens, and testosterone, as well as other factors. Diagnosing PCOS can be difficult because the clinical manifestations do not appear the same from one person to the next.

Reports of breastfeeding with PCOS show a wide range of outcomes. Some people find that they can produce a sufficient milk supply without any problems. Others find that they have insufficient milk production, especially in the presence of little to no breast size changes during pregnancy (Vanky et al., 2012). Still, other people with PCOS report having an oversupply of milk. A research team discovered a correlation between lack of breast size changes during pregnancy and more intense PCOS hallmarks of obesity, higher blood pressure levels, higher triglycerides, and higher fasting insulin levels (Vanky et al., 2012). In addition, this group of people with PCOS who reported minimal breast size change during pregnancy showed more metabolic dysfunction and had a shorter duration of exclusive breastfeeding and a shorter duration of any breastfeeding (Vanky et al., 2012). These results suggest that even among people with PCOS, breastfeeding outcomes are varied, linked to the intensity of PCOS symptoms and the intensity of metabolic disturbance.

Some medications and therapies improve breastfeeding outcomes for those with PCOS. These can be compatible with lactation. Still, as each case is different, people affected by PCOS must work with a knowledgeable caregiver to find the best solution. One size does not fit al, in this case. Even with a treatment regime, boosting milk production for someone with PCOS experiencing low supply will require the same techniques that are always useful for increasing supply: frequently bringing the baby to the breast for cue-based feeding, breast compression and massage while nursing or pumping, skin-to-skin contact with the baby, extra milk expression (pump or hand expression), sensible and informed use of galactagogues, and nighttime nursing. In addition, babies need to be monitored frequently for weight gain, and sometimes, supplementation is necessary.

Thyroid Problems, Hashimoto's, Grave's Disease

Like all hormones, thyroid hormones exist in a delicate balance. Having too much or too little hormone of any kind can create downstream ripples for other hormones and bodily functions. Thyroid disorders are endocrine-related and, when out of balance, can cause milk production issues and a host of other health problems. There are severalstypes of thyroid disorders, including 1) hypothyroidism, 2) hyperthyroidism, and 3) postpartum thyroiditis. In addition, many thyroid conditions exist in conjunction with autoimmunity. Women are more affected by thyroid conditions than men.

Underactive Thyroid

Hypothyroidism is the lack of adequate thyroid hormone production. This condition can impact milk production for some people. One of the tricky problems with identifying hypothyroid conditions during lactation is that many of the symptoms of low thyroid function look and feel like the same symptoms typically present for many people in the postpartum period. These signs can include fatigue, hair loss, sleep disturbances, and decreased energy levels. If you experience these and other symptoms of hypothyroidism during the postpartum period in conjunction with low milk supply, request a thorough evaluation and blood test to check thyroid hormone levels. Many practitioners mistakenly check the TSH level (thyroid-stimulating hormone) without checking your actual thyroid hormones, but this is not a thorough evaluation. Instead, request a full thyroid panel including, at the minimum, TSH, T3, T4, and the two main antibody markers (TPO and Tg). If a hypothyroid condition is confirmed and medication is recommended, it is safe to take thyroid medication during lactation. Work to optimize your thyroid hormone levels and keep in mind that "within range" levels are not necessarily optimal. For example, the current lab reference range in the U.S. for TSH is .45 to 4.5 mIU/ml. This range is a wide range of values, and the extremes values on this spectrum may not be optimal. TSH values closer to 1 mIU/ml are considered more optimal. (Many people feel symptoms of hypothyroidism when TSH values approach 4 or 4.5, even though many doctors would consider those values normal.) Be sure to normalize T3 levels, as this is the active thyroid hormone.

If you are experiencing symptoms of low thyroid production or receive a diagnosis of hypothyroidism or Hashimoto's disease, there are alternatives to conventional treatment. Read Dr. Izabella Wentz's books about uncovering the root cause of your thyroid problems. Her books include:

- Hashimoto's Thyroiditis: Lifestyle Interventions for Finding and Treating the Root Cause
- Hashimoto's Protocol: A 90-Day Plan for Reversing Thyroid Symptoms and Getting Your Life Back
- Hashimoto's Food Pharmacology: Nutrition Protocols and Healing Recipes to Take Charge of Your Thyroid Health

Overactive Thyroid

Hyperthyroidism, the overproduction of thyroid hormones, is also problematic for lactation. Some people who have an overactive thyroid condition can produce milk earlier than expected during postpartum and experience problems with the milk ejection reflex. In some cases, hyperthyroidism may generate an oversupply of milk. In addition, an overactive thyroid can exist in conjunction with Graves' Disease, an autoimmune condition, and conventional treatment can impact lactation.

Treatment for hyperthyroid conditions is usually more complex than treating low thyroid conditions. Be sure to verify that all recommended medication is safe to take while breastfeeding. Consult the Infant Risk Center for more information on medications. If you go through thyroid ablation using radioactive iodine (iodine-131), complete weaning is recommended

Similar to hypothyroidism, there are alternatives to conventional treatment for Graves' disease and hyperthyroidism. Work with a Functional Medicine practitioner, an Integrative Medicine practitioner, or a naturopath who can help you discover the root of your thyroid issues. Most mainstream primary care doctors are not currently offering treatment that deviates from the conventional approach. Read *The Autoimmune Solution* and *The Thyroid Connection* by Dr. Amy Myers. She suffered from Graves' Disease and received conventional treatment before discovering alternatives to thyroid ablation.

Tips for Breastfeeding with Thyroid Conditions

- Seek help from an IBCLC and a knowledgeable physician who can help you preserve lactation.
- Optimize your thyroid hormones with medication if necessary.
- Manage low supply with skin-to-skin, multiple opportunities for daily breastfeeding or pumping, breast compression and massage techniques, at-breast supplementation device, or donor milk.
- Manage oversupply with block feeding (not longer than one week), cool compresses, and cabbage leaves in the case of dramatic oversupply. Work with an LC to manage oversupply.
- Work with an experienced lactation consultant and knowledgeable physician. In this case, many people have discovered that endocrinologists are not the right fit for care with thyroid complications. Remember, endocrinologists often lack the training to support thyroid conditions holistically. They will likely only offer pharmaceutical and conventional treatments. However, there are excellent alternatives. Find the right practitioner to suit your needs and your goals.

- Find online support groups for thyroid conditions. Connecting with others who have similar conditions can open new avenues for support and education.

Maternal Diabetes

Diabetes is a condition in which blood glucose values are higher than normal and are not well-controlled by the body. Diabetes manifests in several forms, including Type 1 diabetes, Type 2 diabetes, prediabetes, and gestational diabetes. Type 1 diabetes is a condition in which the pancreas does not produce enough insulin. Type 2 diabetes is a chronic condition that leads to poorly controlled blood glucose levels. Prediabetes is a state of chronically high blood sugar markers but not high enough to be classified as Type 2 diabetes. Finally, gestational diabetes is a temporary blood sugar condition during pregnancy. Because all forms of diabetes can impact endocrine function, there is the potential for downstream effects concerning lactation and milk production.

Breastfeeding is an important health choice for many reasons (see Chapter 2, Move the Needle, for more information). However, it is vital for people with diabetic conditions because lactation has been shown to improve glucose metabolism (Much et al., 2014). However, some known obstacles for breastfeeding with diabetes may affect milk production or have other downstream outcomes. Consider these findings:

- People with gestational diabetes (GD) are at risk of delayed lactogenesis II, or the onset of/transition to mature milk (Much et al., 2014). In a 2014 study, risk factors for delayed onset of mature milk for those with GD included suboptimal care, lactation care, and support at the hospital after birth (Much et al., 2014). Therefore, if you have diabetes or gestational diabetes, be sure to alert your caregiver and request the most robust lactation care the hospital or birth center offers.
- Like GD, there is evidence that those with type 1 diabetes are also at risk for delayed lactogenesis II, which means it takes longer for the onset of the copious milk supply to appear. This delay puts infants at risk for supplementation. Be sure to put

the baby to the breast about ten times in 24 hours. Practice skin-to-skin as frequently as you can. Add pumping if necessary. If you must supplement, try using donor milk first.

- Breastfeeding with diabetes increases risks for candidiasis and thrush, especially if blood sugar is not well controlled. Watch for signs of oral thrush in your bab, and be aware of your own signs for yeast imbalance. Thrush overgrowth can impact the nipples and become painful. In addition, thrush can create sore spots in the baby's mouth and a rash on the baby's bottom.
- Infants born to diabetic mothers can be at risk for hypoglycemia (Wight & Marinelli, 2014). This connection is important because formula supplements are often recommended for infants when their blood sugar levels drop. If you have expressed and stored colostrum, supplement the baby with colostrum first and provide skin-to-skin care. If you use formula for supplementing, be sure to express milk (use a hospital-grade double electric pump) and plan to eliminate the formula supplements if possible.
- Nighttime feedings for those with maternal diabetes can present challenges with blood sugar drops. You may need to test glucose levels and consider eating a snack at night to prevent swings in blood sugar levels. Work with a knowledgeable LC or diabetes coach to develop your best strategy.
- Diabetes can raise the risk of developing mastitis (Yu et al., 2018).
- Metformin and insulin appear to be compatible with breastfeeding and lactation.

Breastfeeding with diabetes is a complex issue. If you have diabetes, plan ahead, and work with your primary caregiver and a lactation consultant. Know your risk factors and obstacles and watch for possible outcomes like the delayed onset of mature milk, infant hypoglycemia, supplement recommendations, yeast infections, and breast infections. You may want to consider speaking with a lactation counselor before birth to get information on expressing and storing colostrum. Human milk and colostrum supplements are better than formula supplements in most cases for healthy, full-term infants.

Maternal Metabolic Impairment, Overweight and Obesity

For many years, research has shown a relationship between a high degree of pre-pregnancy maternal obesity and a shorter duration of breastfeeding (Rasmussen & Kjolhede, 2004). In addition, people who were highly overweight or obese before pregnancy are less likely to begin breastfeeding on the first day of life (Rasmussen & Kjolhede, 2004). There have been many theories put forth to explain this trend. Some include psychological or behavioral factors, and some point to cultural and biological factors (Amir & Donath, 2007) but lack of proper support may be part of the missing link here as well. Some factors in this scenario are specifically related to the metabolic impairment that can be associated with overweight conditions. Other pieces of this puzzle, specifically the lack of breastfeeding support for overweight parents, could be driven by a mix of social and cultural factors.

Overweight Parents Are Less Likely to Receive the Support They Need

Many overweight parents face hidden challenges. I call them hidden because the obstacles that overweight parents encounter are not always obvious and therefore, they are often not addressed. Studies have shown that caregivers may not perceive an overweight person as someone who needs special lactation care, thus not meeting the needs of this at-risk group with more robust and appropriate support. For example, one study found that healthcare providers did not recognize that overweight people have lower breastfeeding success rates and did not modify their counseling methods for overweight parents (Rasmussen et al., 2006). Another study found that parents with higher BMI had a lower chance of encountering breastfeeding promotion practices during the hospital stay (Kair & Colaizy, 2016). That same study identified all of the following pro-breastfeeding practices that were *less likely to occur for overweight parents* than other parents (Kair & Colaizy, 2016):

- Less likely to have practical help with breastfeeding during the hospital stay
- Less likely to accomplish the first feed within an hour after birth
- Less likely to be given information about breastfeeding

- Less likely to be taught about on-demand feeding
- Less likely to room-in with their babies
- Less likely to be given information about local breastfeeding resources
- Less likely to avoid pacifier use

Why are overweight parents less likely to receive the lactation support they need? This question is complex, and likely has a multitude of answers. I cannot pretend to know all the reasons why this phenomenon exists. Nonetheless, I can help people understand that those with higher BMI may need more robust lactation care with several key aspects of infant feeding: positioning, latch, supporting the breast while feeding, education on delayed lactogenesis II, and maintaining infant hydration if there is a delay in lactogenesis.

Physical Challenges Are Present for Metabolically Impaired, Overweight, and Obese Parents

In addition to the practical challenges mentioned above, overweight people with metabolic impairment may also experience physiological challenges as obstacles to breastfeeding. When colostrum is switching to mature milk in the first days after birth, your body requires significant amounts of prolactin. A study of prolactin response in the first days of breastfeeding revealed that people overweight or obese before pregnancy (BMI greater than 26) had a diminished prolactin response to infant suckling from 48 hours postpartum through the first week (Rasmussen & Kjolhede, 2004). The authors conclude that this is significant because this is a critical time and many overweight people abandon breastfeeding before day 7, when thr prolactin response is somewhat diminished (Rasmussen & Kjolhede, 2004). Prolactin response does improve for those who have metabolic irregularities, but this can take extra time and dedication from parents. Because this diminished prolactin response can delay the onset of mature milk, the baby will be getting an extended colostrum phase. In this period, colostrum is available in smaller quantities than mature milk. Because of the lower volume of milk available, infants must frequently come to the breast to maintain hydration (Walker, 2017).

Overweight and obese conditions often exist in conjunction with many metabolic factors that can potentially impact lactation. For example, overweight conditions during pregnancy are often associated with insulin resistance, hypertension (high blood pressure), gestational diabetes, and preeclampsia. Each of these conditions has its own set of unique factors and circumstances that can potentially cause negative impacts on lactation.

One of the major concerns for breastfeeding outcomes among those with metabolic impairment is delayed onset of lactogenesis II. The onset of abundant milk supply usually occurs between two and three days after birth. Often, overweight parents experience a delay in the onset of the abundant milk supply (sometimes called *milk coming in*). Several mechanisms at work could contribute to the delay in the start of the abundant milk supply. One theory relates to the diminished prolactin response mentioned above. Another theory suggests that latch can be difficult with large breasts, larger nipple-areolar complex, and potentially flatter nipples, leading to poor milk transfer (Walker, 2017).

Early management of breastfeeding can help. Incorporate these strategies to improve infant feeding outcomes in the first two weeks and beyond:

- Communicate your feeding goals to your caregivers during your hospital stay. Be sure that your physician, midwife, and nurses know that you intend to breastfeed.
- Ask for help with positioning if you feel the traditional cradle hold is not optimal.
- Aim for feeding or pumping at least ten times daily, until the onset of your abundant milk supply. After that time, follow your baby's feeding cues but be sure to feed your baby 8 12 times every day. For newborns, err on the side of more feeding, not less.
- Use a nipple everter for flat or shy nipples.
- Use a small pillow or a rolled-up towel under the breast to support larger breasts during feeding.
- Try multiple positions, including traditional cradle holds, football or clutch hold, laid-back feeding, and side-lying. Experiment

with each one and see what works best for you. Many people with larger breasts find the football hold works well.

- Practice skin-to-skin care if there is a delay in the onset of abundant milk. Practice skin-to-skin car, even if your mature milk arrives on time
- If you have had gastric bypass, you are already aware that you need extra vitamin B12. Talk to your caregiver about supplementing with a multivitamin and B12 during lactation.
- Find local support from breastfeeding groups online and in person.

Breastfeeding Problems

Lactation complications can arise during breastfeeding, even when one takes all the necessary precautions to avoid known issues. It is likely that during the journey from the first latch until a child weans that you may encounter some common problems associated with breastfeeding and the use of human milk. Although complications while breastfeeding can be frustrating, irritating, and sometimes painful, they are usually not a cause for abandoning lactation. As lactation consultants like to say, breastfeeding problems have breastfeeding solutions. In other words, one can resolve most of these issues while keeping lactation and breastfeeding intact without resorting to weaning. However, many people who experience complications and difficulties often wean early. One of the main reasons for this is the lack of breastfeeding support. Consider the following. One study of early weaning showed that the reasons cited for abandoning breastfeeding were all complications that parents could remedy with supportive, knowledgeable lactation care during and after the hospital stay (Lewallen et al., 2006).

What are Common Breastfeeding Problems?

There are quite a few common problems that can create difficulties, but there are almost always solutions, as mentioned above. Some of the common lactation issues include:

- Painful, sore nipples or nipple trauma
- Latch difficulties

- Plugged ducts
- Oral thrush (yeast overgrowth)
- Mastitis
- Engorgement
- Low supply and perceived low supply
- Oversupply

Breastfeeding problems have breastfeeding solutions. One can overcome each of these complications by using a variety of treatment approaches. I recommend that anyone experiencing issues mentioned on this list (or other difficult complications) seek skilled care to explore treatment options. Many times, peer-to-peer breastfeeding counselors and volunteer lactation counselors can help you explore your options for treating these common issues. Other times, an IBCLC is the best support (as with mastitis and severe engorgement). The chart on the next page outlines basic action steps for treatment in these situations. Any time you feel that issues are overwhelming, seek help immediately. With skilled care, you can overcome most breastfeeding complications.

Where to Find Skilled Breastfeeding Assistance and Counseling

If you are dealing with infant feeding issues (on this list or not) that are too much to handle and are creating difficulties for you and your baby, talk to someone who can support you with your feeding goals. Most of the time, this will be a trained lactation or breastfeeding counselor, lactation consultant, peer counselor, or IBCLC. There are times when it makes sense to seek care from your primary care physician, but because they often lack training in lactation, it is more effective to talk to someone with professional lactation training. Many people I have spoken to find that when they seek care from a health professional who does not have lactation training, they do not get support for their infant feeding goals. For example, your primary care doctor or the baby's pediatrician may recommend weaning, even if that does not support your feeding goals because they do not have the skills and knowledge to treat your existing issues. Remember, you would not ask an electrician to install the plumbing fixtures in your new house. By that same logic, do not assume that your doctor (or obstetrician) or the baby's pediatrician has the skills to help you with infant feeding. There is no judgment here. It is a simple fact. I am not criticizing pediatricians or other doctors for lacking training in lactation, just as I would not criticize an electrician for not having plumbing skills.

Table 10.1: Common Breastfeeding Problems

Sore nipples or nipple trauma	Try changing positions. Work on mastering a good latch. Be sure the chin touches the breast, and the baby gets an asymmetrical latch. Seek help with LLL, or Breastfeeding USA (or other volunteers). See an IBCLC for severe nipple trauma. Be aware of the signs of tongue-tie.
Latch difficulties	Try the laid-back position, football hold, and other alternative positions.
Plugged ducts	Nurse often. Apply warm compress, gently massage the plug, and use vibration. Do not allow this to fester. It can lead to mastitis.
Oral thrush	You and the baby need treatment. See your doctor.
Mastitis	Never self-treat mastitis. See your doctor and feed the baby/express milk as often as you can. Get lots of rest.
Engorgement	Express milk. If latching is ineffective, use reverse pressure softening to create more pliable breast tissue. Nurse or express milk as often as possible to relieve the engorgement. Cabbage leaves applied to the breast can help but do not overuse this remedy. (Do not confuse engorgement with edema.) Seek help from a lactation consultant.
Low supply	Express milk or nurse 10 -12 times in 24 hours. Consider power pumping. Find the cause of low supply and treat that specific cause.
Oversupply	Apply short-term block feeding (no more than one week) when the baby is nursing from one breast in 3-hour blocks of time before switching sides. (Do not overuse this strategy.) Seek skilled lactation care from peer counselors or a lactation consultant.

Complex and Challenging Cases

Many people will encounter some bumps in the road on the infant feeding journey. (Most parents do, whether feeding the baby human milk or formula. Infant feeding is not always an easy task.) You may have to deal with latch or positioning issues, maybe a bout of thrush or mastitis. You might have a delay in lactogenesis II or even struggle to feed your preemie. But what happens when all the complications seem to come on at once? My suggestions are to find the proper support, work on the issues that seem fixable, and remember that infant feeding takes a different path for each one of us. Do what you can to reach your infant feeding goals and modify your goals if that feels right. Here is the true story of a complex case.

TRUE STORY

Kate was four weeks postpartum, dealing with a low milk supply. She was breastfeeding her daughter despite the low supply, and the baby was also receiving donor milk supplements after every feeding. Her goal was to increase her milk supply and discontinue the supplements. The road leading to low supply included several essential factors known to impact milk supply negatively. It is hard to say in hindsight what the exact causes were. As you read her story, can you spot the red flags?

When Kate's labor showed no signs of starting, she was getting increasingly worried, and her caregiver suggested induction. She received induction of labor using Pitocin and epidural analgesia. In addition, she had all the requisite gear: electronic fetal monitor, catheter, and IV fluids. She was not eating food and was limited to slight position changes in the bed but no real movement. She endured a long labor, lasting 18 hours. She also had severe postpartum hemorrhage with 1.7 liters of blood loss (remember, the average vaginal delivery is associated with only about ½ a liter of blood loss.) Her milk had not come in by day five, and she suspected that something was wrong. During a follow-up evaluation with her caregiver, they identified Kate as having retained placenta. After removing the retained placenta fragment, she assumed that her milk would finally reach full volume, but it continued as low supply. Her doctor prescribed Reglan and sent her home. Over the next few days, she worked with her lactation consultant to investigate all sorts of angles. Was it poor latch and positioning? Was there a tongue tie present? Was the baby not effectively transferring milk?

The lactation consultant at the hospital thought the baby's latch *looked good*. Her pediatrician saw no concerns with latch or milk transfer, and a follow-up visit with another LC revealed no issues. Kate was pumping milk during the day to try to increase supply. It is unusual, but her baby was sleeping eight-nine hours at night at four weeks. Kate did pump twice at night but planned to wean off the nighttime pumping when she returned to work at two months postpartum. She hoped the baby would continue to sleep all night.

Finally, she spoke to another lactation consultant who saw a different picture. Her baby had a nursing blister on the upper lip, lips not flanged out, high palate, and recessed chin. In addition, Kate had slight nipple trauma and lingering pain. Some of these could be signs that the baby uses the lips too aggressively. Although no one had seen evidence of a tongue-tie, could there be more to the picture? Kate had to seek another opinion before she finally discovered that poor milk removal due to tongue-tie was likely contributing to her issues.

What Other Interventions, Situations, and Conditions in This Scenario Could Contribute to Low Milk Supply?

Kate's factors that could impact lactogenesis II and milk supply: induction with Pitocin, epidural analgesia, IV fluid, long stressful labor, postpartum blood loss, and retained placenta.

Infant factors that could impact supply: signs of a poor latch (lips not flanged, nursing blister), high palate, or not waking at night to nurse.

This scenario may sound extreme, but it is a true story. Unfortunately, this perfect storm for breastfeeding difficulties happens more frequently than it should. It might seem impossible to put the finger on one thing in Kate's story that caused her low supply. However, many red flags in this scenario deserve further investigation. Several of the possible causes of low supply may not have been preventable; some were preventable or avoidable if she had known in advance what the possible impact on breastfeeding could be.

Main Points From Kate's Story

- Kate opted for induction, but it was not medically necessary. Kate and her partner may not have felt this was optional because of information she received from her doctor, but it is always a good idea to question this overused intervention. Induction of labor is one piece that could have been avoided and quite possibly could have influenced several other birth factors on her list. Labor induction is also associated with great risk for postpartum hemorrhage (Ainsworth et al., 2017).

- Postpartum hemorrhage is a known risk for low milk supply.
- Pediatricians usually have no training in lactation support. Most pediatricians will not have the skills to accurately diagnose tongue, lip, or buccal ties (tethered oral tissues, TOTS).
- Some lactation consultants or counselors won't have the skills to identify tongue ties either. However, a skilled LC can perform an oral evaluation for your baby and describe the oral function or limitations of function that are present. If you have questions about oral restrictions and if they are impacting your baby's oral motor function, seek care with an expert who diagnoses and treats TOTS. You may need a second opinion, or a third.
- If you experience more than two or three birth interventions or other situations that could cause low milk supply, be aware of your increased risk for low milk supply. Be aggressive about getting the breastfeeding support you need to get started.
- Nighttime breastfeeding is essential. Even though Kate was pumping at night, she was missing out on the sensory input from her baby. Remember, breastfeeding is a sensory experience for the parent and the infant. Also, the baby is a much more effective milk removal system than the pump is. If the baby is available, choose direct breastfeeding, if possible.
- Four weeks old is generally too young for a breastfed baby to sleep eight hours. Infants can consume as much as one-third of their total daily intake at nighttime. This consumption is essential for proper growth and brain development.

Suppose you have multiple risk factors that may impact lactation (e.g., maternal diabetes, cesarean delivery, and premature infant). In that case, you will need to advocate for yourself from the moment your baby is born. Ask for the most robust breastfeeding support that is available. You may need to request more than one meeting with a lactation consultant during the hospital or birth center stay. Ask about local peer-to-peer breastfeeding support groups. Find out if your pediatrician's office has a lactation consultant on staff or if they recommend anyone. Practice skin-to-skin care several times a day or Kangaroo for 72. Remove milk 8-12 times every 24 hours. It may take time to bring your milk to full volume. If you need to supplement, remember that feeding your baby with any amount of human milk is a gift. Be proud of your hard work.

Dieting During Lactation

By the end of pregnancy, most people are ready to shed some weight and return to normal but the early postpartum period is not a good time to initiate any weight loss or calorie restriction. Most recommendations suggest waiting at least six to eight weeks before starting any weight loss strategies. Restricting your caloric intake or efforts to lose weight too soon could compromise milk production.

Slow Weight Loss is Best During Lactation

The good news is that you will lose several pounds during childbirth and the first few days after birth. Weight loss as a direct result of childbirth is estimated to be about seven pounds (3.17 kg) of baby weight and about three more pounds (1.36 kg) for the placenta and amniotic fluid. Over the next several days, maternal weight loss slowly continues due to shedding excess fluid.

It is important to feed yourself well during the immediate postpartum phase (and the entire postpartum year). Your physical and mental health *and milk supply depend on adequate nutrition,* specifically sufficient calorie intake. Many recommendations state that the low end of caloric intake during lactation is 1800 calories per day. This recommendation seems to be the minimum energy intake that one would aim for during lactation and would not be enough to support an active lifestyle or exercise routine while nursing. Specifically, 1800 calories per day may not be enough for many people to satisfy all the energy and nutrition requirements of maternal health and milk production.

Plan for slow weight loss in the first few weeks postpartum. Do not take any drastic measures to lose weight, restrict calories, or burn fat until after you and your baby firmly establish breastfeeding. Even then, be sure to plan weight loss with the slow and steady approach. A good rule of thumb is to lose only about 1 to 1.5 pounds (.45 - .68 kg) per week. Restricting calories to accelerate weight loss can put your milk production at risk, potentially lowering milk supply.

A slow and sensible approach to postpartum weight loss must take into that the entire body must recover from pregnancy and childbirth during a time when you're also lactating. Therefore, be vigilant about avoiding obvious junk food and junk drinks to maximize your intake of nutrient-dense foods. Here are some good recommendations:

- Eat well-balanced meals and snacks consisting of real, whole foods.
- Eat high-quality protein and organic vegetables. Lots of vegetables.Include healthy fats in your diet (omega-3 fatty acids are essential). Fats are essential building blocks for all hormone production in the body. In addition, fats are necessary to absorb vitamins A, D, E, and K. Fats are also essential for insulating your nerves. Don't buy into the outdated idea that all fat is bad. (Sugar and excessive intake of carbs are the real culprits of weight gain and ill health.) Be sure to avoid inflammatory oils.
- Eat foods rich in magnesium, calcium (leafy greens), and zinc.
- Be sure to include adequate sources of B vitamins, especially folate (B9) and B12. In addition, take the methyl versions of these two important vitamins, methyl folate, and methyl cobalamin.
- If you are a vegetarian or vegan, be sure to take a B complex with methyl cobalamin (B12). You will have to supplement because there are no good vegetable sources of B12.
- Drink plenty of water to quench your thirst (but no need to over hydrate).
- Avoid sugar, excess carbohydrates, and processed foods. These can lead to inflammation and accumulation of body fat.
- Limit caffeine to small amounts and watch your baby for reactions.

- Avoid alcohol. (It's unnecessary to pump and dump if you have a glass of wine, but it's a good idea to avoid all alcohol in the early weeks. Alcohol causes you dehydration and some does pass into your milk.)
- Avoid sweets, pastries, deep-fried foods, and processed snack foods.
- Avoid soda of all types. Soda is detrimental to blood sugar regulation. Even diet soda is unhealthy for you and gives you zero nutrients. It will not benefit your health or your milk supply. Giving up soda is a great way to improve your health.

Other Foods to Avoid

Lots of questions come up about what foods to avoid during lactation. Many anecdotal reports suggest that certain vegetables in the maternal diet cause gas or colic in infants. Most lactation consultants say that the idea that some foods cause gas for infants is just a myth. Some babies will, indeed, react to foods in the maternal diet. It is individual for everyone, and the only way to know if your baby is sensitive to your diet is to pay attention. If you discover a pattern of fussy infant behavior, loose stool, or even constipation, it may be worth it to eliminate the offending foods from your diet temporarily. Sometimes, it can be challenging to narrow down the foods causing irritation but start with the most popular offenders: dairy and eggs are the top allergens, but corn, fish, nuts, and soy can also cause problems. These foods can cause reactions in some sensitive babies. Reactions can range from crying and fussiness to more allergy-like symptoms. For example, babies with true allergies may exhibit a runny nose, itchy eyes, a skin rash or eczema, diaper rash, or even blood in the stool. If you suspect your baby is reacting to some foods in your diet, eliminate that food for three full weeks to determine if there is an improvement.

Does Exercise Impact Milk Production?

Most people can exercise without any impact on their milk supply. Again, use caution in getting started. You may want to wait until your body's milk supply is well established and your body has had some time to heal from the birth experience. Follow up with your caregiver at least one time before starting exercise. Also, be aware that it can be best to postpone exercise until after the lochia (bleeding and discharge after childbirth) has stopped, usually a few weeks after delivery. If you begin exercise after the lochia has stopped but you suddenly start bleeding again, you may be doing too much, too soon. Take another week or two to rest and recover.

Some people recommend wearing a looser-fitting sports bra than they might use if not lactating. Also, consider the timing of feeding your baby or pumping before exercise. You may find it uncomfortable to workout, go for a jog, or even do an hour of yoga with breasts full of milk. Nurse your baby just before you plan to exercise. This practice will allow for a more comfortable fit for your sports bra and less chance of leaking milk.

TRUE STORY

In 2019, ultrarunner Jasmin Paris won the Montane Spine Race, a 268-mile trek along the Pennine Way National Trail in England and Scotland. Her race time was just over 83 hours. At the time, she was nursing her 14-month-old baby. She stopped along the run to express milk for her baby and still beat everyone else in the race.

CHAPTER 11

Lactation Interference: Breastfeeding Management Factors

In the introduction of this book, I suggested that lactation is like a card game. Your strategy depends not only on the hand you were dealt but also on the cards you pick up as you play. Breastfeeding management is one of the most important cards that you pick up along the lactation journey. Breastfeeding management refers to the professional consultations you seek, the advice you receive, and your management of milk production, milk removal, and feeding.

The first feeding management you will encounter will likely be during the first hours after birth. Nursing staff, some with lactation training and some without it, are usually ready to assist with positioning and basic breastfeeding skills. Some hospitals have highly trained lactation consultants who meet with families for early breastfeeding consultations. Some hospitals, however, do not have board-certified lactation consultants (IBCLCs) on staff but may have RNs who provide basic lactation care in the early postpartum hours.

After leaving the hospital, however, getting the proper lactation care and support can be challenging. Sometimes lactation care is delivered in a suitable timeframe by the right person with the appropriate training and experience. However, that scenario is likely the exception, not the rule. Because of various reasons, getting the most appropriate lactation support is often difficult. In my opinion, it is often because of the ambiguous nature of breastfeeding support. To a new parent, the labor and delivery nurse and the baby's pediatrician both might seem like knowledgeable options for seeking lactation care. In reality, it is unlikely that either one has significant training in lactation management. Because these professionals are in allied health fields that revolve around infants, it would be easy to assume they have a high degree of lactation knowledge but they usually do not. This ambiguity leads to many people unknowingly seeking care from the wrong professional and often leads to mismanagement of lactation.

Inaccurate information and bad advice can often lead to poor lactation management as well. Sometimes, people can unintentionally prolong breastfeeding issues because they unknowingly followed bad advice. For example, trying to remedy or resolve complicated breastfeeding problems at home without professional help can often escalate pain, infection, and feeding issues. Likewise, following the advice of family and friends can sometimes lead to mismanagement.

It is important to remember that there is variation among providers within the field of trained lactation professionals, just like any other specialization in healthcare. Sometimes, it is best to seek a second opinion if the lactation support you are getting does not feel right or meet your family's needs, even if it comes from someone with appropriate training.

This section highlights some of the ways that poor lactation management can negatively affect breastfeeding.

Bad Advice

You probably already know that once you are pregnant, looking to adopt, and considering breastfeeding, the unsolicited advice starts flowing to you from everywhere. People want to share their personal stories, struggles, and information about parenting and breastfeeding. Some of the advice is valid and may work for you, but some may not. There are several things to keep in mind when you get solicited or unsolicited lactation advice from anyone:

- Consider the source. Is this person a breastfeeding expert? Does this person have any personal experience with lactation, infant feeding, nighttime feeding, or the issues they are talking about? Sometimes, family and friends can be trusted sources of information but be careful and trust your gut. Do research when necessary. Taking advice from healthcare professionals without lactation training can be risky. Unless they have lactation credentials, they are likely not trained in the management and care for the breastfeeding dyad.

- When did this person have their experience with infant feeding? Was it a few years ago? Was it in the 1970s or 1980s? If it has been more than a few years, consider that breastfeeding "wisdom" may have shifted and changed a bit since then. For example, a friend told me that in the 1970s her mother was advised by her child's pediatrician to put the baby to bed with a bottle in one corner of the crib and a hardboiled egg in the other. This would allow the baby to quench thirst or hunger without bothering the parents during the night. For a breastfeeding parent, this is terrible advice because nighttime nursing is essential for maintaining a full milk supply. Further, a hardboiled egg is a terrible idea for an infant; this a choking hazard! Be *skeptical* about taking advice that involves limitations. For example, you may hear, "Only nurse for ten minutes on each side" or "Be sure to feed the baby only every three hours – not before." These two gems are actual quotes my clients have heard from their doctors. Breastfeeding, especially preemies and new babies (and probably older), cannot functionally feed within a set of arbitrary limitations. The baby does not know that he should finish each side in ten minutes. Infants don't operate on our schedule. Several books recommend strict time limits for breastfeeding and arbitrary time guidelines accompanied by strict routines (wake, feed, nap on a rigid cycle). *Be careful with this type of advice.* Know that unlimited access to the breast and feeding on demand form the basis of building and maintaining your milk supply. This practice also allows you to meet your baby's needs in a timely manner. The American Academy of Pediatrics has come out against these rigid, prescriptive methods. Avoid this advice at all costs.
- Be wary of any method or book that advises that their way is the best way or the right way to breastfeed. *Forget that right now.* There are many ways to make human milk work in your baby's life. There is no one way to get it right. There is no one

way to latch, feed, or position your baby for pain-free nursing. So, do not buy into these programs and methods. There are many ways to get it right.

- The internet. This option can be a true lifesaver or a source of terrible infant-feeding information, depending on where you look. Even information coming from sources that *appear valid* can be outdated, wrong, and even detrimental to the breastfeeding relationship. How do you know who to trust? Start with organizations that make breastfeeding their only focus and do not have any other agenda. They should not be trying to make sales or market products. This means that getting breastfeeding advice from Enfamil, Similac, Medela, Spectra, or any manufacturers of feeding products or devices is not a good idea. Their main goal is to sell you their product, not to provide sound, unbiased lactation advice.
- Breastfeeding support organizations are available to help. La Leche League (worldwide), Breastfeeding USA, Baby Café USA, Black Mothers Breastfeeding Association, ROSE (Reaching Our Sisters Everywhere), Australian Breastfeeding Association, National Breastfeeding Helpline (UK), The Breastfeeding Network (UK), and many others like them are groups and organizations that offer breastfeeding support. Many of these organizations provide help lines you can call. In addition, many offer online and in-person support groups.
- Remember books? We're all so connected electronically these days that it can be easy to overlook books as your source of breastfeeding info but don't discount this option. There are so many good books available about lactation and making milk. Head to your local library if you don't want to invest any money but consider buying or borrowing at least one excellent breastfeeding book as a resource.

Scheduled Feeds

When a baby is born, parents routinely ask a set of similar questions concerning infant feeding:

- When do we feed the baby?
- How often does the baby need to nurse?

There are two schools of thought on feeding times for new babies: responsive/cue-based feeding and scheduled feeding.

The infant governs responsive feeding (i.e., cue-based or on-demand feeding). This approach involves watching the baby for feeding cues and responding promptly, allowing the baby access to the breast whenever he displays feeding cues.

Scheduled feeding is quite different. This approach has preset times for feeding. Specifically, each day is the same, with feedings occurring only on the schedule. This approach does not account for growth spurts, cluster feeding, non-nutritive comfort nursing, extra feeding during infant illness, or other off-schedule feeding needs. This approach is likely a hangover from formula feeding.

Scheduled feeds can negatively impact breastfeeding and milk supply. Hormones drive the milk supply in the first hours and days of breastfeeding. Quickly, a shift occurs to allow the infant to determine the milk volume by *frequency of breastfeeding and how much milk is removed* from the breast. Scheduled feeding directly impacts this system; if not enough milk is removed or not removed frequently enough, the body will down-regulate the amount of milk production, lowering milk supply. Cue-based feeding is the best practice for generating a full milk supply and maintaining it. Respond to the baby whenever you see feeding cues.

Responsive cue-based feeding has several advantages:

- Encourages initiation and maintenance of full milk supply
- Allows the baby to accurately set the volume of milk that your body will make. (This is why one person can safely feed twins without worrying about over or under supply.)
- Ensures that the baby's needs for milk, nutrition, antibodies, and immune factors, for being held, warmth, and comfort are being met.
- Allows the baby to boost milk supply for growth spurts and receive tailor-made antibodies during an illness without restriction.

The American Academy of Pediatrics states that following birth in a hospital, "infants must be continuously accessible to the mother by rooming-in arrangements that facilitate around-the-clock, on-demand feeding for the healthy infant" (AAP & ACOG, 2017). Further, the Academy of Breastfeeding Medicine recommends on-demand (cue-based) feeding and states that restricting feeding times may be harmful (Holmes et al., 2013).

Scheduled feeding is associated with slow weight gain and early weaning. Responsive cue-based feeding is associated with a longer duration (in terms of months) of breastfeeding than scheduled feeding, more exclusive breastfeeding in the first six months of life, and more frequent feeds during the day (Little et al., 2018).

Word of Caution

There are many books, blogs, and "experts" promoting the idea of scheduled feeds and rigorous parenting approaches that don't consider that the infant's needs change from day to day and week to week throughout the first year. Be cautious when following advice that involves restricting feeds and creating a heavily scheduled routine of infant wake-feed-sleep times. These methods will not meet infant needs and are not supportive of breastfeeding. Rather, their design is to suit parents' needs and lifestyles.

Pacifier Use

There is some controversy over pacifiers (dummies) for exclusively breastfed babies. Babies are born with a strong suck reflex. The sucking reflex ensures that the baby will feed effectively – an essential innate life skill for your newborn. From a pro-breastfeeding standpoint, it makes sense that the newborns meet all their sucking needs at the breast, not with a breast substitute. This practice ensures that feeding on demand can occur. The parent receives the sensory input from suckling that releases oxytocin and prolactin, which develop and maintain the maternal milk supply. Introducing a pacifier can supplant the breast to meet sucking needs (but not the need for food). The overuse of pacifiers can lead to the risk of missing or sleeping through feedings and not enough time at the breast. Studies show that breastfed babies who use a pacifier may breastfeed, on average, slightly less than those who do not use a pacifier –

one less feeding in 24 hours (Aarts et al., 1999). While one skipped feeding may not seem like much, it is an incredible amount when added up over the days of the first year. It could mean fewer calories for your baby and lowered milk supply for you.

The American Academy of Pediatrics recommends that breastfed babies not use pacifiers until the dyad firmly establishes breastfeeding. The Baby-Friendly Hospital Initiative does not allow the use of pacifiers in Baby-Friendly hospitals, as the early use of pacifiers may interfere with breastfeeding behaviors and intentions in the early days of lactation. Babies need to meet all their sucking needs at the breast in the first few weeks of life. This practice ensures that the infant has access to milk necessary for growth and development. In addition, on-demand breastfeeding instead of pacifier use provides sufficient sensory nipple stimulation that is important for milk production. Some studies have found that pacifiers contribute to the interruption of exclusive breastfeeding (Buccini et al., 2016, 2017).

There are some known benefits of pacifiers for therapeutic purposes. For example, pacifiers can be useful therapy and oral training for premature infants. In addition, there may be benefits associated with reducing the SIDS risk when used at bedtime only.

Apart from the possible interference with breastfeeding, there are other known risks. Pacifier use is associated with an increase in ear infections (otitis media) during the second six months of life. For older babies (24+ months), there is an increased risk of dental problems. Bacteria and fungi can also colonize pacifiers.

The use of a pacifier may be helpful for some people. For those experiencing little or no issues with milk supply, infant latch, or other breastfeeding issues, using a pacifier may be of no harm whatsoever. If you are already experiencing breastfeeding difficulties or low milk supply, you may want to avoid pacifier use. Limited use of the pacifier may be an excellent middle-ground approach. Also, remember to eliminate it if your baby has recurrent ear infections. Bottom line, wait until you firmly establish breastfeeding before introducing a pacifier (four to six weeks) and then use it conservatively. Eliminate it if breastfeeding issues or ear infections increase.

Most Important Reasons to Avoid Pacifiers

- The pacifier does not feed your baby. Instead, it allows your baby to meet his/her sucking needs at a great cost.
- Using a pacifier does not stimulate the breast. When an infant uses a pacifier, she meets her sucking needs without providing your breast's vital input to continue milk production. In nature's design, infants meet their sucking needs *at the breast*. This connection ensures continued input for the breast to maintain production of the milk supply.

Respond to feeding cues by offering the breast, not a substitute.

TRUE STORY

Jeena and her newborn got breastfeeding off to a great start. Things were going well for the first two months. Then, a week or two into the baby's third month, Jeena noticed a decline in her milk supply, and suddenly, her baby was not gaining weight. During a visit with a lactation consultant, they discussed all possibilities for the drop in milk production. Jeena had started no new medications or routines with her baby except one. She had introduced a pacifier. The baby took the pacifier primarily at night, and Jeena also offered it to her baby sometimes during the day. Unfortunately, the pacifier use caused enough lactation interference that the baby missed feedings and caused Jeena to miss feeding cues. This resulted in fewer feeding sessions and subsequently caused a drop in milk production.

Tech-Based Separation

Here's one you have likely not heard of before: tech-based separation. This concept refers to the separation that exists when parents use tech-based gadgets or interventions to promote "happy solitude" for their baby. For example, any type of technology such as an infant seat, swing, smart bassinet, automated crib, or white noise machine that promotes long stretches of sleep or long periods of solitude for infants is a method of tech-based separation. Your baby may be in the same room with you, but if he is in a smart bassinet sleeping through his feeding time because he has been artificially lulled into a deep sleep, he will not be at the breast. The same goes for any tech that promotes solitary situations for your baby. Unfortunately, Mother Nature does not have an alternative safety net for solitary infants. Infants should never spend time alone or experience long stretches without parental contact. Their safety net is you.

For most of human history, infants existed in societies where everyone inherently knew the dangers of leaving an infant alone. Consider this: while we may be close to the baby sitting in the infant seat, this is only a modern illusion of togetherness. Infants need close bodily contact, night and day, with their parents. Using tech-based separation tools often interferes with breastfeeding because infants are encouraged to be quiet, solitary, happily entertained, or asleep for much longer periods than they might otherwise be. This can cause missed feeding times, suppression of feeding cues, over-sleeping, lack of sufficient human contact (which is truly essential for babies), loneliness, and frustration. It can also lead to lowered milk production because feeding cannot happen when the baby is separated from the parent. When milk is not removed from the breast, milk production breaks down.

Many of the tech-based separation tools are high-tech but some are low-tech as well. Consider all these tools that have the potential to contribute to separation:

Table 11.1: Tools that Promote Parent/Infant Separation

High-tech separation tools	Low-tech separation tools
Smart bassinet	Sleep suits
Swings	Pacifier
White noise	Tight swaddling
Automated bouncer seat	Contoured foam infant seat Improper use of car seat

You may be thinking that this list is too extreme. After all, who doesn't have a few of the items on this list? We are conditioned to believe that these gadgets are safe and necessary for modern parenting, right? The reality is that we have lost touch (literally) with the ways of traditional human parenting. Human touch is an integral part of the infant survival system. There are no substitutions or alternatives.

Having said all that, I also want to express my deep understanding that we all long for some helpful solutions when it comes to parenting. It is a job that is nearly impossible to achieve for an individual. No doubt, the solitary nature of being the primary caregiver-parent gave rise to these kinds of separation tools in the first place. So, what is the solution?

Finding Balance

First, focus on holding your baby and meeting your baby's human contact needs, and *nurturing at the breast*. Practice skin-to-skin care when you can. Follow your baby's feeding cues and respond by offering the breast every time. Keep your baby in your room at night, in a nearby crib, or a safe sleep situation in the adult bed.

Second, use your high-tech (and low-tech) tools with moderation. You will need to find safe ways to put your baby down when you do something that does not allow you to hold her safely. For example, you will have to find a safe place for your baby while you take a shower or cook a hot meal. You may need to put your baby down to help your toddler. There are times when parents need a safe place, besides a good infant carrier, to securely place the baby for short periods. In these instances, it is acceptable to place your baby safely in a bouncy seat or another seat that safely holds infants. The key is to use these in moderation. Like the car seat, these tools are necessary, but overusing them is a mistake. Do not allow your baby to stay too long in any infant bassinet, swing, crib, seat, or other product that promotes separation and solitude for your baby. Do not overuse pacifiers, sleepsuits, or other low-tech products that promote prolonged sleep periods or allow for skipped feedings. Use your best judgment with these tech-based solutions.

As always, if you suddenly realize that you are relying on these solutions because you have met your limit and you feel completely (or even partially) overwhelmed, please reach out to your support network and look for help. You need human connection, too, just like your baby. Parenting is too big of a job for one person with limited support.

Nipple Shield - Double-Edged Sword?

The nipple shield, a thin silicone sheath that covers the nipple during feeding, has a long and colorful history in lactation. According to the authors of *Breastfeeding and Human Lactation*, nipple shields have been in use for hundreds of years and have had varying degrees of impact on breastfeeding (Wambach & Riordan, 2016). The authors also report that nipple shields of the past were made of "lead (which caused brain damage in babies), wax, wood, gum elastic, pewter, tin, horn, bone, ivory, silver and glass" (Wambach & Riordan, 2016). Fortunately, things have changed for the better. Today's nipple shields are thin, pliable silicone. Nipple shields can be beneficial for some, even making breastfeeding possible when nothing else helps. For others, the nipple shield can be a trap that prevents successful breastfeeding. This tool is a classic case of a double-edged sword. As such, it is wise to use caution with the nipple shield.

Who Needs a Nipple Shield? How Will it Help With Infant Feeding?

Using a nipple shield can be advantageous in certain situations. For example, nipple shields can provide the structure that some nipples lack and help the nipple maintain its shape inside the shield. This additional help can be useful for people with flat nipples, nipples that do not evert easily, or inelastic nipples. Under normal conditions, the baby is responding to the stimulation of the nipple inside his mouth. The baby feeds well when he can easily detect the nipple at the juncture of the hard and soft palate. Sometimes, as in the case of flat nipples, the nipple may lack the structure needed to stimulate this part of the baby's palate. A nipple shield can provide that structure. In addition, even when the nipple is everted and has good structure, some infants have oral anatomy complications that make using the nipple shield advantageous. For example, a nipple shield can be useful if the baby has palate anomalies (bubble palate), recessed lower jaw, weak suck (especially preterm infants or babies with neurological problems), or low muscle tone. There are other reasons people may choose to use a nipple shield, including overcoming nipple damage or when an infant is demonstrating great difficulty trying to latch onto the breast. In many of these instances, the nipple shield can provide the therapeutic assistance the baby needs to make a successful latch and maintain the latch for a full feeding.

Disadvantages of Using a Nipple Shield

As I mentioned earlier, using this tool can also have unintended consequences. Most of the unintended negative effects come from using a nipple shield when there is another, more infant-friendly solution for the feeding problem. For example, suppose an infant appears to have excessive difficulty latching in the hours after birth. In that case, a well-meaning caregiver who lacks the skills for assisting with latch difficulties may hastily propose using a nipple shield. This solution may appear to be a quick fix because it can enable the baby to latch onto the breast successfully. However, nipple shields do not come with advice or a how-to-manual for resolving underlying problems. Further, how does one eliminate the shield once the dyad resolves breastfeeding complications? This can cause undue stress for parents, realizing days later that they would like to nurse without the shield but lack the informational resources to make that happen. Many times, this is an entirely avoidable situation. Parents can make changes that elicit more of the baby's innate breast-seeking skills and reflexes with the proper guidance from a skilled lactation consultant. This assistance can facilitate a pathway forward for the infant to latch well and avoid the nipple shield altogether.

One concern with nipple shields is that unless the shield is applied correctly or is overused when not truly necessary, it could lead to breastfeeding problems and obstacles. Some of the difficulties include suboptimal milk transfer, nipple trauma such as abrasion or pinching, and creating unintended infant preference for nursing with the shield (in other words, the baby refuses to nurse without the shield in place). In addition, in the case of suboptimal milk transfer, immediate downstream consequences can negatively impact infant health. For instance, if the baby cannot extract an optimal amount of milk from the breast during every feeding, the breast begins to decrease milk output, which causes lowered supply. Lowered supply can quickly lead to slow or insufficient infant weight gain, recommendations for formula supplementation, and even weaning.

What is the Solution for Nipple Shields?

My recommendations align with what most lactation resources and consultants suggest. Only use the nipple shield if you truly need one. More importantly, it must provide an improved quality of infant feeding when other options do not. How can you tell if you genuinely need a nipple shield? That answer will be different for everyone. Only you can be the judge. One good rule of thumb is to try several things before introducing a nipple shield. Think of it as a last resort. That said, I also see the nipple shield as a practical step on the feeding journey for someone likely to throw in the towel without using the shield. If you are on the verge of abandoning breastfeeding because of nipple trauma or other feeding difficulties and the shield helps you, then use it. Just be cautious and work with lactation support to correct the problems and to create a plan for eliminating the shield.

General Tips for Using a Nipple Shield

- Try latch adjustments, position changes, and lots skin-to-skin before introducing the nipple shield in the first days after birth.
- Think of it as a temporary step on your infant feeding journey if you use a shield.
- Correct the underlying problems if you can (correct poor latch, allow damaged nipples to heal, give your preemie time to grow and gain feeding skills) before eliminating the shield.
- Have a plan for weaning from the shield when you and the baby are ready.
- To wean from the shield, start feedings with the shield and remove it during the feeding, sometime after the letdown.
- Try a skin-to-skin day, where you and the baby stay skin-to-skin all day and allow the baby to use innate feeding skills without the shield.
- Use a nipple everter instead of the nipple shield to draw out flat nipples before nursing. Some people recommend applying ice to help the nipple achieve good structure before nursing.
- Most LCs recommend close monitoring of infants who use a nipple shield. Count wet and dirty diapers, watch for signs of dehydration and slow weight gain, check the baby's weight more often *at the doctor's office* with a professional-grade scale (not a home scale).

- Clean your nipple shield consistently.
- Be aware of inadequate milk transfer. Be sure your breasts are much less full after feeding. Also, watch for plugged ducts, which could indicate that the breast is not draining fully during feeding.
- Some LCs recommend pumping after feeding with the nipple shield. Again, if you choose to pump or hand express milk after feeding with the shield, have a plan for gradually eliminating these extra pumping sessions after issues resolve.
- Don't ever cut the nipple shield. This practice is an outdated and potentially dangerous concept. Instead, always leave the shield in its original shape and condition.
- My best advice for nipple shields is to work with skilled lactation care, especially if you feel you need help while using it or when trying to eliminate it.

Nighttime Feeding and Sleep Training

Oh, sleep! This topic could fill an entire book. However, in the interest of brevity, I will include information here related to sleep and lactation. For more general information on breastfeeding and sleep, three books I recommend are *Sweet Sleep* by Diana West, *Sleeping with Your Baby: A Parent's Guide to Co-Sleeping* by Dr. James McKenna, and *Safe Infant Sleep*, also by Dr. James McKenna.

As adults (teenagers not included), we prefer our waking hours to occur during the day and reserve our sleeping hours for overnight. For newborns, there is no distinct night and day. New babies sleep and wake without a clear pattern for the first few weeks of life. If your baby could make an agenda for each day, sleeping would be high on the priority list, but not necessarily sleeping through the night. Why? Feeding is also a high priority, and babies accomplish this throughout the night at the breast.

Baby's Agenda

- Eating
- Snuggling, being held

- Sleeping and growing
- Peeing and pooping
- Repeat, night and day

From a strictly mechanical point of view, breastfeeding a new baby works well when infants are fed on-demand, including nighttime. Remember, breasts make milk in response to milk removal. If milk sits in the breast without being removed, feedback is initiated that tells the breast to slow or stop production, even during the overnight hours. This message is not one you want to send to the breast overnight, or at any time while the baby is young. So, in developing and maintaining a full milk supply, *you must remove milk in the overnight hours*.

In addition to keeping up milk production, nighttime breastfeeding is essential for calorie intake for your newborn. Human milk digests in about two hours in the infant's stomach. This easy digestion allows for frequent refueling, which gives the breast the round-the-clock message to keep up milk production. It also provides the baby with the necessary calories to do the most important job of the first year: grow. Babies grow while they are asleep, so it makes sense that they need to keep a steady supply of calories on board throughout the night.

Restricting nighttime feeding can be *disastrous for your milk supply*. Human parents are not meant to take extended breaks from breastfeeding until well into the first year after the baby starts solid food. Further, human infants should not go for long stretches without food, ever. Keep in mind that breastfeeding a new baby is much different than breastfeeding a five- or seven-month-old. Older babies are more efficient and can nurse more quickly, getting what they need in less time, and this means less nighttime nursing for most older babies. Some babies will sleep for a long stretch at the beginning of the night, but in the early weeks and months, it is not advisable to let newborns go more than three hours without feeding. When breastfeeding is well established, after six to eight weeks, you may consider letting the baby stretch the first sleep period to about four hours. After one long stretch at the beginning of the night, babies usually wake every two to three hours during the rest of the night for feeding. This period is also the time of day when milk production is at its highest. Restricting feeding at this time could cause engorgement, plugged ducts, a decrease in milk supply, and painful breasts that prevent latching. Again, restricting nighttime feeding for small babies, preemies, and jaundice babies can be problematic. Feed them around the clock.

Many people are interested in sleep training to get their baby to sleep through the night. It is tempting to think that this is a solution. I have been there – my oldest child did not sleep through the night until she was 19 months old. Rest assured, it does not usually take that long. We had some unusual circumstances. Trust me, I know you are exhausted and wishing for a good night's rest, and sleep training *sounds* like a good solution but it isn't.

Allowing your baby to cry him or herself to sleep will raise cortisol levels and bring babies from protest (e.g., active crying, high-stress levels) to despair (e.g., no crying to conserve valuable energy reserves but cortisol stress levels are still high). Actively meeting your baby's needs by nighttime feeding is not always easy, but it is part of the compassionate care you provide as a parent. Please read about the risks associated with sleep training.

Fortunately, breastfeeding provides a calming response. As you know, breastfeeding is a sensory experience. Mother Nature intended breastfeeding to be an exchange of the senses between parent and baby. This sensory input directs our hormones, primarily oxytocin and prolactin, to produce milk and enhance loving responses when the baby shows signs of readiness to feed or neediness for cuddling, holding, and warmth (or whatever the reason). Oxytocin is also the hormone of tranquility and bonding. These hormones are in place to make milk and help you feel good about breastfeeding and parenting. In addition, these relaxing hormones can help people cope with some factors (like nighttime feedings) that may be frustrating at first. Of course, by bringing your baby to the breast throughout the night, you're feeding him. In addition, you're also giving yourself a dose of the oxytocin cocktail that will help facilitate feelings of calmness, enhance your parenting behaviors, help you bond with the baby, and of course, help keep milk production at a high volume.

Aside from the great potential for decreasing your milk supply, there are other risks of not feeding at night as well. First, breastfeeding is protective against sudden infant death syndrome (SIDS). The nighttime waking could be the mechanism that offers this protection. Formula-fed infants wake less often and have a higher risk of dying from SIDS than breastfed infants. Second, nighttime nursing is important for stalling the return of fertility. Long stretches between nursing sessions will likely bring fertility faster than short durations between feedings. For breastfeeding to help control your fertility, it is essential to nurse around the clock. Third, breast milk can contribute to sleep patterns in infants. Breast milk contains tryptophan, an amino acid that is a precursor to melatonin. The body uses melatonin to induce sleep onset in the evenings and regulate sleep. Research shows that melatonin is abundant in nocturnal breast milk and may improve infant sleep (Cohen-Engler et al., 2012). Melatonin is not present in infant formula (Cohen-Engler et al., 2012). Finally, breastfed babies can take in as much as 20-30% of their total daily calories during the overnight hours. This intake represents a substantial share of their total milk consumption.

Final Thoughts on Sleep Training and Nighttime Feeding

I strongly recommend against sleep training. It is not biologically sound, not supportive of your milk production, not compassionate care for your baby, and represents a misguided approach to nighttime infant care and infant feeding. The bottom line is this: babies need to eat during the night. Your milk must move out of the breast overnight. There are no magical solutions for a workaround.

Use extreme caution with any book, method, app, program, class, or sleep coach who promises that babies will sleep or should sleep 8-12 hours by the time they reach two months or three months old. Be skeptical of any program that suggests that babies should sleep according to a prescribed pattern of sleep and waking, even including the number of minutes for waking and sleeping. Every single baby is different and has different physical and emotional needs. The infant sleep apps and training methods do not account for individual differences and needs. Therefore, sleep training apps, books, strategies, and programs are generally far off base for meeting your baby's needs and for supporting milk production. Nighttime feeding is not always easy, but it is an optimal way to meet your infant's biological needs.

While researching sleep training and infant sleep apps online, I found many comments from lactation consultants (in an LC forum) about their clients' experiences with sleep training programs and apps. Many lactation consultants notice a negative impact on milk production when their clients use sleep training. Some LCs even notice that their clients have more negative mental health outcomes when they use sleep training and apps. Here is what other LCs say about many popular but harsh sleep training programs and apps:

- (This sleep training app) is a fast track to weaning and supplementing.
- Many sleep programs are not sleep programs. They are scheduled "underfeeding" methods.
- Every one of my clients who used (this particular) sleep program has had milk supply issues.
- These newer programs are all a variation of the old cry-it-out method.
- Denying food to your baby during the night is irresponsible.
- These sleep training programs are *incompatible* with healthy infant feeding.
- Many babies end up failing to thrive due to sleep training.
- This (particular) app suggests that night waking for infants is due to parental associations. Blaming parents for infant waking is not ethical. Night waking is a normal biological function for infants. It's protective.
- Some of my clients followed all the "wake windows" (from this sleep training app), and their babies did not sleep. This was a major contributor to parental postpartum anxiety.
- I counsel my clients to stop over-tracking, follow the baby's cues, and use their own parental instincts. Stop watching the clock and let go of the sleep obsession.
- My recommendation is to delete the app.
- An overwhelming percent of my clients using sleep programs and apps are struggling with anxiety, and using the apps intensifies their worry and uneasiness.
- Some of my clients feel their babies fail when they are awake longer than the app suggests; they wonder what is wrong

with their baby because he doesn't follow the rules. Infants do not know the rules.

Misinterpretation of Infant Behavior

Sometimes, when parents perceive that their baby is not satisfied with breastfeeding, they tend to give up breastfeeding before reaching their own breastfeeding goals. Several studies show that the parent's perception about whether their baby is satisfied by breastfeeding plays into the decision to abandon lactation (Gatti, 2008; Neifert & Bunik, 2013). Furthermore, many parents base these decisions on the misinterpretation of infant behavior. In other words, even when the available milk supply adequately nourishes an infant, parents can misread infant behavior, which leads them to conclude that something is wrong with breastfeeding.

The Infant Feeding and Practice Study II (Fein et al., 2008) was a longitudinal study that followed hundreds of families throughout their baby's first year. This study questioned over 1,000 people why they weaned during the first year. The most frequent response for weaning the baby from the breast was, "the baby was not satisfied." According to Jan Tedder, a board-certified lactation consultant, parents might observe behaviors such as "crying, hard to calm, difficult to wake up to feed, 'restless' sleeping, frequent awakenings at night, or seemingly inattentive to or uninterested in his or her mother" (Tedder, 2015) and interpret them as a sign of breastfeeding insufficiency. All of these actions are normal infant behavior that does not necessarily signal infant hunger or breast milk insufficiency.

Part of the learning curve for parents is reading their baby's signals. Every parent must go through a period of trial and error to understand their baby's needs. If your baby is not calmed by feeding or does not seem satisfied after feeding, offer the breast again. In addition, try these strategies:

- Allow the baby to determine when each feeding is over. Specifically, let the baby release the breast on his own.
- Do not limit feeding to an arbitrary time (for example, eight minutes on each side). This is not conducive to milk production or healthy feeding practices.

- Use massage and compression techniques while breastfeeding and pumping to help your body move more milk toward the nipple.
- Wear your baby in a sling or infant carrier.
- Practice Kangaroo Care before and after feeding.
- Pay attention to your baby's fussy times of the day. Many babies have a specific time when they are temperamental. This is not always a signal that they are hungry. It could simply be a pattern. Many call these "the witching hours." Offer the breasts or use other calming techniques.
- Try co-bathing. Taking a warm bath with your baby is a great way to calm a fussy baby. If your baby is hungry, nurse while in the bath. Read more about this in the section in Part II called *Baby won't latch*.

Early Use of Bottles

Babies can be exclusively fed with human milk, even if the baby is not directly feeding at the breast. In this part of the world, bottle feeding is the most common alternative. However, many lactation professionals caution against the early use of bottles because of the potential to negatively impact breastfeeding.

The breast and the bottle are radically dissimilar. While both "designs" dispense infant food, their delivery mechanisms require the use of different approaches, different facial and oral muscles, and levels of skill. For years, the major criticism of the early use of bottles was attributed to nipple confusion. We define nipple confusion as an infant's frustration by switching between direct breastfeeding and bottle feeding. Because your baby will use distinctly different skills at the breast than with a bottle, he might become irritated and fussy when switching between these two. Many lactation consultants suggest that nipple confusion is not about the nipples (whether natural or artificial). Instead, the confusion centers on flow preference. Bottle flow can vary, but it is usually faster and easier to get milk from the bottle than from the breast. As a result, an infant will have to work a little harder to get the milk to letdown while breastfeeding. For this reason, experts recommend slow-flow nipples for those who use bottles *and* put the baby to the breast.

Some lactation professionals suggest that the early use of bottles can pave the way for a host of breastfeeding problems, including breast refusal and suboptimal sucking skills (Newman, 1990). The Baby-Friendly Ten Steps initiative created by the World Health Organization (WHO) and UNICEF cautions against the use of bottles or pacifiers in the early weeks. Step nine states, "Give no artificial teats or pacifiers (also called dummies or soothers) to breastfeeding infants." The rationale is that the baby's intense need for suckling should be satisfied at the breast and not with artificial nipples (including bottles) because it can interfere with correct suckling techniques and impact the maternal milk supply. In *The Womanly Art of Breastfeeding*, La Leche League International recommends waiting several weeks until breastfeeding is well established before introducing any artificial nipples or bottle feeding (Wiessinger et al., 2010).

Alternative feeding methods include bottle feeding with slow flow nipples, cup feeding, spoon-feeding, an oral syringe, or dropper.

Too Much Technology

For thousands of years, infant feeding and baby care have been essential human skills. Indeed, for most of those years, people have had success with breastfeeding unaccompanied by the technology, gadgets, and gear we use today for breastfeeding and infant care. While there are clear benefits from using some of the tools and tech available today, there is a point at which the overuse or misuse of gadgets can interfere with the breastfeeding relationship and even negatively impact your milk supply. In addition, some of the technology that today's families use can compromise parenting skills and create a separation of the dyad that is not conducive to breastfeeding.

Before I begin, I would like to clarify that *I am not fundamentally opposed to using technology and gadgets, especially if these can help preserve the breastfeeding relationship when it might otherwise be abandoned.* I do not specifically recommend that you avoid all the products addressed in this discussion. My goal here is to give you some warning that the tools and gadgets you might want to use can sometimes create problems for breastfeeding. Often, these products and tools appear to help or benefit parents with situations that seem otherwise overwhelming. Be warned that product manufacturers will not report that their products could compromise or interfere with lactation and the parent-child relationship.

Many times (but not always), parenting skills can be a more baby-friendly solution to infant feeding and baby care issues. Developing your parenting skills involves more time and effort, but the advantages far outweigh the use of gadgets and tools to meet your baby's needs. Once you have developed the skills of parenting and breastfeeding, you and your child develop deeply connected bonds. Your baby learns to trust you and other humans, which is the basis for forming relationships. Without the interference of technology, you and your baby are biochemically connected, always sensing the cues from each other. This connection enables parents to intuitively tune into their infant's cues and behavior and provide the right environment for meeting their needs. Most of the time, tools and tech are a poor substitute for human interaction, human touch, and human connection, all of which your baby craves.

Overuse or improper use of infant tech can include the following:

1. *Using an infant weight scale at home is a recipe for trouble.* This tool sounds like a great idea that may even assist parents by monitoring a baby's weight gain without having to go to the pediatrician's office or by doing weighted feeds. The downsides of the home baby scale are numerous. Most at-home infant weight scales are not sensitive enough to perform weighted feeds, and they can generally be quite inaccurate as well. One parent told me she supplemented after a weighted feed because the scale only reflected a small gain. Her baby promptly spit up what she thought to be the entire volume of the supplement. I caution parents not to use at-home infant scales (at all) for several reasons, including a lack of sensitivity and inaccuracy. In addition, it is beneficial to develop other skills for monitoring your baby's milk intake, like observing diaper output, watching your baby for signs of satiation, and checking your breasts to assess whether they feel less full after feeding. Finally, I caution parents not to use only one measurement (i.e., weight) and instead, consider the whole picture when evaluating the baby. If it's possible, only monitor

your baby's weight at well-check appointments throughout the first months of life. The truth is that many parents can focus too much on the numbers (infant weight gain, in this case) and not enough on the baby and comprehensive observation of infant wellness. Develop your parenting skills and unless your baby has special needs, let go of the desire to weigh your baby at home.

2. *Using "Smart" infant bassinets, motion sleeping devices, and auto-rocking cribs/infant seats are also a bad idea*. These bassinets or cribs are popular with parents but not with lactation consultants. In numerous online discussions, I have seen only one out of hundreds of LCs express support for these kinds of cribs. The Smart bassinet restrains the infant in a tight swaddle, and the crib provides motion. These bassinets also provide sound to lull the baby to sleep and help keep him asleep. The major problem with this type of crib is that when your baby sleeps through his normal feeding times at night, he is not taking in all the calories he needs for growth. In addition, he is not removing milk from the breast (which you know is the quickest way to tell your breasts to slow and stop milk production). Using this tool has major consequences. First, by tightly swaddling the baby, he cannot access his innate reflexes. These reflexes help your baby wake during the night for feeding and because *night waking is protective*. Missing feedings during the night means your baby will not stimulate the breast and keep milk production steady. Encouraging an infant to sleep too long can quickly impact your milk supply because of a delicate feedback loop built into the breast. When the baby is not removing milk and the breasts become full, your body signals milk production to slow down. Over a few days, this same input causes a drop in milk supply. This type of crib may also encourage plagiocephaly (flat head syndrome). Be wary of any seat, bassinet, or crib that uses motion and white noise. These types of bassinets and cribs can disrupt night feeding, quickly and negatively impacting milk supply.

3. *Infant tracking apps are problematic*. Have you ever wondered how cavepeople got along without infant gear and gadgets? The simple answer is that most baby gear and gadgets are unnecessary, including infant tracking apps for your smartphone. Cavepeople did not need any tracking apps because they lived in constant contact with their infants. Most modern families do not require high-intensity infant tracking either. There is no substitute for closely observing your baby's cues, habits, and daily rhythms. You can become a more responsive, tuned-in parent by developing these skills. Of course, there are times when you may need to be extra attentive to some measurement of your baby's daily rhythms (number of feedings, wake-sleep cycle, or dirty diapers). Even so, unless the tracking is incredibly simplistic, there is always the chance that parents could focus more on the numbers, graphs, and charts in the tracking app than on physical observation of the baby. If you choose to use a tracking app for your baby's daily habits, be sure it is simple, easy to use, and only use it if necessary. Otherwise, let your senses and intuition take over. Tune into your baby, not your phone.
4. *Breast pumps are a mixed bag of outcomes*. You may be thinking that I have made a terrible mistake by including the breast pump on this list. Be assured that this is not a mistake. The breast pump can be an incredible tool for bringing in a full milk supply when the infant cannot, pumping milk while you are separated or working, helping boost supply, and many other positive uses. But lately, I have heard from so many people who are *pumping unnecessarily*. When asked why they are pumping, people usually tell me they were told to pump to establish a good milk supply. This advice is genuinely terrible unless a diagnosis exists regarding a breastfeeding problem, and pumping represents the best solution. Otherwise, establishing a good milk supply works best when the infant removes milk from the breast. If you recall, breastfeeding is a whole-body experience. Your body responds to numerous sensory cues (seeing and holding your baby, smelling your baby, touching the baby) while you are breastfeeding. Even though we can try to mimic those experiences when we pump, the baby is better at stimulating the breast (and

whole body) to bring in your milk. I have seen many people in recent years who are directly breastfeeding their infants all day in addition to pumping several times a day. Some people state that this is to build their stash in the freezer to go back to work or be away from home. Again, this is usually completely unnecessary. There is no need to have thousands of ounces of expressed milk in your freezer. Suppose you are going back to work; delay pumping until a week or two before you begin working. You can have some milk available, perhaps enough for a few days away, but you will not need much more than that. Once you are back at work, you will pump on Monday what the baby will eat on Tuesday. Essentially, you will always be one day ahead of your baby. Of course, you can have a little extra in the freezer, but a colossal stash is unnecessary in most situations. Use the breast pump wisely. Pumping too much can cause your body to produce more milk than your baby needs.

5. *Breast-like bottle nipples are not the real thing*. Manufacturers market some nipples claiming to mimic the breast better than other, more traditional bottle nipples. This distinction may not matter for people who exclusively use bottles, but for those who are breastfeeding and bottle feeding, this marketing ploy might sound perfect. But is it? First, no bottle on the market can truly mimic the humanness of your breast. It just is not possible. While many manufacturers claim these nipples are more life-like, lactation consultants often disagree. One LC told me that she never sees an infant latch onto the breast-like nipples with a proper latch. In many breast-like bottle nipples, the nipple can be too narrow, and the part that mimics the areola is too broad, causing a baby to practice nursing with a poor latch. These suboptimal latch skills will not translate well for switching back to the breast. The other obvious problem with any of these breast-like nipples is that they can never match the pliability of the human nipple-areolar complex. Babies create a vacuum once they latch onto the breast with a tight seal. This pressure changes the shape of the human nipple and areola. One cannot achieve this type of simulation with a bottle. Instead of breast-like nipples, focus on slow-flow nipples

and paced bottle feeding. If you are going to use bottles in addition to direct breastfeeding, be sure that the person who feeds your baby understands the technique of paced feeding and why it is important.

6. *Pacifiers, dummies, soothers, and binkies can be equally problematic.* Like many items on this list, the pacifier can be friend or foe. Be aware: one should only introduce a pacifier after the milk supply and breastfeeding are well established (about four to six weeks if breastfeeding is going well). There are therapeutic uses of the pacifier, and if your baby needs this type of therapy, do not be alarmed. Use it for therapy and then allow the baby to meet all other sucking needs at the breast. The major disadvantage for the pacifier is that it can be overused and thus, puts the baby at risk for skipping feedings. In the early weeks, I recommend avoiding the pacifier altogether. Later, it can be used but be cautious not to rely on the pacifier when your baby needs to come to the breast. Remember, there are numerous reasons babies come to the breast, not just for calorie intake. If the baby needs nursing, comfort, closeness, and food, offer the breast first.

7. *The sleepsuit and infant swaddling can be overly constraining.* These suits have been around for many generations if you include swaddling as a type of sleepsuit. The allure of the enchanted suit that helps your baby sleep is quite attractive but is it safe? There are several concerns for sleepsuits and breastfeeding. One of the main problems with the sleepsuits and swaddling is the potential for discouraging infants from accessing their innate reflexes. In addition, the swaddling and sleeper suits can promote too much sleep, which means that your baby will likely sleep through her natural feeding time. Though this sounds advantageous to an exhausted parent, it can be detrimental to your milk supply. Nighttime waking to feed is beneficial for maintaining a full milk supply. It helps your baby take in the necessary calories for the day, and nighttime waking is protective against SIDS. Avoid or use sleepsuits with caution.

This list is only a small sample of the breastfeeding tools and infant gear available for new parents. Other gadgets you may encounter could also be harmful to breastfeeding and your milk supply. Be careful with the items and gadgets you use along the breastfeeding (and parenting) journey. Many of the available tools are completely unnecessary. Many of them are helpful but only in moderation. Use your best judgment – only you know what is best for your family. Be careful not to overuse any one tool. Take time to learn skills that help meet your baby's needs without gadgets.

Final Thoughts on Tools and Gadgets

Parenting tools can be your friends or enemies; it depends on how you use them. I do not recommend you avoid all these tools, but I highly suggest that you use them with care and in the most responsible way. As a final example, consider the infant car seat. The car seat is 100% necessary if you travel by car with your baby. In other words, it is not optional. It is essential to use the infant car seat responsibly. The baby must be restrained properly in the car seat at all times, otherwise, it can quickly become an unsafe situation. Make sure to check the usage guidelines for harness straps and chest clips for your infant seat. Many times, these are not correctly adjusted. In addition, overuse of the infant seat can cause problems as well. You have probably heard that you should not allow your baby to sit in the car seat or sleep in the car seat unless the seat and the baby are traveling in the car. There are avoidable risks of overusing car seats. These risks include hypoxia (restricted airway causing a drop in oxygen saturation), exacerbation of reflux, and temporary circulation problems from staying in the same position for too long. In addition, there can be problems with plagiocephaly (flat head syndrome), and other positional problems, like torticollis, may occur. The American Academy of Pediatrics recommends restraining infants in car seats only when traveling and not at other times (Durbin et al., 2018).

While the car seat may not interfere with breastfeeding (unless your child is sleeping through normal feeding times in the car seat), it is clear that the improper use of this necessary tool can cause harm. This same logic applies to most parenting and breastfeeding tools. Use them with care.

Unnecessary Supplementation

For healthy, exclusively breastfed infants, human milk is the only item on the menu. Everything else, including water, sugar water, ready-to-use infant formula, and powdered formula, is unnecessary, and some are dangerous, especially for preemies. Be sure you are clear about your intention to breastfeed your baby exclusively, so there is no risk of inappropriate use of supplements during your hospital stay.

Studies show that newborns receive supplementation at the hospital frequently and often during the first day of life. This extraneous feeding happens so regularly that there are established guidelines from the WHO for using supplements. In addition, The Academy of Breastfeeding Medicine has a protocol established (Protocol #3) for the appropriate use of supplements with full-term newborns (Kellams et al., 2017).

A study conducted with 342 breastfeeding dyads found that 62.8% of the infants received supplements (mostly with formula) during the hospital stay. Interestingly, 5.9% of the families did not receive any information about the supplements until after they were administered (Boban & Zakarija-Grković, 2016). Some of the reasons for the use of early supplementation in this study include:

- Lack of milk
- Crying baby
- Birth by cesarean
- Newborn weight loss
- Sore nipples

(Boban & Zakarija-Grković, 2016)

The authors state that only 24.6% of the supplements given during the study period were deemed medically necessary (Boban & Zakarija-Grković, 2016). Let us consider these common reasons for the use of supplements.

Are Supplements Indicated Because of the Lack of Mother's Milk?

Colostrum is present in small amounts in the first two days postpartum. Copious quantities of mature milk do not usually appear until later (sometime between 36 and 96 hours postpartum), usually after the family has gone home from the hospital. Supplementing with formula in the first two days of life is counter-productive because if the baby fails to breastfeed, the breast does not get the necessary stimulus for colostrum removal and milk production. If supplementation becomes necessary, pumping the breasts is required to stimulate milk production. Begin pumping with a hospital-grade double electric pump within two hours of birth. Pump at least eight times per day, including overnight.

Are Supplements Indicated With a Crying Baby?

Infants cry to signal their needs to caregivers. Whatever the need is, breastfeeding can usually be the answer. If the baby needs holding, breastfeeding provides for that. If the baby needs nourishment, effective breastfeeding with good milk transfer is the answer. If the baby needs warmth, skin-to-skin time will facilitate increased temperature and provide opportunities for breastfeeding. In the absence of other compelling factors, crying is not a signal for supplementation.

Are Supplements Necessary After Birth by Cesarean?

Please know that breastfeeding after a cesarean birth is entirely possible. It may be necessary to have help from OR nursing staff, but one can often initiate breastfeeding soon after cesarean birth. Some hospitals have adopted policies that support early skin-to-skin care and breastfeeding after cesarean birth. Since the onset of a copious milk supply is often delayed after a cesarean, it is best to nurse early and often stimulate milk production. Breastfeeding after cesarean surgery can be facilitated by using modified positions, including the clutch position (also called football hold), where the baby's legs stretch out toward your side, not toward the other breast. Bring your baby to the breast often and try lots of skin-to-skin time after cesarean to help stimulate milk production.

Are Supplements Necessary in the Case of Newborn Weight Loss?

This issue is complex and can sometimes be the indicator for supplements (but not always). Keep in mind that if supplements are indicated, consider using human milk before formula. Pumping your own milk can be an option (so is donor milk). See the sections on Infant Weight Loss and IV fluids for more information on newborn weight loss.

Are Supplements Useful in the Case of Sore Nipples?

Breastfeeding with sore nipples is often traumatic for the parent. Continued breastfeeding when nipple pain is present can further damage nipple tissue. The most important and best way to treat sore nipples is not supplements. Instead, the most effective way to treat sore nipples is to discover the source of the problem and eliminate it. If sore nipples are persistent, investigate better latch techniques, deeper latch techniques, and laid-back breastfeeding. In addition, allow the infant to self-attach while providing skin-to-skin. Observe the baby for oral anatomy issues (tongue tie, lip tie, high arching palate). Pumping (temporarily) and feeding your milk can be an effective way to heal cracked or sore nipples. This strategy keeps the demand and supply system intact while you are healing, but make sure to investigate the source of nipple pain. Using formula and not pumping your milk will cause a breakdown in the demand and supply system and cause a serious supply drop. Remember, introducing supplements in the hospital is correlated with early weaning (Chantry et al., 2014).

An important study on how routine maternity care practices affect breastfeeding duration shows that people who experience effective breastfeeding are exposed to several protective factors in the early postpartum period. The six factors are, 1) breastfeeding initiation within one hour of birth, 2) giving only breast milk, 3) rooming in, 4) breastfeeding on demand, 5) no pacifiers, and 6) fostering breastfeeding support groups (DiGirolamo et al., 2008). One of the key protective factors of breastfeeding is "giving only breast milk," no supplements of any kind (DiGirolamo et al., 2008). The other two factors that were highly associated with breastfeeding duration beyond six weeks were: initiating the first breastfeeding session within one hour of birth and avoiding pacifiers (DiGirolamo et al., 2008). This fascinating study also compared breastfeeding duration between mothers who experienced the six protective factors that support breastfeeding and mothers who experienced none of the protective factors. The people who did not experience or receive protective breastfeeding support were 13 times more likely to end breastfeeding early (DiGirolamo et al., 2008).

One of the biggest concerns that LCs and parents have about using formula supplements, even temporarily, is that often, new parents don't receive specific instructions about how to protect breastfeeding during the supplementation period. In addition, many people state that they receive no information about stopping the supplement or how to transition back to breastfeeding full time. This lack of information is a major complication of the use of formula supplements. It is akin to providing stitches to a wound, but no instructions on removing them. Many times, parents who have used formula supplements often call in help from an LC because they cannot see a clear pathway back to exclusive breastfeeding. If caregivers recommend formula supplements, you will need a plan of care to protect the milk supply for the duration of supplementation and another plan for returning to exclusive use of human milk. Without these two plans in place, the return to exclusive breastfeeding could be in jeopardy.

General Guidelines for Weaning Off Formula Supplements

Work with a lactation consultant to develop a plan that is best suited for your current situation. Here are some general things to keep in mind as you transition from mixed feeding (some human milk and some formula) to exclusively using human milk.

- Work to build your milk supply. Consider adding power pumping. Try breast compression and massage while feeding at the breast and while pumping. Remove as much milk as you can during each feeding or pumping session.
- *Gradually* transition away from the formula supplements. This transition gives you time to build up your supply to meet your baby's needs. This strategy may take two weeks (or more). Be patient and keep working to increase your milk supply. Working with a lactation consultant may be necessary.
- Hold your baby skin-to-skin.
- Monitor your baby's wet and dirty diapers closely. This observation will be one good indicator that your baby is getting the amount of milk she needs.
- Monitor your baby's weight gain at your pediatrician's office.

This process can take time. Be persistent with milk removal. Read *Making More Milk* by Lisa Marasco and Diana West for more information on building your milk supply.

You Receive Advice to Wean

So many people (wrongly) receive advice to wean their newborns, older babies, and toddlers. This advice not only comes from poorly informed friends or family members but also from doctors. The advice to wean is so common that most LCs can recite lengthy lists of reasons why their clients have been told to abandon breastfeeding. One problem with this scenario is that most people trust their doctor's advice, and advice to wean can sometimes lead to the early and unnecessary abandonment of breastfeeding. The truth is that most situations you encounter during lactation are compatible with lactation, even most medications, and medical procedures.

I consulted with a few LCs about why their clients receive advice to wean. Here is why some health care professionals have recommended (unnecessary) weaning:

- Baby is gaining weight too fast
- Baby is gaining weight too slowly
- Weaning during pregnancy is "necessary"
- Baby is not sleeping through the night
- Baby wakes "too much" to nurse
- People who are sick with the flu (or other viral infection) should not breastfeed
- Must wean after mastitis (or other breast infection)
- Baby is experiencing jaundice
- Baby is experiencing allergies
- Baby has reflux
- Baby is teething
- Baby is 12 months old (or some other arbitrary number)
- Baby is over 20 lbs. (or some other arbitrary number)
- Teen parents should not breastfeed
- Parent is returning to work
- Human milk has no nutritional value after 12 months
- Small-breasted people can't produce adequate milk

- People of your race don't breastfeed
- Baby needs cow's milk now
- Mammogram is necessary
- People with mental health issues should not breastfeed
- Infant needs medications
- Parent needs medications
- Infant needs surgery or parent needs surgery
- People using topical medications should not breastfeed
- People getting teeth whitened should not breastfeed
- People getting dental work or root canal should not breastfeed
- *People who do their laundry on Monday should not breastfeed*

The laundry comment is a joke, but most of the reasons detailed above are equally ridiculous. Can you imagine that someone believes that human milk has no nutritional value after 12 months? All of these recommendations came from healthcare professionals. However, none of the reasons above are legitimate reasons for weaning.

If you receive advice to wean, for any reason, and this does not align with your infant feeding goals, get a second opinion. Remember to consider the source of the recommendation. Did it come from someone with lactation training? Consult with a lactation expert before weaning. Contact the Infant Risk Center in Amarillo, Texas about medications. Contact them Monday through Friday, 8am-5pm central time, (806) 352-2519, or on the web at infantrisk.com.

Please know that there are some valid reasons for weaning. This list is not exhaustive. There are likely other reasons as well.

- You want to wean.
- If you need to take iodine-131, you must wean (several weeks before taking I-131).
- According to Hale's Lactation risk assessment, you should consider weaning if your medication is L4 or L5, potentially hazardous or not compatible with lactation. Call the Infant Risk Center for more information. Alternatively, investigate taking something else or postponing the medication if possible.

- If you need to take cancer treatment with chemotherapy medications, you must wean.

If weaning is indicated, please read about gradually weaning if there is time for it. It is better for you and better for your baby (in most cases). In addition, if you find that you must wean and weaning does not align with your infant feeding goals, you may experience a significant amount of grief over the weaning process. Even people who are ready to wean sometimes experience weaning as grieving. Seek help and support for yourself and your mental health. You do not have to go down this path alone. Ask your primary care doctor or lactation consultant for local mental health resources.

Mismanagement of Lactation and Feeding

There are gray areas for lactation support. For example, many professionals offer lactation education and support, but they have varying levels of expertise and training. Oddly enough, it is highly likely that you will encounter substantial lactation counseling from people who possess no training in lactation management. This advice may arrive from friends, coworkers, family members, and even healthcare providers. Many people have found that the healthcare professional they see most often in the postpartum year is their baby's pediatrician. Still, as we have discussed, pediatricians are usually not trained in lactation support and management. You may also see your own primary care doctor, an OB-GYN, or midwife during the postpartum year, and while it may be convenient or tempting to seek lactation care from these providers, it is not always wise. Seeking care or even receiving inadvertent lactation advice from healthcare professionals without proper skills and training in lactation opens the door for a great deal of mismanagement.

Lactation mismanagement can impact milk production and infant feeding in a variety of ways. Sometimes, bad advice or outdated recommendations barely make an impact because milk production is already robust, and the infant is nursing well. But when the breastfeeding dyad is already in a vulnerable situation (latch issues, pain, low milk supply, nipple trauma, etc.), poor lactation management can negatively impact the feeding experience and milk supply.

What Does Mismanagement of Lactation Look Like?

When I teach breastfeeding education classes, my clients are intrigued by the idea of lactation mismanagement but often cannot visualize how it looks. Many people have asked me how to recognize the mismanagement of lactation, especially if it impacts their breastfeeding journey. Always use caution when you get advice and recommendations from people lacking training in lactation. This advice seems obvious when we receive tips and information from friends and family. However, it can get confusing when the advice and recommendations come from a respected and trusted healthcare provider.

The doorways for lactation mismanagement open when we receive the wrong diagnosis, recommendations for inappropriate treatments or outdated techniques, recommendations based on erroneous information, and any strategies that facilitate poor maternal and infant outcomes for milk production, lactation, and feeding. Below are some examples of scenarios that happen with regularity. Each of these represents some type of lactation mismanagement.

After birth in the immediate postpartum period, there are numerous opportunities for mismanagement of milk supply and infant feeding. Consider the following:

- Unnecessary supplementation with formula while the baby is still in the hospital. This situation happens so frequently that the Academy of Breastfeeding Medicine created a protocol (ABM Protocol #3) to outline the appropriate uses for supplementation while breastfeeding.
- Supplementing with formula without first considering the mother's own milk or donor milk.
- Parents receive recommendations for pumping in the first days postpartum without clear indicators signifying that pumping is the solution to a real problem.
- Over feeding formula supplements in hospital. Infants feeding at the breast are transferring only small amounts of colostrum in the first few days of life. This is nature's design. Often, when infants are bottle-fed formula supplements, they are overfed.

- Hospitals often encourage or administer nipple shields and pacifiers without clear indicators that these are the tools to solve real feeding problems. Be cautious with both.
- Failure to provide guidance for breastfeeding infants with oral anomalies (cleft palate and lip, TOTS, low muscle tone).
- Rapid Arm Movement (RAM) method or "open and shove." These are outdated concepts. The RAM method (this is a fictious name made up by lactation consultants) is a terrible technique. The parent waits to see a wide-open mouth and then uses Rapid Arm Movement (RAM) to bring the baby in quickly, face to nipple, hoping that the baby will grasp hold of the nipple in just the right way. The "open and shove" technique is similar. Be wary of any advice that instructs you to use these approaches to achieve the latch.
- Testing for hypoglycemia without regard for timing. Testing in the first two hours of life will likely result in low blood sugar readings because this is a time when infants typically experience a physiologic drop in blood sugar. In other words, lower blood sugar readings can be considered normal in the first two hours after birth. Read more in the ABM Protocol for Hypoglycemia (#1) (Wight & Marinelli, 2014).
- Teaching poor positioning or prescribing rigid positioning techniques. Caregivers provide this advice more often than they should. There are many ways to hold an infant to optimize feeding. Each dyad is an individual unit with unique anatomy and features. It pays to experiment with various positions for holding the baby while feeding.
- Giving the wrong flange size for pumping, if necessary, in the hospital.

You may receive advice or recommendations at the pediatrician's office that can negatively influence infant feeding. Below are examples of mismanagement of lactation you may encounter at the doctor's office.

- Your pediatrician gives time-limiting recommendations for feeding. For example, "Only feed ten minutes on each side" (or eight minutes). Another classic example is, "Your baby gets all the nutrition he needs in the first seven minutes at the breast." Both of these recommendations are not only incorrect but could be dangerous. Some babies, especially those requiring extra care, need additional time at the breast.

- Recommending triple feeding without a full evaluation of lactation.
- Poor weight gain that is not closely monitored and remedied. One LC told me, "Weight checks are not the same as lactation support." A weight check is simply a data point. Without a complete evaluation of multiple factors, the weight check alone has little value.
- The doctor recommends night weaning because the baby should be sleeping through the night by 12 weeks (or 15 pounds, or another arbitrary measure). This advice is nonsense and completely erroneous.
- Recommendations for scheduled feeding. This recommendation is almost always suspicious advice.
- Misidentifying a real problem. For example, the doctor assumes a low milk supply when the problem is milk transfer, not milk supply. You are making enough milk, but your baby cannot extract enough milk.
- Recommending supplements or triple feeding without telling parents exactly how and when to discontinue the protocol.
- Failure to refer to qualified and trained lactation care.
- Assuming that all pain in the nipple is thrush. There are many diverse causes of nipple pain. It requires a full breast evaluation, oral exam for the infant, and feeding evaluation.
- Recommendations for weaning at six months or 12 months because the milk has no value after this arbitrary time frame. Obviously, this is false. Your milk is extremely valuable at every age.
- Over diagnosing and over-treating reflux. Unfortunately, over-treating for reflux is quite common. Try an elimination diet of the most common allergens first (eggs, dairy, corn, soy, nuts) before giving your baby prescription meds for reflux.

- Recommending the switch to formula for CMPA (cow's milk protein allergy). Eliminating cow's milk products from the maternal diet is a perfectly acceptable way to treat CMPA.
- Universal recommendations for iron and vitamin D supplementation for the infant. This advice is not sound advice.
- Recommending the pump and dump strategy for all meds, anesthesia, and alcohol. Do your research, but I view this as outdated advice. There might be times when pump and dump is called for, but in most cases, it is usually unnecessary.
- Recommending any type of sleep training or limiting breastfeeding at night. This advice is dangerous, even if your doctor seems to think it is acceptable.
- Prescribing the wrong antibiotics for mastitis.
- Recommending warm compress for engorgement. (Use a cool compress for engorgement. You can use warmth or moist heat to help move milk right before nursing but only momentarily. Too much heat will promote more inflammation.)
- Practitioners offering tongue-tie release without high level training. Go to a trained professional who specializes in tongue-tie release.

Applying advice from friends or adhering to cultural norms can create breastfeeding mismanagement. Unfortunately, you might be engaging in some of these without realizing that they can negatively impact lactation.

- Sleep training
- Overusing a manual silicone natural suction pump
- Following a rigid feeding schedule
- Overusing the pacifier
- Over pumping
- Neglecting to utilize the baby's innate feeding instincts
- Failure to recognize when your own mental health is fragile, and you need immediate supportAssuming that the amount you can pump is the amount of milk your baby takes inTaking herbs, using coconut water, Gatorade, and lactation cookies instead of seeking professional help for low milk supply

- Not pumping/removing milk during overnight hours if the baby takes a bottle with your partner at night
- Seeking care from the wrong professional. Your doula may be highly trained and knowledgeable about many aspects of pregnancy and support during labor but is likely not trained as a lactation consultant. Seek care from the right specialist.

To maximize your odds of receiving the best possible lactation care, follow these guidelines:

1. Seek lactation services from qualified and/or certified professionals. Ask about their training and background in supporting the breastfeeding dyad.
2. Seek a second or third opinion if you receive suspicious recommendations.
3. Advice from untrained people comes with a grain of salt. Do your own research.

Doctor Recommended Switching to Toddler Formula or Cow's Milk

Many people who intend to breastfeed set their initial nursing goal for 12 months. However, when the baby's first birthday rolls around, some are surprised to find that their babies are not ready to wean. Further, in many cases, the parent is not prepared to abandon breastfeeding either. Even more surprising is that at about 12 months, some pediatricians begin to counsel families to transition away from human milk. Some doctors suggest switching to cow's milk. In recent years, toddler milk has become an increasingly popular recommendation after weaning from human milk or infant formula.

Bad Advice

That advice is completely counter to the World Health Organization (WHO) advice. In its recommendations, the WHO clearly states that infants should be exclusively fed human milk under the age of six months and continue to consume human milk in addition to complementary foods up to age two and beyond. The American Academy of Pediatrics (AAP) recommends human milk for two years and beyond, with continued maternal and infant benefits. The WHO and AAP make no recommendation for switching to toddler formula. They do not recommend toddler formula because it is completely unnecessary.

Not long ago, toddler formula did not exist. People fed their infants with either human milk or formula (and sometimes both) until their baby outgrew the need for either one. By that time, children are already eating solid food of all kinds. A healthy toddler consumes a solid food diet with various vegetables, meats or fish (or other protein), and some fruit. Human milk consumption can continue well beyond 12 months and has many benefits for toddlers. Infant formula is not necessary after 12 months, and many who have used formula find that this is a good time to switch to cow's milk, but again, that is not necessary. Humans are not designed to consume cow's milk, so it is optional; choose that if it is right for you but remember that people don't need to consume cow's milk at all. Consumption of cow's milk is heavily promoted in the U.S., but it is not the right choice for many people. Some people choose this and some do not, but cow's milk is unnecessary (same for toddler formula).

The toddler milk industry is the fastest-growing segment of the artificial formula industry. In recent years, this has become a niche market for formula manufacturers seeking to boost revenue from the already saturated infant formula market. Make no mistake, the infant formula industry is a multi-billion-dollar industry, but in recent years, formula sales have lagged somewhat. To cover these losses, infant food brands have promoted toddler milk as a healthy option for children ages 1-4.

While this might appeal to busy families looking for nutritious options for their toddlers, it is anything but healthy. One popular brand heavily marketed in the U.S. has nonfat milk, corn syrup solids, and a variety of vegetable oils as the top three ingredients. Frankly, none of these are whole food and healthy options for humans, much less for growing toddlers. What's worse is that these products often come with a substantial dose of sugar. The product label won't reflect added sugar; manufacturers mask these sugars as corn syrup solids (a dehydrated form of corn syrup added to dry powdered products).

Because toddler milk is not infant formula, the WHO Code (The International Code of Marketing of Breastmilk Substitutes) does not apply. Manufacturers in the U.S. (and likely elsewhere) market these products as the next step after infant formula. The reality is that these "follow-on formulas" are simply the next step for the infant formula manufacturers to create revenue and keep toddlers and children consuming their products.

How Should I Feed My Toddler?

Skip the recommendation to use toddler formula. Consider this a trend or a marketing gimmick rather than a healthy food option. Toddlers can continue with human milk well beyond their first birthday. Most breastfeeding toddlers eat solid foods and continue nursing several times a day. Read about baby-led weaning for more information on slowly weaning throughout the toddler years.

Cow's milk is certainly an option for toddlers. Again, it is not necessary for good health or adequate nutrition for toddlers. If your baby's pediatrician recommends that you begin feeding your baby with cow's milk because it's a convenient source of calcium and vitamin D, please know that you have plenty of other options.

Nondairy Sources of Calcium and Vitamin D

Even if you are giving your baby some cow's milk, it is a great idea to introduce food sources of calcium as well. Calcium is plentiful in dark green vegetables and leafy vegetables. Some excellent options are broccoli, brussels sprouts, and leafy greens (e.g., dark lettuce greens or kale). Avoid heavy consumption of spinach because it contains high amounts of oxalic acid, which interferes with calcium absorption. One can also find calcium in some types of beans, nut butters, seed butters, oily fish with bones, and some sea vegetables.

Vitamin D (which acts as a hormone, not a vitamin) comes in its optimal form from direct sunlight. While it is a good idea to avoid excessive sunlight that can burn the skin, getting some direct sunlight on your skin is healthy and essential. Humans should not avoid the sun. Use good judgment and keep your baby out of direct sunlight in the hottest part of the day when the sun's rays are most direct. Expose your baby's skin to sunlight in the early part of the day and the afternoon a few times a week, if possible. Not much sunlight is required, but some sun is necessary. Dark skin requires longer exposure times to acquire adequate amounts of vitamin D. If you choose to supplement vitamin D for you or the baby, be sure to use vitamin

D3 (not D2) and take it in conjunction with vitamin K2. Vitamin K2 works with vitamin D3 and calcium to optimize bone health. K2 tells your body where to put calcium, for example, in bones and teeth and not in soft tissue like blood vessels.

Other Benefits of Sun Exposure

Getting sunlight in the early morning has benefits beyond vitamin D. Early morning sunlight activates the retina in the eye, helping to optimize your circadian rhythm. This early morning exposure to sunlight helps set up daytime alertness, boosts serotonin, regulates cortisol, and contributes to healthy sleep cycles. If you are interested in helping your baby establish a good wake and sleep cycle, bring your baby outdoors in the morning for a few minutes to enable sunlight to activate the retina. Practice this every morning, if possible, to help establish a healthy circadian rhythm.

CHAPTER 12

Lactation Interference: Healthcare Factors

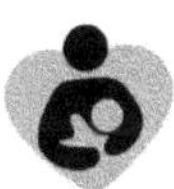

It seems odd that the healthcare system itself could play a role in lactation interference but for many people, this is the largest lactation interference factor they will encounter. The factors outlined in this section deal specifically with elements of the healthcare system or healthcare delivery that negatively affect breastfeeding care and support. For more information on lactation interference that is related more to the doctor-patient relationship, see Chapter 11: Breastfeeding Management.

Lactation Care Conundrum - Where to Seek Care for the Breastfeeding Dyad

In the United States, most people usually seek care from an OB-GYN (doctor of obstetrics and gynecology) for prenatal care and birth. After the delivery, the OB-GYN provides postpartum follow-up care for the parent, and a pediatrician provides care for the baby. The parent can also seek healthcare from a primary care physician (PCP) or family doctor. Unfortunately, none of these physicians have any regular training in lactation and care of the breastfeeding dyad. If none of these doctors can provide skilled lactation care to both members of the breastfeeding dyad, how can healthcare providers ensure continuity of care for lactation and both partners in the breastfeeding relationship? Unfortunately, the short answer is they cannot, and they do not (most of the time). This lack of qualified lactation care for both parent and baby makes breastfeeding support highly fragmented in the U.S.

In the U.S., the best option for highly skilled lactation care is an international board-certified lactation consultant (IBCLC). Certified lactation consultants (CLC) and other lactation counselors are also good options. However, unless the IBCLC or CLC is also an MD or nurse practitioner, they cannot write prescriptions. Exceptions to this are physician assistants and family physicians, *who also have a lactation credential*. This profile is likely a rare combination. In some states, certified midwives and certified nurse-midwives can also write prescriptions and provide care for both the mother and baby. However, a midwife is usually not also credentialed as a lactation consultant, but certainly, some are.

It is the parent's responsibility to coordinate care for breastfeeding by finding a certified and skilled lactation counselor. However, it becomes problematic when the breastfeeding dyad faces problems that require high level lactation care, need prescriptions for both parent and baby, or are dealing with feeding complications that affect both parent and baby. Here are two examples:

- Thrush. This condition is an overgrowth of yeast in the infant's mouth and genitals. This condition also affects the nipples, making breastfeeding more difficult and painful for the parent. The pediatrician can diagnose thrush and write a prescription for the baby, but not the parent. The parent needs to see their own physician, who then must examine the breast, nipple, and areola, diagnose thrush, and write a prescription. The process is cumbersome, complicated, requiring two separate office visits and two copays. Just getting a new parent and newborn to one doctor can be exhausting and time-consuming. The lack of continuity of care makes breastfeeding care complicated for many people. Because of the way our system currently works in the U.S., it can be difficult or nearly impossible to find a one-stop shop for all lactation care needs for both parent and baby.
- Ankyloglossia (tongue-tie) accompanied by plugged ducts and mastitis or nipple damage. Tongue-tie can lead to poor breast drainage, plugged ducts, mastitis, and nipple damage. These conditions are complex and require high-level care for both parent and baby. To resolve the mastitis, the parent needs immediate care and may need prescription medication. The baby needs high-level care to diagnose and release the oral restrictions and resolve the tongue tie. It is improbable that the parent and baby in this situation will seek care from the same physician.

Strategies for Finding Care

- Find a *supportive, breastfeeding-friendly pediatrician*. This provider is *extremely* important for everyone breastfeeding, but essential if you are interested in breastfeeding beyond one year. Ask friends, read online reviews, or schedule a consultation/interview with the doctor before committing to that practice.
- Find a pediatrician's office that has an IBCLC or CLC on staff.
- Skip the pediatrician and seek care from a family doctor. The family doctor can provide care for both parent and baby, write prescriptions, and see the whole family in one office. The downside is that this provider (just like primary care docs and pediatricians) may not have lactation experience.
- Seek primary care from a doctor who is knowledgeable or at least supportive of breastfeeding and willing to learn.
- Seek perinatal care from independent midwives, homebirth midwives, or birth centers.
- Seek lactation care from an IBCLC when needed. In theory, this will ensure that your lactation consultant and your pediatrician are communicating. (The IBCLC will send reports from your consultation to your pediatrician.)

Where to go for Skilled Lactation Care

In the U.S., lactation care during the baby's first year can be quite fragmented. Sometimes, it is difficult to know where to get the best care. Currently, we have a system that requires parents and babies to seek lactation care from two or more caregivers/doctors because there are no comprehensive lactation physicians who care for both parent and baby. Each of the caregivers is limited by their training in lactation, who they are qualified to provide care for, or by whether they can write prescriptions or not. However, since most breastfeeding care and guidance does not involve prescription medicine, seeing an IBCLC or a CLC is generally a suitable option. If the need for prescription medication becomes necessary for either the parent or baby, seek care from a breastfeeding-friendly physician.

Table 12.1: A Typology of Caregivers

Caregiver	Cares for	Lactation Training	Write Prescriptions
Midwife	perinatal care	sometimes	depends on training
OB-GYN	perinatal care	likely none	for parents
Pediatrician	infants and children	likely none	for babies & children
Family doctor	all ages	likely none	for all ages
Primary Care doctor	adults	likely none	for adults
Pediatric dentist	children	*	limited to dental care
IBCLC	breastfeeding dyad	fully trained	none

**Pediatric dentists have limited training in lactation, and their background is usually only related to infant oral anatomy. However, they are experts regarding oral anatomy function and dysfunction. Many can diagnose tongue and lip ties and provide treatment. Dentists can only write prescriptions related to dental procedures.*

Not Being Heard and Not Being Seen

Validation is a major key to lactation support. Validation is a way for others (partners, family members, healthcare providers) to recognize and affirm our feelings and concerns, giving these concerns validity and confirming the feelings as real. Problems with lactation may occur when the support team is not validating concerns or feelings, which many people describe as "not being heard" or "not being seen."

Who is at risk for not being heard? In theory, anyone could be a victim of being dismissed or disrespected. The reality is that it may be much more likely for those already marginalized in society to experience the lack of validation in the healthcare setting. For example, this could apply to people who identify as minorities, speak a native language other than English, people in the LGBTQ+ community, overweight parents, and people at either end of the childbearing age spectrum.

What does this anti-validation look like? It can take many forms, but you know it when you encounter it. Consider the following situations. If anything rings a bell for you, you may have already experienced a lack of validation, disrespect from healthcare workers, or not being heard or seen:

- Is your doctor ignoring your concerns?
- Has someone on your support team dismissed your feelings?

- Have you been belittled, made to feel stupid, or even ridiculed for being overly anxious about any aspect of infant feeding, your health, or the health of the baby?
- Have your questions and concerns been belittled or rejected?
- Have you had a feeling that your healthcare team doesn't trust that your concerns are valid or real?
- Do you feel that others think you are exaggerating your health concerns?
- Have you ever felt that your age, gender identity, race/ethnicity, or even your weight has contributed to a situation where you're not heard or seen by your healthcare provider?
- Have you been disrespected by your healthcare team?

All of these situations are examples of invalidation or dismissal. All of these situations are evidence of unsupportive care. However, there are ways to remedy this situation. Consider the following suggestions:

- Get a second opinion immediately if you have high-level physical or mental health concerns that are ignored, brushed off, or dismissed.
- If you feel that your doctor doesn't trust you, thinks you're exaggerating, or consistently brushes you off, find a new supportive care provider who will listen to you.
- Be sure you present your most important concerns first and state them clearly. For example, instead of simply saying that you're experiencing difficulties with latching and feeding, you might say, "I want to talk to you about my concerns with the baby's ability to latch. He can latch, but it is painful. He makes many clicking sounds and then unlatches and relatches several times. This cycle continues, and it's hard to feed him. I need assistance getting a good latch." Again, be specific and state your concerns clearly.
- Advocate for yourself. Sometimes, compassionate, caring doctors, and nurses are overwhelmed. It can help to remind your caregiver of your highest priority concerns several times. Remember, the squeaky wheel gets the grease.

- If you are overwhelmed with infant care and feeding, experiencing exhaustion and fatigue, it can be helpful to write a list of your concerns ahead of time so that you don't forget to discuss specific things with your doctor. Alternatively, you can bring another adult with you to your appointment to help you. The other adult can be there to support you as you advocate for yourself and your baby. They can also help you remember everything you discussed with your caregiver.
- Communicate your feelings. Instead of simply saying, "I am having trouble getting a good latch." You might consider adding some information about how this makes you feel. Consider this instead: "I am having trouble getting a good latch, and I am so frustrated about this. I want this to work but I am now considering giving up breastfeeding. I just don't know what to do. I have tried everything."
- If you receive unsound advice that appears to lack evidence and feels biased, find a new caregiver. For example, I met a woman years ago who told me she had her first baby when she was 17. She told the pediatrician that she was breastfeeding, and the doctor responded in this way; "You should not worry yourself with breastfeeding. You're so young. Focus on finishing school and staying active with friends. Then, you can worry about breastfeeding your next child." Obviously, the doctor was actively dismissing her. There is zero validation here and zero support for her goals. She eventually found a new pediatrician who was supportive of her goal to breastfeed and did not dismiss her because of her age.
- Talk to friends and ask other parents in your community about where they find supportive care. Word travels fast and other parents in your community may already know where to find trustworthy, supportive, and informed care.

TRUE STORY

In the first weeks of breastfeeding, Janell had considerable nipple and breast pain while nursing. There was no nipple damage, only sore nipples, and breast discomfort. She asked her baby's pediatrician about the pain. The doctor quickly examined the baby's mouth but saw nothing unusual. The baby appeared to be thriving and was gaining weight well. She casually asked Janell about any nipple damage or trauma, but because pediatricians are caregivers for infants and children, the doctor could not examine the nipple or breast. The pediatrician told Janell, "Keep working on the latch. The pain will likely resolve on its own."

This example is a good illustration of dismissing a parent's concern about pain. Also, recall from Part I of this book that pain indicates something is wrong. Pain is a signal; it's the body's way of communicating that adjustments are necessary. Do not ignore pain. In this case, the suggestion that the pain might resolve independently is simply nonsense. (Janell may have also been better off speaking to someone who is a trained lactation professional.)

Seek care from someone who listens to your concerns. If you feel that you are not being taken seriously, you are not being seen or heard, look for a new caregiver. It can make a substantial impact on your breastfeeding journey.

Growth Charts

At no other time in the human life span is weight gain as vital as it is in the first year of life. Infants who are well-nourished and thriving gain weight consistently throughout their first year. Growth patterns can vary widely due to many factors: the feeding method, the baby's sex, genetics, and introduction of solid foods all play a role in infant weight gain and growth from birth onward. Your baby's pediatrician will measure and weigh the baby at each visit and plot that information on a graph. This practice can be one indicator to demonstrate if the baby is growing as expected or not. Weight gain and infant growth patterns are two clues that show the relative health of infants. Because of this, the baby's growth pattern will be of keen interest to you and the pediatrician. But what happens when a baby appears to be slipping off the growth curve for their age?

When infant growth patterns slow down more than expected, we can examine two things: the infant's nutrition and feeding patterns *OR* the chart used to plot the data that showed the slowing patterns.

Sometimes, slowed growth can reveal nutritional deficiencies and signal the need for a different dietary approach. Other times, it is a function of using a faulty growth chart that only makes it appear that the infant is not growing as expected.

What? Are there faulty growth charts? Yes, friends, there are faulty growth charts. In 1977, the National Center for Health and Statistics in the U.S. developed growth charts for doctors to determine the relative health of infant growth patterns. There are several problems with these growth charts. First, they are outdated. The charts use data from 1929-1975 from Ohio, USA. These data reflect only the people living in a certain part of the world long ago. This tool is not a good measure for today's infant growth. The second and perhaps most prominent problem with the 1977 growth charts was the data used in developing the charts. The growth charts were developed using data from a time when breastfeeding reached its lowest point in the U.S., and formula use was at its peak. This means that most of the infants whose recorded weight and length measurements went into developing those charts were formula-fed babies.

The implications of these biases are far-reaching. First, it is inappropriate and inaccurate to compare an exclusively-breastfed baby to charts with data from formula-fed infants as the norm. Breastfed and formula-fed babies exhibit different weight gain and growth patterns in the first 18 months to two years (and, as some argue, throughout the rest of life). If you exclusively breastfeed your baby, providing no solids and no other food supplements of any kind, be sure the pediatrician is using the appropriate growth chart for breastfed babies. Otherwise, the doctor could wrongly conclude that the baby is not gaining well and recommend unnecessary breast milk, formula, or other food supplements. Unnecessary formula supplements for your baby equals less breast milk for your baby.

In my work with breastfeeding families in the Philadelphia area in the early 2000s, a client told me that her 18-month-old was flagged as underweight and had slow growth patterns. The baby was breastfeeding and eating an array of complimentary family food. Their pediatrician recommended adding butter to all her meals where appropriate (e.g., on vegetables and bread.) Was this necessary? Perhaps different patterns would have emerged if they were charting the baby's weight on the World Health Organization (WHO) growth chart (WHO, 2000), which used breastfed infants as the norm.

In 2006, the WHO developed growth charts superior to the 1977 (or even 2000 updated) CDC growth charts. They are superior for several reasons: the CDC had a limited sample size and no access to infant weight for the smallest babies in the sample. According to the CDC, "weight data were not available between birth and three months of age" (CDC, 2010). How was the growth chart for infants developed without having access to weight data for babies under three months old? The WHO growth charts are superior for breastfed babies because they are normed using data from breastfed babies. The infants in the WHO study were all predominately breastfed through four months old, and all were breastfed for at least a year (CHTI, 2021). The WHO growth chart is much more appropriate for infants receiving breast milk than the CDC charts. Do not use the CDC charts for children under the age of two.

Prevention and Protection Strategy

Ask your pediatrician's office what growth chart they use. Be sure that your baby's weight gain is plotted on the newest WHO growth chart for breastfed infants.

Lack of Skilled Care or Access to Skilled Care

Imagine a team of athletes or a group of talented musicians who all have fantastic potential. However, they cannot attract a coach or teacher for many reasons. They want to play, compete, and perform, but they are all flying blind without a coach, and success is unlikely. Breastfeeding is similar, but the stakes are much higher.Several factors come together to foster breastfeeding success and access to skilled lactation care is an essential piece of the puzzle. Finding professional care can be a complex issue for some of us. First, and maybe the most damning part of our model of care in the U.S., most medical schools do not teach much about human lactation if anything. It may surprise you to learn that breastfeeding competencies rarely accompany medical training for any health professionals (Watkins et al., 2017). This means that your pediatrician had little lactation education in med school and likely has no formal training in the care of the breastfeeding dyad. Would you take piano lessons from someone with no background or training in music? Would you take driver's education classes from someone with no background or training in driving? Pediatricians are highly trained and skilled to care for infants and children, but they rarely receive training on human lactation in medical school. As a result, it is up to each doctor to attain that knowledge for themselves. Because it is not required, most pediatricians don't seek lactation training. Likewise, most other healthcare professionals have no additional training in lactation, although some doctors and nurses do. Be aware that you may be getting outdated, anecdotal, or even harmful advice when you get advice from your baby's pediatrician or your own physician about infant feeding.

For many new parents, the pediatrician's advice carries more weight than advice from friends, the internet, books, and even lactation consultants. People tend to trust their doctor and pediatrician because they are reliable sources of healthcare information for most issues. For years, I have been hearing from parents who share their stories about receiving breastfeeding advice from a pediatrician whose recommendations lead to unnecessary supplementation with infant formula, no nighttime breastfeeding, poor latching techniques, lack of effective milk transfer, and on and on.

A wise La Leche League leader told me that parents get two kinds of advice from pediatricians: parenting advice and medical advice. While it may make sense to follow the doctor's recommendations for medical advice, it is totally optional to follow recommendations for parenting advice. Of course, the key to success with this strategy is to know what constitutes medical advice and what does not. Sometimes, determining what is medical advice and what is parenting advice can be difficult for new parents. Essentially, every parent must go with their gut on this one. A general rule might be this: if the recommendations or advice is not directly related to the baby's health and safety, it might be parenting advice (or worse yet, outdated or unsound breastfeeding advice). Here are some examples of parenting advice from pediatricians:

- Advising you to sleep when the baby sleeps
- Comments on how long the baby should be sleeping (all night, at least a four-hour stretch, at least six hours before waking, or some other arbitrary number)

- Suggestions to use a white noise machine
- Comments about what solid food to feed
- Suggestions to use cow's milk or toddler milk
- Comments non-therapeutic pacifier use
- General recommendations about weaning by a certain age

Some of this may be reasonable advice but all of it is optional. In the end, you are the person who decides how to feed your baby, where the baby will sleep and when, what solids the baby will eat, and ultimately, the duration of human milk feeding for your baby. Bottom line, if you think that you are getting parenting advice instead of medical advice from your baby's doctor, think of it as optional. Their recommendations may not fit with your lifestyle, your cultural beliefs, or support your choices for breastfeeding.

Another reason it can be hard to find skilled care for breastfeeding is the steep entry fee for seeing a lactation consultant unless insurance covers your appointments. Since August 2012, the Affordable Care Act (ACA) has required that insurance companies cover lactation supplies, education, and breastfeeding support with a qualified professional. Unfortunately, because the language in the law is vague, insurance companies that were just a few years ago providing coverage for lactation visits are now denying coverage in some instances. In some instances, such as rural areas, there are no skilled lactation professionals such as IBCLCs, lactation educators, or certified lactation counselors (Grubesic & Durbin, 2020)including those provided by Baby-Friendly Hospitals, International Board Certified Lactation Consultants, breastfeeding counselors and educators, and volunteer-based mother-to-mother support organizations, such as La Leche League, are critically important for influencing breastfeeding initiation and continuation for the mother-child dyad. In addition, the emergence of community support options via information and communication technologies such as Skype and Facetime, social media (e.g., Facebook. In the case of rural Ohio and likely other states, breastfeeding support in rural areas may be only available by the Special Supplemental Nutrition Program for Women, Infants, and Children (WIC) program. Because there is an income threshold required to access WIC, some families will not qualify for services (Grubesic & Durbin, 2017).

Strategies for Finding Skilled Care

- Seek care from pediatricians with in-office lactation professionals on staff.
- Check to see what your insurance covers for breastfeeding education services and lactation consultants.
- If you qualify, make use of WIC classes and support.
- Get information and education from free, local breastfeeding support groups like La Leche League, Breastfeeding USA, and Baby Café USA. There are local and regional groups as well.
- Consult a second opinion when your gut tells you that something is off.
- Consider telehealth for seeing a lactation consultant if one is not available in your area. Since the COVID-19 pandemic, some companies have expanded services to include online or phone appointments with an LC. Many times, this is covered by insurance and may be a better option than seeing a local healthcare provider who has limited or no lactation training.

TRUE STORY

At a 10-month check-up with her baby's pediatrician, Nicole discussed breastfeeding with the doctor. The pediatrician told her that at 12 months, she would need to begin adding cow's milk to all the human milk that she feeds her baby. According to this doctor, during the second year of life, infants in the U.S. need to wean from breast milk to whole cow's milk. He stated that even though the World Health Organization (WHO) recommends breastfeeding for a full two years, that recommendation is only for people living in countries with lower nutrition status. Nicole believed that the WHO recommendations for breastfeeding for two years included her baby, not just infants in low-income nations. Therefore, she dismissed the pediatrician's advice and continued with breastfeeding.

This information came from a pediatrician in Texas (USA) in 2020. What I find so striking about this terrible and misguided advice is that no human needs cow's milk. It is optional. Human bodies are built to drink and process human milk, not cow's milk. Where did this advice come from? It is likely a holdover from formula feeding because infant formula is unnecessary for babies after one year. Does this doctor have any training in human lactation? I believe that the answer to that question is a resounding no, but some new parents may believe this person is an authority on breastfeeding and take this advice. Why does the doctor think that at 12 months, there is a sudden need for cow's milk and that human milk is now somehow deficient and even unnecessary? Why would infants in the U.S. have a reduced need for good nutrition compared to other nations? With obesity and diabetes rates soaring in the U.S., doesn't it make sense to recommend human milk for more than one year? There are so many red flags in this story. It doesn't take much background knowledge in lactation to recognize that this pediatrician was offering (unsound) parenting advice and not medical advice.

Healthcare System Infant Formula Giveaways

In 1981, the World Health Organization ratified the International Code of Marketing of Breast-milk Substitutes (also called the WHO code by lactation professionals) to regulate the infant formula marketing industry and curb years of sleazy and dangerous marketing practices that have systematically undermined breastfeeding all over the world. Unfortunately, although it has been over four decades since the WHO developed the code, the U.S. never adopted any provisions of the code, and numerous U.S.-based companies and many physicians violate the code every day. Some of those violations include in-office promotion of formula, free samples, giveaways, and coupons at hospitals and doctor's offices nationwide. This problem is so widespread that the Academy of Breastfeeding Medicine created a protocol to provide supplementary guidelines to physicians (in addition to the WHO code) outlining best practices for in-office breastfeeding promotion (ABM Clinical Protocol #14 Breastfeeding-Friendly Physician's Office – Optimizing Care for Infants and Children) (Vanguri et al., 2021).

Risks Associated with the Promotion of Formula Within the Healthcare System

First, the promotion of formula from within the healthcare system suggests that formula is a healthy or optimal choice. If it comes from the hospital or a doctor's office, the formula will appear to be *endorsed* by and approved by the healthcare community. This appearance of endorsement of infant formula is particularly significant because it can lead new parents to make conclusions about their caregiver's attitude toward infant feeding methods. In fact, caregivers' attitudes about infant feeding can profoundly influence parental choices. Consider this:

- Data from the Infant Feeding Practices Study II of over 1600 people showed a significant correlation between maternal perception of their caregiver's attitude toward exclusive breastfeeding and their own breastfeeding outcomes. In this study, exclusive breastfeeding rates were higher at one and three months when people perceived that their caregiver preferred exclusive breastfeeding (Ramakrishnan et al., 2014). Another study showed that breastfeeding failure at six weeks postpartum could be predicted by maternal perceptions of the hospital staff's attitude toward breastfeeding (Radzyminski & Callister, 2016). In other words, people are substantially influenced by what they perceive about their caregiver's belief about infant feeding. The appearance of endorsement matters, whether the caregiver appears to support breastfeeding or whether they support formula. It amounts to influence either way.

Before the Code

Before the introduction of the WHO code, hospital and doctor's offices were actively marketing formula. Formula companies provided physicians with free formula samples to give to new families, distributing them at the time of discharge from the hospital. Pediatricians also participated in free formula giveaways. In addition, pediatrician's offices of the past would prominently display in-office advertising with literature and posters promoting infant formula. Doctors themselves were often recipients of giveaways, receiving swag from formula companies (pens, stationery, and even medical equipment) with the company logo blatantly displayed. Doctor's offices also received financial incentives for staff training, conferences, or meetings. These gifts and incentives created a certain feeling of indebtedness and brand loyalty to formula manufacturers among the families who received the free samples and doctors who received the swag and incentives.

Since 1981 and the Introduction of the WHO Code

In the U.S., the scenario described above about the past is problematic because it is not confined to the past. Formula marketing today remains in many hospitals and doctor's offices in much the same way because the U.S. never formally adopted the WHO code. There certainly are hospitals, companies, and individual physicians who are code compliant, but they are uncommon in the U.S. However, there have been some significant improvements over the last few decades. Below are some examples of important developments to ban the promotion of formula in healthcare settings.

Ban the Bags

Ban the Bags is a national campaign in the U.S. seeking to combat aggressive and predatory marketing of infant formula, particularly, the free formula gift bag distribution at hospital discharge. Originally, Ban the Bags was an effort by the Massachusetts Breastfeeding Coalition to stop the in-hospital distribution of free formula gift bags to all new families. Since 2007, this campaign has spread to many other states and cities across the U.S. Several states are bag-free, including Delaware, Maryland, Massachusetts, New Hampshire, Rhode Island, and West Virginia. All hospitals operating in Indian Services are bag-free. The cities of Philadelphia and Washington, D.C. have also stopped the distribution of free formula gift bags.

Baby-Friendly Hospital Initiative

The Baby-Friendly Hospital Initiative was established in 1991 by WHO and UNICEF. The Baby-Friendly Hospital initiative supports the WHO code. Hospitals seeking to achieve Baby-Friendly status also must agree to implement the Ten Steps to Successful Breastfeeding.

Ten Steps to Successful Breastfeeding (World Health Organization, 2018b):

1a. Comply fully with the International Code of Marketing of Breast-milk Substitutes and relevant World Health Assembly resolutions.

1b. Have a written infant feeding policy and routinely communicate it to all staff and parents.

1c. Establish ongoing monitoring and data-management systems.

2. Ensure that staff have sufficient knowledge, competence, and skills to support breastfeeding.

3. Discuss the importance and management of breastfeeding with pregnant women and their families.

4. Facilitate immediate and uninterrupted skin-to-skin contact and support mothers to initiate breastfeeding as soon as possible after birth.

5. Support mothers to initiate and maintain breastfeeding and manage common difficulties.

6. Do not provide breastfed newborns any food or fluids other than breast milk, unless medically indicated.

7. Enable mothers and their infants to remain together and to practice rooming-in 24 hours a day.

8. Support mothers to recognize and respond to their infants' cues for feeding.

9. Counsel mothers on the use and risks of feeding bottles, teats, and pacifiers.

10. Coordinate discharge so that parents and their infants have timely access to ongoing support and care.

Steps 3 through 10 are particularly related to care and support for the breastfeeding dyad. If you give birth at a Baby-Friendly Hospital, these steps will likely be in place. If you are giving birth at a facility that does not have Baby-Friendly status, you may need to request immediate postpartum skin-to-skin care and rooming-in.

You might also need to remind caregivers to refrain from feeding your baby anything other than your own milk, and to avoid giving pacifiers.

There is mounting evidence that giving birth in a Baby-Friendly hospital protects the breastfeeding relationship. For example, in the U.S., studies show that infants born at Baby-Friendly hospitals are more likely to initiate breastfeeding than babies born at other hospitals (Merewood et al., 2005). In addition, Baby-Friendly hospitals report higher exclusive breastfeeding rates during the hospital stay (Merewood et al., 2005).

By implementing the ten steps listed above, Baby-Friendly hospitals never promote formula, give free samples or display images that idealize formula use. They also cannot accept sponsorships or incentives from formula manufacturers. This creates an atmosphere of human milk promotion and protection instead of fostering brand loyalty to infant formula.

CHAPTER 13

Lactation Interference: Social and Cultural Factors

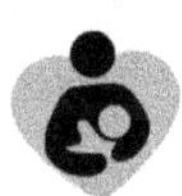

Social and Cultural Factors

In the introduction of this book, I claim that some of the lactation interference factors are not just random situations or events that exist on the fringe that you *might* encounter. Many of these lactation interference factors are social and cultural elements that are woven into our lives. They are part of the fabric of society, and many of these factors are truly unavoidable. For example, in the United States, it is perfectly legal for formula manufacturers to market their products directly to consumers in all types of media (print, TV commercials, online advertisements, and other types of marketing). These advertisements are so commonplace in the U.S. that virtually no one is surprised to see persuasive formula ads featuring happy families, babies, and toddlers consuming industrially-produced baby formula. It does not shock anyone because it is so normal. It is essentially part of U.S. society and culture. That normalcy is what makes this category of lactation interference factors so insidious.

In this section, we will cover a range of ubiquitous lactation interference factors. These factors exist in many facets of life and are unavoidable because they are omnipresent and accepted as culturally normal. Culturally "normal" does not always mean the best option, healthy, or even *acceptable*. The good news is that challenges are emerging to counteract some of these social and cultural factors. For example, in the Unsupportive Workplace section, I outline several ways a return to work/job can interfere with lactation and infant feeding. I have also included important information about three companies leading the way to make the workplace parenting friendly and human milk friendly.

Some of the factors in this section are quite difficult to avoid or ignore. These factors include *formula marketing, feeding babies in public*, and an *unsupportive workplace*. However, the tide may be turning on these and other interference factors. To create a more optimal environment for feeding our babies, we, the families who choose to feed infants with human milk, must initiate the change. We can substantially impact the social and cultural "normalcy" of authentic, biologically normal infant feeding.

Partner Support is Critical

Breastfeeding is not just for the breastfeeding dyad; it is a family affair. Research shows that one of the single most important factors regarding the maternal choice to breastfeed and confidence in breastfeeding is the attitude or opinion of the partner (Arora et al., 2000; Pavill, 2002; Rempel & Rempel, 2011). Fascinating research shows that when the partner receives prenatal education about breastfeeding, initiation rates go up. For example, Wolfberg et al. (2004) found that the breastfeeding initiation rate was 74% for people whose partner had attended a 2-hour breastfeeding education class, compared to only 41% for people whose partner did not attend a breastfeeding education class. Clearly, the opinion of partners has a dramatic impact on our infant feeding choices. Partners are sometimes unclear of their role regarding infant feeding, especially if breastfeeding is the preferred choice. Often, partners are confused about how they can help with breastfeeding, be supportive of the dyad, bond with the baby, or interact with a newborn. However, there are many ways partners can support the choice to breastfeed and support the breastfeeding parent. One can usually characterize this into two types of support: *emotional support* and *functional support*. Providing both types of support is critical to breastfeeding success.

Emotional Support is the Key to Being a Supportive Partner:

- Be available for discussions about infant feeding, infant wellness, and baby care.
- Listen attentively and actively.
- Use encouraging words and body language. For example, "You're doing great! This is incredible!"

- Know that sometimes, your best response is to validate feelings and concerns. You might say, "Yes, I know this is tough, but we can get through this. I am here to help whatever way I can."
- Acknowledge your partner's feelings and frustrations. "You are having a hard day. I can tell that you're tired."
- Ask genuine questions about your partner and the new baby. For example, "How is it going? Are you feeling burned out? What can I do? Was this feeding easier than yesterday? Is your nipple pain feeling better? Is the baby's latch improving? Has pumping at work been going well?"

Functional support is absolutely necessary, no matter how your family plans to feed the baby. Functional support is what you can physically do to support infant feeding and care in your household.

- Learn your baby's feeding cues.
- Help your partner find comfortable positions for nursing.
- Learn to soothe your baby with infant calming techniques.
- Bathe your baby.
- Change your baby's clothing.
- Change diapers.
- Prepare a healthy snack or provide a water refill for your partner while the baby is at the breast.
- Do other household tasks like caring for older children, meal prep, pet care, dishes, and laundry.
- Functional support can also be about finding information about breastfeeding to help support your partner and the baby.
- Functional support also entails advocating for the family and your breastfeeding rights. For example, you may need to explain to a waiter, a lifeguard, or a shop owner that breastfeeding is legal, and your family has the right to breastfeed in any location where your presence is legal. You might also be the mediator when it comes to unsupportive family members. As the partner, you may need to explain to an aunt or your mother that breastfeeding is your choice as a family and is a healthy and safe way

to feed a baby. Be ready to defend your choices as a family instead of putting the weight of your choices (and their defense) on one partner.

Here are some essential strategies to help partners take the initiative and participate in breastfeeding and support in the prenatal period and beyond:

- Define your role as breastfeeding supporter. How will you help emotionally and functionally?
- Find classes and online education that directly address partners and their role in supporting breastfeeding.
- Partners can become knowledgeable about breastfeeding by learning about lactation, reading books, or finding reputable online information.
- Help identify and locate breastfeeding-friendly care from pediatricians, primary care doctors, and lactation counselors/consultants.
- Attend doctor visits, if possible (especially for infant care), in the early weeks.
- Be ready to adjust household chores and take an active part in things that were not necessarily part of your routine before.
- Learn to be an advocate for breastfeeding; learn about your rights and know your local laws.
- Speak of your family choices as a team. Use *we* when you find that you need to explain your choices. For example, "We decided this is our best approach to infant feeding and for maternal health." Avoid putting the credit (or blame) all on the breastfeeding parent. The family is a team.
- Know that you don't always have to explain or justify your choices, but a little explanation goes a long way with those closest to us. Strangers need no answers.

Formula Marketing

The marketing of infant formula has dramatic and detrimental effects on breastfeeding initiation and duration. The world of breast milk substitute marketing has a controversial and scandalous past in the U.S. and abroad. The infamous Nestlé Boycott, dating from July 1977, has taken many forms and exists in different organizations globally. It originated because of the alleged ill-effects of the Nestlé infant formula marketing campaigns in developing countries. People in developed nations are at no less risk of being influenced by the marketing of breast milk substitutes than people in developing nations. Consider these facts:

- Studies show that women exposed to industry-generated formula advertising are less likely to be breastfeeding at the time of hospital discharge (Howard, 2000).
- Receiving samples of infant formula (discharge gift bags) from the hospital at the time of delivery significantly decreases breastfeeding exclusively at ten weeks of age and six months (Feldman-Winter et al., 2012; Sadacharan et al., 2014).
- Abbott Labs, makers of Similac, has been collecting data about breastfeeding and formula use since 1954 with fake research "institutes," using a survey tool to gather data directly from families about infant feeding practices. Abbott was fined $50,000 in New York for this deceptive practice (Johns, 2018).
- Marketing can take many forms: print advertising, TV and online marketing, social media platforms and campaigns, in-office marketing at pediatrician's and family doctor offices, hospital discharge gift bags, and targeted coupon campaigns. This marketing aims to make it appear that using breast milk substitutes is ubiquitous, safe, and easy – *and endorsed by your hospital and pediatrician.* Unfortunately, this endorsement serves to legitimize formula feeding. As a result, breastfeeding rates drop with exposure to aggressive formula marketing tactics.
- The infant formula industry is a highly profitable sector of the food market, worth $70 billion per year (Hastings et al., 2020).

It is nearly impossible to avoid exposure to formula advertising during pregnancy and as a new parent in the U.S. and other developed nations. Although the World Health Organization (WHO) created a document outlining safer ways to market breast milk substitutes (commonly called the WHO Code), many companies violate the Code every day. In this context, U.S.-based companies are some of the biggest offenders. Many countries worldwide have signed on to the Code and pledged to adhere to safer marketing practices for formula marketing but the U.S. is not one of them. In addition, in 2018, the U.S. refused to back a U.N. breastfeeding support resolution that had language that the U.S. officials deemed offensive. The language in the resolution included a call for nations to "protect, promote and support breastfeeding" (New York Times, 2018). Are corporate profits more worthy of promotion than breastfeeding and child health? Unfortunately, this decision fosters a climate and culture where formula feeding is the norm and breastfeeding is still considered the alternative.

Until genuine and effective policy changes are in place to end the marketing of infant formula, it may be impossible to counterbalance the ill effects of the marketing of breastmilk substitutes. This task may seem impossible, but policy activism dramatically changed marketing tactics from various industries in the past. For example, the Public Health Cigarette Smoking Act of 1970 banned the advertising of cigarettes on TV and radio in U.S. markets. Similarly, there are regulations for alcohol marketing, and as a result, alcohol ads will not air when kids watch children's programs or preschool programs. So, why not regulate the marketing of infant formula?

The authors of a recent exposé on the infant formula industry sum up the main point in this way:

"The problem is not the product but rather out-of-control marketing, which is driving dangerous over-consumption in the interests of corporate profits" (Hastings et al., 2020).

In other words, corporate profits are driving infant formula marketing, and there are no limitations or boundaries on this corner of the marketing industry in the U.S. That said, there are situations where infant formula is necessary and even lifesaving. However, promoting it at the cost of human milk is irresponsible and damaging for human and environmental health. We are long overdue for a complete reckoning (and revision) of the formula marketing industry.

Grandmothers: Help or Hindrance?

In the long view of human history, grandmothers were integral in helping new mothers navigate the transition to parenthood and learn about infant feeding. Grandmothers could teach breastfeeding wisdom because, presumably, they had years of experience breastfeeding. However, the skills of feeding an infant at the breast were lost to most people in formula feeding societies, beginning in earnest in the 1950s and lasting through today. Many grandmothers of the 1970s, 80s, and 90s (and beyond) could not advise their grown children with breastfeeding because they had no experience with lactation. Formula feeding practices, knowledge, and skills do not translate well to breastfeeding. The rules and logic are different. Many grandmothers find it hard to support breastfeeding because they lack the skills and knowledge. In addition, some grandmothers may perceive the idea of their daughter choosing to breastfeed as a rejection of the choices they made with their own children.

It can be tricky to navigate the unexpected emotions and attitudes that reveal themselves among family members regarding infant feeding. A client told me about her own mother gently pushing her to try formula with her first child. The grandmother's intent was not to sabotage breastfeeding. She recommended that her daughter try formula because she thought this would give her a break from all the work of lactation and childcare. Her thought was that another person could feed the baby if she needed to step away. The grandmother intended to be supportive, and because formula feeding was the majority of her experience, she thought this would help. In reality, this was not supportive of my client's intention to use only human milk.

Recent research suggests that grandmother support can be helpful to new parents learning to breastfeed, but only if the grandmothers "had had their own breastfeeding experience or were positively inclined toward breastfeeding" (Negin et al., 2016). Cultural differences must be accounted for as well. Negin et al. (2016) showed that among highly educated Chinese populations, grandmother support was associated with lower rates of exclusive breastfeeding (Negin et al., 2016).

Types of Grandparent Help

When it comes to grandparents offering to help, the type of support they can offer generally falls into three categories: *financial*, *practical*, and *emotional*. For this discussion, we are concerned with practical support and emotional support.

Getting the most out of your support team is essential in the early days of breastfeeding and childrearing. To do that, you must know what type of support you need, and you may have to ask for it. Both can be stumbling blocks for people. As new parents, only you will be able to assess if your family and friends will be reliable breastfeeding supporters, either practical or emotional. Let's look at what each type of support entails.

Emotional Support

- Loving, patient, and kind encouragement without judgment
- Validation of concerns, feelings, emotions
- Active listening and support without negative feedback
- Listening *without* always providing solutions
- Encouragement, cheerleading, reassurance, praise
- Phone call or texting to check-in
- Being emotionally available and focused
- Genuinely ask how new parents are managing
- Ask what support is needed; identify ways to help

Practical/Functional Support

- Cooking, making meals and snacks for today or the freezer
- Laundry
- Driving the parent to an appointment
- Housekeeping chores
- Grocery shopping
- Helping with infant bathing, changing diapers
- Watching the baby for short periods so a parent can rest, take a shower, eat a meal
- Childcare

Be honest about your needs and ask for help from caregivers, friends, and family when you know they can be reliable. Don't ask for breastfeeding help from the baby's grandmother unless you know that she has the skills and knowledge to help you. It can be highly advantageous to tell your close family and friends what your infant feeding goals are so they can be supportive. After all, if they don't know your breastfeeding goals, they may unknowingly give unsupportive advice or do things to sabotage your efforts. There are many stories in parenting and lactation communities of grandparents feeding formula (or feeding solids) to an exclusively breastfed baby without asking the parents first. Just because you choose to breastfeed doesn't mean that everyone will assume you're not also using formula. If you are using some formula, let others know your routines so that you maximize the time your baby spends at the breast.

Asking for help is not always easy, but it is an essential skill of parenting. No one can do it alone. First, make a list of your crew, your network of people you feel you can rely on most. You'll feel less like a burden asking them for help than approaching a neighbor you hardly know. Of course, if that neighbor offers to help, take them up on it. Second, be sure what you're asking is within the limits or skills of the person you've asked. For example, do not ask your 11-year-old niece to make you a meal; that may not be a skill she has acquired yet. Third, ask your partner, a good friend, confidant, cousin, or sister to act as your advocate in finding support. This person can set up a meal train or ask others in your network to offer support if you're overwhelmed or uncomfortable asking for help. Fourth, find parenting support groups for emotional support if you find you're in need. This support may include local breastfeeding support groups or online groups for breastfeeding advice. Finally, do not hesitate to reach out if you believe you are experiencing any kind of postpartum mood or anxiety disorder. Right now, even if you're still pregnant or doing well after the birth, find out who or where to call if you need help. Keep the contact information handy in case you need it. In the U.S., Postpartum Support International has a helpline: 1-800-944-4773 in English or Spanish.

TRUE STORY (SOME DETAILS WERE CHANGED FOR PRIVACY)

Casey, a breastfeeding mother in Raleigh, North Carolina, had her first baby in 2021. Her mother and grandmother, living in South Carolina, were excited to meet the new grandbaby. They scheduled a seven-day visit when the baby was just one week old. When they arrived, they fully expected to spend their week holding the baby, bonding with their new grandchild, and being waited on as special guests. On the other hand, Casey was in the first days of breastfeeding, getting the hang of the latch process and feeding the baby on demand. She spent much of her time feeding the baby, napping when the baby was asleep, and focused on her own self-care (essential in the first weeks postpartum). Casey's mother and grandmother were disappointed that they got so little time to hold the baby, and were surprised that they never had the opportunity to feed the baby a bottle. They also told Casey that they felt unwelcomed by the family because no one was looking after their needs. Casey's mother even reminded her about her grandmother's age and health. "It wasn't easy for grandma to make the trip here to see you!" They rescheduled their return to South Carolina, leaving three days early in disappointment.

Casey told me that this incident forever changed her relationship with her mother and grandmother. I asked her about more details of the grandmothers' lives and infant feeding experiences. She revealed that both women had used formula exclusively with their children and knew nothing about the routines and practices of breastfeeding. It is unfortunate that Casey, her mother, and grandmother all had significantly different expectations for the week of their visit. Casey was expecting some help, even if it was just emotional support. She was reasonably close to her mother and thought that she could rely on her for support. However, the mother and grandmother had expectations of holding and feeding the baby and being catered to as out-of-town guests. It's nearly impossible to know how life will go with your new baby, but one can avoid these types of situations. For example, Casey and her mother should have discussed what might happen during the visit and Casey's limitations for catering to their needs. Further, there should have been a discussion of the needs for an exclusively breastfed baby and who would be taking care of Casey while she cared for the baby. Granted, these types of conversations are not always easy. However, setting expectations is essential for these types of family visits.

Unsupportive Workplace Without Guaranteed Paid Leave

It is *shocking* that, today in the U.S., hundreds of people will stop breastfeeding well before they had planned to because of an unsupportive employer.

Think about this scenario: Jayne and her newborn get breastfeeding off to a good start. Because Jayne is the breadwinner for the family, she returns to work after four weeks. At work, there are difficulties in securing a private space to pump. Her boss tells her to pump in the restroom. In addition, the employer will not always allow breaks when Jayne needs to express milk. Because she cannot regularly remove milk from her breasts, she develops engorgement, plugged ducts, and, eventually, mastitis. She ultimately switches to mixed feeding with formula. She goes hours each day without removing milk, and soon, her milk supply substantially decreases. Finally, she is feeding formula exclusively.

This scenario is not fictional. It happens to people in every state, every week, at hundreds of places of employment throughout the U.S., not just hourly-wage jobs. So, let's talk about why this is an entirely unacceptable outcome for the mother and her baby.

- First, it is unconscionable that the United States does not guarantee paid maternity leave. The U.S. is the only industrialized nation that offers none. Canada gives 15 weeks paid leave for birth or adoption. The U. K. gives 39 weeks paid leave. In Sweden, it's 52 paid weeks, sharable between the parents.
- In the U.S., the Affordable Care Act (ACA) has some provisions to guarantee a clean, private place to pump that is not a restroom. Unfortunately, every day, some employers across the country break the law by not providing this space.
- Only allowing pumping breaks when it's convenient for the employer is not conducive for lactation.
- Many parents who return to work and wish to continue breast-

feeding are forced into choosing between keeping their job and feeding their new baby at the breast. This choice is discriminatory.

- Some people have been demoted, lost pay, or lost their jobs after asserting their rights to breastfeed when their bosses push back against the provisions of the law.
- In 2019, Huffington Post investigated several cases of failed pumping at work. They found that employers often do not know the law, and even when they do, some are not making efforts to comply (Jamieson, 2019).
- The ACA only provides for pump breaks at companies with over 50 people and some types of hourly workers. The law makes no provisions for salaried workers.
- At the time of this writing, congressional lawmakers in the U.S. are working to pass legislation to guarantee paid maternity/parental leave, but as of yet, it has not happened. So far, this is proving to be difficult.

In the U.S., it is often difficult to find knowledgeable and supportive employers. Still, some forward-thinking companies are at the forefront of this issue, setting the example for others. Here are several companies leading the way for families when it comes to mixing breastfeeding with employment:

Amazon: In their Seattle headquarters, Amazon boasts 100 lactation rooms to accommodate pumping while working. Each room offers hospital-grade pumps and refrigerators for storing pumped milk. If people prefer to bring their own pumps, the lactation room has storage for personal equipment.

Facebook: In the U.S., Facebook offers over 100 nursing rooms at their offices throughout the country. These rooms also offer refrigerators, pumps, and facilities for cleaning equipment.

Deloitte: This accounting firm offers private nursing rooms at all of its U.S. offices. Deloitte provides each breastfeeding employee with a pump and a generous six months of phone counseling with a lactation consultant.

Strategies for Dealing with Your Employer

- Don't wait. Talk to your employer while you're pregnant.
- Become informed about your rights under the ACA and what you are entitled to. Visit the United States Breastfeeding Committee webpage and read about Federal Workplace Law. On this page, you will find explanations for the ACA Break Time for Nursing Mothers Law. In addition, there are useful links about all aspects of the law, including one page from The Office on Women's Health, which is specifically for employers. It has information and guidelines for employers on how to support nursing mothers at work.
- File complaints when companies fail to meet the required accommodations. Sometimes, this is uncomfortable, but this is the only way we can move forward. If companies are never penalized for failure to meet their legal requirements, the culture of pumping at work will not change.

Incarceration

Many socially and economically marginalized groups lack opportunities for breastfeeding education and support. However, there are few groups more challenged than incarcerated mothers in the United States. A 2019 report from the Prison Policy Initiative states that there are about 231,000 incarcerated women in the U.S. According to Pregnancy in Prison Statistics (PIPS), about 4% of incarcerated women are pregnant (ARRWIP, 2019). The number of infants born during incarceration is increasing in the U.S. each year. Currently, only nine correctional facilities in the U.S. provide prison nurseries. In these facilities, babies can live with their mother for several months, sometimes up to two years. In these situations, breastfeeding is possible. However, for most infants, separation from the parent is the norm, with babies going to custodial family members or foster care within hours after birth. Recent research from Nova Scotia suggests that barriers to breastfeeding during incarceration are equally high in Canada as well (Paynter, 2018).

Breastfeeding during incarceration is a human rights issue. In many places in the U.S., it is a human rights failure, but some states recognize and provide legal protection under state law. California, for example, provides in California Penal Code 4002.5: "On or before January 1, 2020, the sheriff of each county or the administrator of each county jail shall develop and implement an infant and toddler breast milk feeding policy for lactating inmates detained in or sentenced to county jail. The policy shall be based on currently accepted best practices" (California Penal Code 4002.5, 2018). This law also provides for expression of human milk, and storage of milk for later use.

In 2019, New Mexico legally recognized that inmates have the right to breastfeed or provide milk for their infants. Their laws provide for implementing breastfeeding policies at correctional facilities based on best practices. New Mexico also has a law that requires a court to consider pregnancy or lactation as a condition for release or bond, but these examples appear to be the exception, not the rule.

More support for the rights of incarcerated people who are pregnant and/or breastfeeding is desperately needed. In addition, it may be time to reframe this discussion to protect and preserve parent-baby bonding during incarceration and include infant's rights as well. Whether they are born to a parent who is serving time or not, every baby should have the right to breastmilk from their own parent. It is a monumental injustice that the criminal justice system would seek to separate any newborn from its parent and their milk supply.

While you might think that this does not apply to you because you are not currently in prison, human rights violations regarding infant feeding come at a substantial cost for all of humanity because this guarantees suboptimal feeding and potential future health consequences for some children.

TRUE STORY

In 2021, Rory, a new parent with an 8-week-old infant, was detained by local police. She was arrested and jailed overnight. The facility offered her no breast pump. She was separated from her baby and could not collect and store milk, even if she chose to hand express. This scenario plays out frequently, but we rarely hear about this injustice because of the marginalized nature of incarcerated populations. As a society, we are generally behind the rest of the world on all infant and maternal health measures, and incarceration is no different. Depriving infants of their own mother's milk during incarceration is a massive human rights failure.

Awkward and Embarrassing (for Some People)!

Feelings of embarrassment and awkwardness can be difficult for some people to believe (especially those who live in breastfeeding-friendly communities). However, these feelings contribute to early weaning or not initiating breastfeeding at all. In a formula feeding culture, society rarely associates breasts with infant feeding. For example, there are strong cultural undercurrents in the U.S. that sexually objectify breasts. Exposing the breasts while feeding a baby can cause embarrassment and shame for the mother in some instances (Leahy-Warren et al., 2017). In her fascinating book, *The Politics of Breastfeeding: When Breasts are Bad for Business*, Gabrielle Palmer discusses the taboo of the exposed breast in many industrialized societies. She reasons that because "breastfeeding in industrialized society is closely bound up with perceptions of sexuality," it can cause embarrassment for those who witness breastfeeding, not just those who *are* breastfeeding. It is, indeed, a complex and complicated topic. In the 2011 Call to Action to Support Breastfeeding issued by former U. S. Surgeon General Dr. Regina Benjamin, embarrassment is listed as one of the many barriers to breastfeeding in the United States. The report states, "Embarrassment remains a formidable barrier to breastfeeding in the United States," and is intimately linked to the continued societal tendency of condemnation of public breastfeeding (Office of the Surgeon General (US) et al., 2011). I highly recommend reading the full report.

TRUE STORY

Several years before I had my own children, my friend Lyn had her first baby. I visited her at home during the first week after the birth. While I was there, Lyn's baby displayed classic feeding cues, and she put him to the breast to try breastfeeding. She had initiated breastfeeding on the day of birth. Still, she had little practical support, if any, with latch and positioning. In addition, she was self-conscious about breastfeeding, even at home with me, her good friend, as the only other person in the house. I could tell that she felt awkward and unprepared with her baby at the breast, but at that time, I had zero skills with infants or infant feeding. Consequently, I was no help. During my visit that afternoon, she repeatedly put the baby to the breast but felt unsatisfied about his attempts to nurse. During one of his trips to the breast, her phone rang. She was expecting a call from her sister and asked me to answer it. Instead, it was not her sister but another good (female) friend of ours calling to check in after her birth. I explained that Lyn could not answer the phone because she was "trying to get the hang of breastfeeding." Lyn was thoroughly embarrassed by my comment. "If anyone else calls, just tell them I am unavailable at the moment." She was too embarrassed by the idea of breastfeeding that she did not even want others to hear about it, much less be a witness.

What are the solutions to this complex issue? A recent study in Ireland (a predominantly formula-fed nation) suggests that breastfeeding support groups can provide a sense of normalcy and foster communities of acceptance for breastfeeding (Leahy-Warren, et al., 2017). In addition, general themes that emerged from the study found breastfeeding support groups can:

- Help people build confidence in their breastfeeding skills
- Overcome embarrassment
- Act as a buffer to the negative attitudes they encounter about breastfeeding (Leahy-Warren, et al., 2017)

Other ways to gain confidence in breastfeeding and avoid embarrassment include:

- Practice breastfeeding in front of a mirror at home. This practice gives you a chance to see how little skin is actually exposed and how to position your clothing.
- Buy a few nursing tanks or shirts. Nursing shirts keep your belly covered while allowing easy access to the breast.
- Use a small blanket or nursing cover to make you feel more comfortable (but know that it can attract attention). In contrast, a nursing baby with no cover often appears to onlookers to be sleeping in arms rather than feeding.

- Pick a safe place to practice breastfeeding – a friend's home, a breastfeeding support group meeting, your local library, friendly coffee shop, or cozy bookstore. Don't try your first public breastfeeding session in a busy place where you feel uncomfortable.

Returning to Work

In a family friendly society with high regard for human milk, returning to work does not impact breastfeeding and lactation. Currently, we (in the U.S. and many other places) are not living in that reality. Many parents who return to work struggle to make their work life mesh well with their infant feeding goals. This return to work while breastfeeding can present barriers to the continuation of breastfeeding and pumping. For many people, going back to work can negatively impact breastfeeding duration, leading to early weaning and the inability to reach infant feeding goals (Murtagh & Moulton, 2011; Scott et al., 2019).

Although there are federal laws in the U.S. protecting break time for parents who express milk while working, there are some exceptions to the law, which means that not every worker has guaranteed break time. The law is supposed to provide two specific accommodations for breastfeeding: unpaid break time for workers to pump and a private place for expressing milk other than a bathroom. Recent research on the outcomes of the Affordable Care Act concerning these two specific mandates for breastfeeding revealed that only 40% of parents report having access to break time and a place to pump (Kozhimannil et al., 2016). This research suggests that there is low compliance with the law. In addition, this study showed clear advantages for people who have access to both break time and a private place to pump. The study reports that parents with these accommodations at the workplace were 2.3 times more likely to continue breastfeeding exclusively through six months than those who did not have access to these accommodations (Kozhimannil et al., 2016).

A fascinating study of local regulations examined 151 U.S. cities to determine how many locales protect parents who pump milk while working. Unfortunately, only two cities out of the total 151 had specific legislation in place to provide protections for expressing milk while working (Froh et al., 2018).

There are many benefits f*or employers* who manage to facilitate workplace pumping and help promote the use of human milk among employees. Consider these benefits for the boss when the workplace is highly engaged and supportive of lactation:

- Better employee satisfaction
- Fewer employee absences to care for sick children
- Better recruitment and retention of employees

Basic employer support for breastfeeding involves several essential elements: 1) management's active support, 2) a safe, clean place to pump milk, and 3) an appropriate place to store expressed milk. Frankly, achieving these goals does not seem insurmountable. Yet, the challenges to combining work with successful breastfeeding persist.

TRUE STORY

Leanna was working in a busy dental office. She was pumping milk twice during her workday. After a few months, her manager began to make negative comments about the break time she needed for pumping, once even stating that Leanna's baby should now be weaned. There was confusion over where Leanna could pump as well. Although she used empty exam rooms for pumping after she returned from maternity leave, this option was suddenly frowned upon. When Leanna complained, she was inexplicably transferred to another location, 45 minutes from her home. The longer commute made it difficult for her. She eventually found a part-time job closer to home that would better accommodate her breastfeeding and pumping schedule.

Ironically, studies show that even working at businesses at the forefront of healthcare and health promotion can often present the same issues and challenges for parents who pump/express milk during the workday in non-healthcare related fields (Scott et al., 2019).

Combining Work With Your Infant Feeding Goals

There are ways to reach your infant feeding goals while still working. You may need to be flexible during the year after your baby is born. Be open to temporary changes in your work situation. Consider the following:

- Do not assume anything about your maternity leave and accommodations for expressing milk once you return to work. Speak to your employer before you go on maternity leave, if possible.
- Know your rights. This foundation is critical and could save you a lot of headaches, especially if your employer is unaware of their legal responsibilities. Read about "Workplace Support and Federal Law" on the United States Breastfeeding Committee webpage, usbreastfeeding.org.
- Take the most extended maternity leave that is possible. It can take about six to eight weeks to establish a good breastfeeding routine. Still, many people find that returning to work two months postpartum is too soon. If possible, postpone returning to work until after three months.
- Inquire about going back to work part-time for a few months as a transition back to full-time work.
- Ask about job share opportunities.
- Look into on-site childcare (or childcare that is close to your workplace). This arrangement can allow for at least one in-person feeding session per day in place of expressing and storing your milk.
- Look for a breastfeeding support group. It helps to speak to others who have experienced the challenges of nursing and working.
- You will need to express some milk before your first week of work, but you will not need hundreds of ounces of milk in your freezer. You will only need enough milk for your first day away and probably a little more just as a safety net. After you begin working, you will pump on Monday the milk your baby will drink on Tuesday. Essentially, you will always be pumping one day ahead. Of course, you can have a small supply in your freezer *just in case,* but you do not need a massive stockpile of milk. Remember, too much pumping can interfere with your supply. Only pump what you need.
- Feed your baby just before you walk out the door for work or during the drop-off at daycare. In addition, plan to feed your

baby as soon as you are reunited later that day. This routine may mean that you must alert your baby's caregiver not to give a bottle in the hour just before pick-up. Otherwise, if your baby seems full, he will not be interested in nursing. This approach minimizes the amount of milk you have to provide for daycare and ensures that the baby will come to the breast as much as possible.

The Vulnerable Period

Before initiating lactation, many people set some primary feeding goals. These are usually centered on the duration of months or years that they intend to feed their baby with human milk. Based on my observation, one common goal in the U.S. is to reach at least one year of breastfeeding. Many people who intend to breastfeed do not reach their personal infant feeding goals. The reasons are varied and multi-factored. Some people feel that circumstances that seem out of their control force their hand, causing the early termination of milk production and breastfeeding. Some of these reasons include concerns about 1) infant weight gain, 2) issues with comfortable and effective latch, 3) issues related to parental leave, 4) maternal or infant illness, 5) unsupportive work environment, 6) unsupportive healthcare personnel, 7) unsupportive family, and 8) cultural norms more aligned with formula feeding.

These and other *factors often converge in the first 12 weeks postpartum, causing the early abandonment of human milk infant feeding*. According to the CDC, for infants born in the U.S. during 2019 (data released in 2022), data indicates that 83.2% of all infants initiated breastfeeding. By three months, only 12 short weeks later, that number plummeted to 45.3% for exclusive breastfeeding (CDC, 2020b).

These initial 12 weeks are a definite vulnerable period for infant feeding. Most people giving birth today in the U.S. have a care provider who supports lactation initiation. But what happens when the new family goes home from the hospital or birth center? What happens when the midwife leaves and parents are caring for their newborn full time, without the support of hospital staff, nurses, and LCs?

I have a distinct memory of leaving the (now defunct) Indianapolis Birth Center with my newborn baby in the early morning hours of a lovely October day, 2006. My husband drove home while I sat in the backseat with our new baby. I was stunned that the birth center staff let us leave with this newborn, a tiny person who was totally dependent on us to care for her, and *we had no idea what we were doing*. We left the comforting care of the midwife and birth center staff to arrive at our home without any lactation help at all. Of course, we had family visiting us, but none were experts in infant care and infant feeding. (Fortunately for me, my two sisters had already breastfed their children. I could, (and did) ask for their help and lactation wisdom, but that was not clinical care and support.) The reality is that once people head home after the birth experience, there is no follow-up lactation care built into our current maternity care system. *None*.

If a parent needs care during the postpartum period for lactation, they must seek it and initiate it independently. This gap is a significant one in the chain of breastfeeding support. Further, it can lead to the early termination of lactation.

At Birth: 83.2% initiate human milk feeding. 83.2%

At 12 weeks: 45.3% of infants are exclusively breastfeeding. 45.3%

This vulnerable period can be more extreme or less extreme, depending on your own situation. A typical scenario for lactation support in the U.S. follows this trend:

Stage/Phase	Lactation Support
Prenatal	**Optional -** Local lactation classes, books, online education
Birth	**Likely guaranteed -** In-hospital lactation care, support of some kind
First week	**Not guaranteed -** Infant pediatrician appointment
Six weeks	**No lactation support -** Postpartum OB-GYN follow up
Monthly	**Not guaranteed -** Pediatric care may or may not have lactation support for infant, but not parents

The take-away from the chart above is a simple one. Our current model of care before, during, and after childbirth in the U.S. (and likely elsewhere) is a vulnerable period for lactation that has almost no guaranteed support for lactation. The only time that breastfeeding support is likely is during the birth experience. This type of support varies widely depending on what type of lactation care is available at the hospital or birth center where the birth takes place. Some hospitals are far better than others when it comes to lactation support.

Less Vulnerability, More Protection

How can we move from a highly vulnerable lactation care model to a model of care built on protecting and preserving lactation? In the big picture of holistic infant feeding care and support, it may appear that the changes need to come from global and national health organizations, government agencies, insurance companies, hospitals, and local infant feeding services within our communities. But why should we wait until these organizations and agencies make a move to end the vulnerable approach to supporting lactation in the first few months?

Change can also come from individuals. As a parent, you can write your own story for infant feeding. Your infant feeding care and support are not always limited to tradition or what others usually do. The following are a few options that allow for more progressive care and support of breastfeeding.

- Meet with a lactation consultant or breastfeeding counselor in the prenatal period for lactation counseling and education.
- Take comprehensive breastfeeding classes locally or online.
- Find several LCs in your area. Save their contact information before giving birth.
- Get a good breastfeeding book.
- Find out what lactation support services are available in your area.
- Make it your priority to meet with some kind of lactation support group or lactation consultant at least *two times* during the first two weeks postpartum.
- Locate a breastfeeding support group in your area and attend their meeting. Note: As a long-time breastfeeding support volunteer, I find that people who come with their newborns to support groups early on are more likely to get connected to the resources they need. Local breastfeeding support groups usually have a wealth of information about supportive pediatric

care options like tongue ties and other special needs situations.

- Find several online breastfeeding communities that you feel will suit your needs for infant feeding and parenting support. These groups exist in ways that support diverse communities, including language-specific breastfeeding communities, racial and ethnic communities, LGBTQI+ communities, parents nursing twins, and multiples. These may not be local to you, but you will find online support for virtually any infant feeding and parenting approach that suits your needs.
- Determine if you qualify for free services of any kind (through insurance, WIC, or other agencies).
- Set up a breastfeeding consult with an IBCLC in the *first few days postpartum*. This consultation ensures that you will get early education, care, and intervention if necessary. Set up a follow-up meeting during day 10-14 postpartum.
- Ask your baby's pediatrician whether they offer lactation consultant services in their office. If they do not currently offer LC services, ask if they would consider adding a lactation consultant to their staff.
- Be sure to investigate what lactation services your insurance will cover. Insurance covers lactation services, but the window for coverage may be short. For example, insurance may cover services during the first 12 weeks or some other designated period.
- Do not wait until you visit the baby's pediatrician to seek lactation care. This appointment may be too late. Further, many pediatricians have no training to support lactation or provide clinical lactation care to the breastfeeding dyad.
- Every person who chooses infant feeding with human milk should receive expert, trained lactation care at least twice in the first two weeks. Again, this does not always exist in a typical postpartum care approach, but you can arrange for this yourself. This may not seem ideal, but lactation support, whether from an LC or free breastfeeding support group, is *not optional*. If you want to produce milk and feed it to your

baby, you will need some type of support.

- Bottom line: You must find and arrange for your own breastfeeding support and clinical care (if necessary). In the U.S., there is currently no other viable path.

Dubious Milk Makers: The Unscientific, Anecdotal, Non-Evidence-Based, and Sometimes Purely Mythical Ways People Claim to Increase Milk Supply

Oh, what to do when you *think* you have a low supply? Suppose you frequently read internet blogs or posts from others who have experienced low supply. In that case, you may encounter some bad advice (I talk about this in another section). Unfortunately, there is an abundance of anecdotal (not scientific) information about increasing milk output on the web and much of it is garbage.

First, if you have read Part I of this book, you already know that milk supply is part of a sensitive feedback loop in which demand creates supply. When milk evacuates the breast, immediate hormonal signals begin telling the milk production cells to build up milk supply again. This signal is how your body makes milk. In general, there are no other ways to produce milk. A few techniques, medications, and herbs can enhance milk production, but there are no magic solutions. In fact, focusing too much on quick fixes or magic bullet solutions could take your attention away from the actual technique that works for increasing milk supply: removing milk from the breast.

Suppose you suspect that you are experiencing a low supply. In that case, I caution you not to self-diagnose this condition or find your own treatment. Instead, work with a trained lactation professional or peer-to-peer counselor who can help you. The first thing that will be necessary is to determine whether you have a low milk supply or not. Sometimes, people suspect a decrease in milk production, but in reality, there is not a drop in supply. This false signal can happen in the early weeks when your body regulates milk production to meet the exact demand from your nursling after initially being driven by hormones. It can happen at other times as well. In addition, one might suspect low supply if the baby drops weight or seems hungry. However, this could be driven by factors involving milk transfer instead of supply. Again, work with trained breastfeeding support specialists to help determine if there is a low supply or not.

Next, if you determine that you have low milk supply, the next step is to uncover the cause of low supply. A lactation consultant (LC) would *not* simply acknowledge the low supply and then make random recommendations for increasing production. The recommendations and remedies for increasing supply must be an excellent match for the specific cause of your low supply. Low supply can result from several situations and conditions, so knowing the underlying causes can reveal the best pathway for increasing milk production. For example, suppose low supply is a result of poor milk transfer due to ankyloglossia (tongue tie). In that case, the best path forward might be to remedy the tongue (or lip) restrictions so the baby can extract enough milk. In this scenario, recommending other ways to build supply without fixing the actual cause of the problem will likely not be the best approach. If "low supply" suddenly appears after you go back to work, investigate your pump parts or pumping technique. Is the motor in good working order? Do you have the proper size flange? Perhaps the baby is being fed too fast at daycare, and there is no issue with supply - only the appearance of an issue. Be sure you accurately determine the cause of the low supply before choosing a path to remedy the situation. The remedy you choose for building your milk supply must match well with whatever is causing the decrease in your milk supply.

Now, on to the mythical ways to increase milk production. There are numerous milk-enhancing myths that you might hear from friends, family, a coworker who breastfed, blogs, others posting in lactation forums and online groups, and even from some medical professionals. Here are a few examples of the totally unscientific, wholly anecdotal, and sometimes patently false ways people claimed to have increased milk production.

Herbal Teas

Herbs have a long and sometimes dubious history in lactation, especially in the context of increasing milk production. Indeed, some herbs show promise but most results come from anecdotal evidence (based on personal experience) rather than scientific evidence. In other words, there are not many rigorous scientific studies showing the utility, safety, and effects of herbs for increasing human milk production.

Commercially-produced herbal teas available at the grocery or health food store are almost always available in single-use tea bags. The consumer cannot easily control the dose, except by lengthening the brewing time or using more than one teabag per cup. A few years ago, an experienced LLL leader and IBCLC in Bloomington, Indiana, told me that herbal teas are not usually effective for increasing milk supply. She added that a person would need to consume much larger quantities than generally recommended. For example, Traditional Medicinals Organic Mother's Milk Women's Tea claims the serving size is one teabag per eight fluid ounces of water. Even with a long steeping time, it is unlikely that the small amount of dried herbs in one teabag will be an effective galactagogue (substance used to increase milk production). A quick look at the online reviews of this product reveals that what my LLL leader friend in Indiana told me is true for many people; most are using much more than the recommended amount to see results. One reviewer states that she must brew her tea using two teabags, and one cup a day is not enough. She brews two teabags three times daily – six bags per day to see an increase in her milk supply.

Herbal products *can* have a place in promoting milk production, provided you do some research first. Many people find that loose herbs, herbal tinctures, and capsules help boost milk supply. As with any galactagogue, there are risks. What works for one person may not work for another. Using herbs without first investigating the actual cause of low milk supply is risky and could cause future problems. Be sure to determine the cause of low milk supply before using any herbal teas or herbal tinctures.

Drinking Cow's Milk

With any luck, this fairytale has already been put out to pasture. When I had my second child, I was told to drink an extra glass of milk every day to ensure healthy milk production. At that time, I did not have the heart to say to the doctor that this recommendation was pure make-believe. There is no evidence that drinking cow's milk increases human milk production in any way. Dairy products will not boost your supply and are high on the list of potential allergens for breastfed infants. Be aware of this and watch for signs that your baby tolerates the dairy in your diet. Remember, cow's milk proteins pass into your milk and are much harder to digest than human milk proteins. Signs that your baby is not tolerating dairy in *your* diet include 1) excessive spitting up, 2) colic behavior, 3) bloody stool (sometimes hard to see), 4) vomiting, 5) becoming irritable after feedings, 6) stuffy nose, 7) hives, 8) eczema, or other skin rashes.

Oatmeal (Lactation) Cookies

A few years ago, when this idea was just gaining traction, I knew several people who traded lactation cookie recipes. They claimed the cookies could boost milk production. I recall asking an experienced breastfeeding counselor, "How are people falling for this? These are just oatmeal cookies." She agreed that oatmeal cookies are unlikely to boost milk supply.

Since that time, many creative entrepreneurs have fueled the craze by commercially producing lactation cookies at an incredible retail mark-up. Anecdotally, people claim that oatmeal and brewer's yeast, two of the ingredients in lactation cookie recipes, sometimes help boost milk supply. However, there is no scientific evidence of this. What's more telling is that many people report that although this variation of the classic oatmeal cookie is quite tasty, it does nothing to boost milk production. So, here is the bottom line: if you want to eat a cookie, then do it but do not expect to have a few cookies and wake up to breasts overflowing with milk the next day. It just does not work like that. Instead, if you want to give oats or oatmeal a try, have a bowl of oatmeal for breakfast for several days and see if you notice any differences in your milk production. All in all, do not give too much credence to the idea that lactation cookies boost milk supply. They could help you increase your weight but are not likely to help you increase your milk supply.

Gatorade (blue, red, pink, choose your color)

This fictitious lactation madness, pure myth, needs to end. Please do not take Gatorade for low milk supply or tell others that this works. It doesn't. Gatorade, a sports drink, is not supported by any evidence to increase milk production. None of the ingredients in any color of Gatorade sports drinks can even be casually associated with legitimate galactagogues (substances known to increase milk production). Still, some people claim that Gatorade does, in fact, help with milk production. If there is any truth to this, even for one person, it is not because Gatorade contains any substance that will increase breast milk production. Perhaps a chronically dehydrated person noticed an increase in milk supply after drinking Gatorade. This result was not a direct effect of a galactagogue in the drink. Rather, the resulting increase in milk supply could have stemmed from finally reaching sufficient hydration, thereby increasing milk output. Again, Gatorade is not a solution for increasing milk output. First, find out what is causing your low supply and then choose a solution that is matched well with the cause of low supply. Gatorade is not a galactagogue, and it does not remedy any of the causes of low milk supply.

Coconut Water and Body Armor

This popular myth is similar to Gatorade. Suppose drinking coconut water or Body Armor (a commercially available drink that contains coconut water) does seem to increase your milk supply. In that case, it is not because there are any ingredients in the drink that are galactagogues. Rather, it could be one way to achieve sufficient hydration for a dehydrated person. Falsely, this leads someone to conclude that these drinks increased milk supply. By that same logic, we can speculate that most hydrating fluids, including water, are galactagogues that help increase milk supply. Unfortunately, this conclusion is not necessarily true. What is true is that humans, especially those who are lactating, need to be sufficiently hydrated for bodily systems to perform at peak levels. People who are lactating should drink water, tea, or consume other liquids (soups, broths, other hydrating drinks) to maintain sufficient hydration, but do not obsess over taking in too much water. There is some evidence that overhydration is not advantageous for lactation.

Considerations for Other Drinks

Use caution with caffeinated drinks (e.g., soda, coffee), fruit juices, sports drinks, and alcoholic drinks. Use all of these in moderation to avoid too much sugar and caffeine. If you have a small glass of wine with dinner, no need to pump and dump. However, infant care with a hangover is never fun, and dehydration is not conducive for maintaining your milk supply. So, use your best judgment and limit or avoid alcohol.

Other recommendations I have heard for boosting milk supply (*completely lacking any credible evidence for increasing milk production*) include:

- Algae, spirulina, green smoothies
- Sweet potatoes, spinach, leafy green veggies, carrots, peas
- Figs, dates, and stone fruits (peaches, nectarines, plums, mangoes)
- Whole grains, legumes
- Sesame seeds, pumpkin seeds, black strap molasses
- Olive oil

I find it interesting that this list of foods and supplements recommended for increasing human milk production (except black strap molasses) is incredibly similar to a list of healthy foods that many humans eat. So, take a good look at this list. What do you notice?

There are many vegetables, other greens, and fruits on this list. Of course, this is good advice for supporting a healthy diet, but none of these is a legitimate galactagogue. If you can tolerate whole grains and legumes, feel free to include them in your healthy diet. It is unlikely that they will impact your milk supply. Sesame seeds, pumpkin seeds, black strap molasses, and leafy greens are interesting because they are all considered good sources of iron. An older study (Henly et al., 1995) explores the relationship between iron deficiency and milk production. Their results suggest that iron plays a role in maintaining a healthy milk supply (Henly et al., 1995). Including olive oil (or other healthy fat sources) is also good dietary advice but is not likely to increase your milk production. This list of foods for "boosting milk production" does not include any evidence-based galactagogues. Still, it is a great place to start if you are wondering what to eat during lactation, if only because of the "whole food" nature of the foods on this list.

What I find most interesting about this list of foods are those that are missing. Specifically, there are no mentions of junk foods and junk drinks, which is excellent advice for anyone producing human milk and others in the family. Stay away from highly processed pseudo-foods, processed meats, high sugar snacks, cookies and pastries, and sugary drinks (soda, gourmet coffee drinks from your local barista, sports drinks, fruit juices). This recommendation has nothing to do with milk supply. Rather, these foods are not part of a healthy diet for anyone. As I said earlier, if you really want a cookie, have one but don't expect it to boost your supply. As a rule, choose foods and drinks that support your health, not things that sabotage your health.

Road Map for Low Supply:

1. Work with skilled lactation care to determine if you have a low supply or not. (Maybe it is simply a milk transfer issue.)
2. If a low supply exists, it is necessary to pinpoint the cause. This evidence will enable you to find an appropriate remedy or strategy for improving milk supply.
3. Work with trained breastfeeding support (LC, breastfeeding counselor, peer-to-peer support) to develop strategies that will help rectify or remove the problems. For example, if the problem is weak suck and oral dysfunction, the road to better breastfeeding and increasing milk supply may involve oral-motor therapy for your baby with a qualified physical therapist.
4. After removing or correcting the issues (e.g., tongue-tie release, replacing old pump parts, infant oral therapy), begin using evidence-based strategies to boost milk supply.

Evidence-Based Strategies for Boosting Milk Production:

- Skin-to-skin
- Express more milk
- Increase number of breastfeeding or pumping sessions per day
- Nurse more overnight
- Consider power pumping
- Use hands-on pumping and compression while nursing
- Prescription medication is available, if necessary, for some

people

- Combining strategies may produce the best results

For more resources, read *Making More Milk* by Lisa Marasco and Diana West. They also have a webpage called lowmilksupply.org. They have good information about herbal galactagogues and necessary precautions.

Teen Parents

Breastfeeding rates are typically lower among adolescent parents and compared with adults. Further, adolescents generally breastfeed their children for a shorter duration (Olaiya et al., 2016; Wambach & Cohen, 2009). Adolescent parents experience many of the same barriers to breastfeeding as adult parents do, but they also encounter some unique challenges.

- Caregivers frequently make negative assumptions about a teen parent's interest in breastfeeding (Wambach & Riordan, 2016). This assumption can affect the amount of care and support available for the adolescent parents while in the hospital. Data from the CDC suggests that, like adult parents, teen parents experience better breastfeeding outcomes when they encounter supportive breastfeeding practices in their maternity care experience during childbirth (Olaiya et al., 2016).
- Teen parents often express embarrassment as the main barrier to choosing breastfeeding (Wambach & Koehn, 2004; Woods et al., 2013). Other barriers identified by teens as affecting their decisions about breastfeeding include lack of family support, lack of support from a primary caregiver, other elements of lifestyle and independence, and the complexity of breastfeeding (Woods et al., 2013).
- Adolescent parents may be less likely to ask for assistance and use the available resources (Wambach & Cohen, 2009).
- Breastfeeding education and support can help improve breastfeeding outcomes among teens, including the duration of breastfeeding (Wambach et al., 2011).

If you are a pregnant teen considering breastfeeding, take a good breastfeeding class. Look for an in-depth, independently taught breastfeeding class (generally more than 60 minutes), face-to-face or online. In addition, watch videos of newborns latching onto the breast and learn about breastfeeding support options in your area.

Free Online Videos

Stanford University has a series of good breastfeeding videos on their Stanford University Newborn Nursery website. Start with the video called Breastfeeding in the First Hour. All of these videos are informative, and show laidback breastfeeding and skin-to skin care. These videos can be considered your online breastfeeding class, taught by Dr. Jane Morton, former Director of the Breastfeeding Medicine Program at Stanford University.

Nancy Mohrbacher's YouTube channel is another good resource. Search this YouTube channel for videos about "natural breastfeeding positions," otherwise known as laidback breastfeeding. This YouTube page has a multitude of videos showing people in various reclined positions feeding newborns. You will see that you can use the laidback breastfeeding position on a couch or upholstered chair or more fully reclined on a flat surface (with the use of pillows). Nancy Mohrbacher is an IBCLC and the co-author of *Breastfeeding Made Simple*. Her webpage also has helpful resources for breastfeeding.

Jack Newman's Visual Guide to Breastfeeding is an online video available on YouTube. This video is great for learning many of the concepts of breastfeeding and shows various people of all different shapes and colors. My review of this video is generally positive, except they do not show laidback breastfeeding with newborns. In many scenes, there are too many hands managing the breast. Jack Newman is a Canadian doctor and well-respected IBCLC. He also has a webpage with valuable information for many topics in lactation.

Free Options for Breastfeeding Support

La Leche League (LLL) International offers free in-person meetings, phone support, and online group support (on many Facebook pages). LLL is peer support, facilitated by leaders that LLL has accredited to help other breastfeeding parents. There are LLL chapters all over the world. See their website for more information and locations:

https://www.llli.org/

Breastfeeding USA also offers peer support through in-person meetings, online, phone, and text support. Breastfeeding USA accredits their counselors to provide breastfeeding support. There are Breastfeeding USA chapters in most states, and this group is growing, adding new groups frequently. Check out their webpage for more information: https://breastfeedingusa.org/

WIC is a program in the U.S. that offers many benefits for people who choose to breastfeed. WIC is the common name for The Special Supplemental Nutrition Program for Women, Infants, and Children. It is a federal assistance program offered by the U.S. Department of Agriculture. The main goals for WIC include safeguarding nutrition and providing assistance to low-income pregnant women, breastfeeding women, and children under the age of five. WIC has peer-to-peer breastfeeding counselors on staff and offers support for nursing families. Check with your local WIC office to see what benefits are available for people in your area.

For other options concerning breastfeeding support, check local hospitals and birth centers for breastfeeding support groups, join breastfeeding groups online, check the services offered by your baby's pediatrician.

Racial Disparities for Lactation Outcomes

As you can see by the number of breastfeeding interference factors included in Part II, many people find breastfeeding challenging. For racial minorities in the U.S., the obstacles to successful breastfeeding are more numerous and often more challenging. Generally, there are many risk factors for lowered breastfeeding rates in the U.S. Some of the risk factors include:

- Single parenting
- Low income, income below poverty level
- Low levels of education, less than high school education
- Younger age of parents
- Living in rural locations, isolated from family or resources

Minority parents, including American Indians, Hispanics, African

Americans, Alaskan natives, and Pacific Islanders, are disproportionally and sharply affected by the risk factors listed above. Further, many minorities experience other obstacles in addition to the social determinants listed as risk factors above. Consider these factors that may affect minority breastfeeding rates:

- Lack of culturally appropriate lactation care
- Lack of community support for breastfeeding
- Returning to work sooner than planned
- Offered formula supplements immediately after birth at much higher rates than average (McKinney et al., 2016)

In the introduction of this book, I asked you to consider that the deck is stacked against Black parents (and other minorities) who receive substandard perinatal and lactation care. Evidence supporting this outcome emerges from the maternal and infant outcomes from pregnancy and birth, but it is also apparent when considering breastfeeding outcomes. Breastfeeding can be more complex for some minority groups because of bias among healthcare providers and the lack of support for breastfeeding in minority communities. In addition, there are other factors known to affect lactation that disproportionally affect minorities in the U.S. For example, Black parents in the U.S. experience higher than average cesarean rates (Valdes, 2021), higher than average rates of preterm birth and low birth weight (Burris & Hacker, 2017), and higher rates of type II diabetes. These factors are known to negatively impact lactation and, coupled with socioeconomic factors described above, create more challenges for breastfeeding.

In addition to all the circumstances discussed above, it is crucial to highlight that African Americans, Alaskan natives, and American Indians experience much higher than average pregnancy-related deaths (Oribhabor et al., 2020). When people die due to pregnancy or childbirth complications, the chances that their baby will be fed human milk is likely reduced to zero. In this way, maternity outcomes are intricately tied to breastfeeding outcomes.

Strategies to Eliminate Racial Disparities in Lactation

Although there is likely no simple answer to tackle the complex historical, sociocultural, health, and economic elements that created and continue to sustain suboptimal breastfeeding outcomes for minorities in the U.S., the authors of a recent study on racial disparities in pregnancy outcomes highlighted some crucial factors that need solutions. Their study was specific to maternal morbidity and mortality, but every recommendation the authors made is necessary for eliminating racial disparities in lactation care. They recommend the following:

> ". . . improving access to high-quality preconception, maternity, and postpartum care for minority women, multi-ethnic education for physicians and healthcare providers in a bid to eliminate implicit biases, adequate funding, and improvement of healthcare facilities in minority areas, education of healthcare providers on variation in the incidence of some certain conditions in different ethnic groups so that care is patient-centered and culturally appropriate" (Oribhabor et al., 2020, 1).

In addition to those strategies, guaranteed maternity and parental leave for all parents in the U.S. could be the single most significant step toward removing some obstacles that keep minorities from fully reaching their own breastfeeding goals. If all workers had even two or three months of paid parental leave, families could establish breastfeeding without the worry and stress about going back to work at two weeks postpartum. Recall that some European nations guarantee six to twelve months paid leave. Even if the U.S. could ensure 12 weeks of paid parental leave, that would get families through the vulnerable period and provide time to work through any early lactation challenges. Every family in the U.S. would benefit from paid parental leave, but in my opinion, this could be a significant game-changer for minorities. What are we waiting for?

Recommended Resources for Learning More About Racial Disparities and Improving Outcomes

Full disclosure: I am a trained lactation consultant and an advocate for infant and maternal health, but I am not an expert on racial disparities in maternal and infant health. To better understand the complexities of the social and cultural factors that lead to racial bias in the health-care in the U.S., please get information and education from the people who are the experts. Here are a few experts who do a much better job than I could at defining the problems and explaining the solutions for racial equity in healthcare.

For Parents

Kimberly Seals Allers is an award-winning journalist and a health advocate, who has authored five books, including *The Mocha Manual to a Fir Pregnancy* and *The Mini Mocha Manual to Pregnancy and Childbirth: The Essential Guide for Black Women*. Her latest book, *The Big Let Down*, explores how cultural forces and big business have undermined breastfeeding. Kimberly Seals Allers is the creator and founder of multiple women-centered and Black-centered initiatives and projects, including the Irth app, on a mission to bring equity to pregnancy and childbirth. You can find out more about her and all of her current projects and books at kimberlysealsallers.com.

ROSE - Reaching Our Sisters Everywhere

ROSE is a non-profit organization based in Atlanta, GA with a mission to protect breastfeeding all over the country, with the specific goal of increasing breastfeeding rates for African American women. ROSE offers a multitude of supportive measures, including support groups, trainings and educational opportunities, online forums, and many other offerings. Find out more about ROSE at breastfeedingrose.org.

BreastfeedLA

BreastfeedLA is an organization committed to supporting breastfeeding while focusing on diversity, equity, and inclusion. BreastfeedLA offers a host of lactation resources for parents (and for professionals), including factsheets about breastfeeding, a directory of local lactation support professionals, online resources for lactation education and support, legal resources, and mental health resources. BreastfeedLA is also associated with the Asian Pacific Islander Breastfeeding Task Force, which offers local support meetings open to everyone. Find out more information at breastfeedla.org.

For Lactation Professionals (and those who aspire to be)

The B.L.A.C.K. Course - Birth, Lactation, Accommodation, Culture, Kinship

Are you interested in learning more about lactation in a course that was designed by and for Black people? The team from The B.L.A.C.K. Course has created a comprehensive lactation training program for those who are preparing to become breastfeeding counselors or those preparing to take the IBCLC exam. This course is led by four experts: Ngozi D. Walker-Tibbs, Lydia O. Boyd, TaNefer Camara, and Felisha Brooks-Floyd. Find out more about the course at theblackcourse.com.

The Melanated Mammary Atlas®

Founded by Nekisha Killings, MPH, IBCLC, The Melanated Mammary Atlas® is a tool for professionals who work in lactation and other fields of healthcare that involve breast health and breast care. The Melanated Mammary Atlas® seeks to expand what is known about breast conditions with regard to black and brown skin tones. Too often, conditions of the breast (and other body parts) are depicted in medical texts and the literature using white skin tones and examples. This can lead to misdiagnosis for breast conditions for people with black and brown skin. The Melanated Mammary Atlas® is a database of images showing breast conditions in a range of black and brown skin tones. By providing healthcare professionals with accurate images and representations of breast conditions for black and brown skin, this database contributes to the delivery of more equitable healthcare for all.

Indigenous Lactation Counselor Training

Camie Jae Goldhammer, MSW, LICSW, IBCLC and Kimberly Moore-Salas, IBCLC have created a course called Indigenous Lactation Counselor Training. This course is for those who identify as Native, Indigenous, or First Nations people who wish to expand their knowledge of breastfeeding and gain skills in lactation counseling. These professional lactation consultants take their course on the road into indigenous communities to teach the skills of lactation counseling. For more information, please visit their Facebook page called Indigenous Lactation Counselor.

BreastfeedLA

This organization, mentioned above, also offers training and education opportunities for aspiring professionals in the field of lactation with the goal of addressing the underrepresentation of Black, Indigenous, and people of color in the lactation profession. BreastfeedLA offers a Lactation Education Program for aspiring professionals as well as guidance and resources for becoming an IBCLC. Find them online at breastfeedla.org.

Not Knowing How to Ask for Help

Getting infant feeding off the ground can be a struggle for many people, whether the baby takes human milk or formula. For most first-time parents, there is a steep learning curve with many elements of infant care because these are skills they have never had to use before. In addition, most of us learn about infants by having our own, not by helping aunts, cousins, and family friends as people did in the past in more communal societies. This often puts first-time parents in the position of relative unease with handling a newborn, feeding a baby, and infant care.

What is interesting is that adults who lack knowledge or skills sometimes do not ask for the help and support they need for various reasons. For example, in an earlier section of this chapter, I noted that teen parents who initiate breastfeeding might be less likely to ask for help (Wambach & Cohen, 2009). In my experience, teens are not the only parents who are unlikely to ask for help. For example, I have known several people who switched to formula because they felt uncomfortable asking for the support they needed.

Imagine the following scenarios. Do you think it would be easy to ask for help in all of these situations?

- Until now, everyone in your family has always used formula. Your mother and sisters lack the knowledge and skill to help you. You are the only person in your family to choose breastfeeding.
- You are a minority, giving birth at a hospital where no attending caregivers share your racial or ethnic background. You would feel better talking to someone in your cultural community about breastfeeding.
- You are a younger first-time parent. You are somewhat shy, and the whole idea of feeding a baby at the breast sounds daunting.
- You are a quiet person, and you prefer not to ask for help. Instead, you would choose to read about breastfeeding online or in a book.
- You need to talk to your boss about pumping, but you feel embarrassed about bringing it up. You don't know how to approach the conversation because your boss is a man, and it seems strange talking to him about pumping human milk.
- The whole idea of going to a lactation consultant who might examine your breasts or touch your breasts is off-limits for you.
- You are a survivor of sexual violence and trauma. You would rather not seek care because that might mean having to explain your history.

Asking for help can be difficult for many adults in a multitude of different situations. Some people feel that they would be burdening others if they ask for help or assistance. However, during the early postpartum phase, it is highly likely that you will need help from someone, whether it is your mother, sister, friend, or even a neighbor. It is one specific time in life when relying on your network of community support truly becomes necessary. Most people are happy to help, especially when they realize that you have just had a baby. Alternatively, if asking for support from friends and family is not possible or uncomfortable for you, you can hire support as well. Postpartum support is available in many forms, some of which are free support and some for hire, including postpartum doulas, peer-to-peer volunteer breastfeeding support, local babysitters, family members who support you and your choices, WIC, friends, and neighbors.

Independent people can find it challenging to ask for help because they prefer not to rely on others. They prefer to meet their own needs, reinforcing their beliefs in their resilience and independence. For some people, asking for help shows inherent weakness. Before cellphones and GPS, there was a running joke in parts of the world about a person who drives around lost, recognizes that he is lost but refuses to pull over and ask for directions. This "lost traveler" situation no longer exists for most of us because of the magic of cellphone maps and other apps for finding your way but this situation persists in other forms. For example, this situation plays out for many families with newborns because they are suddenly thrown into a new world of infant life, and they feel lost for a while during the adjustment period. When you feel like the lost traveler in baby land, it is perfectly acceptable and even necessary to pull over sometimes and ask for directions.

In other instances, some people find it difficult to ask for help because they have a deep-seated fear of losing control of their own choices, autonomy, and the decision-making process. In this case, it can be helpful to reframe the way you think about asking for help and how it genuinely affects your decision-making. For example, imagine asking for breastfeeding help from a peer-to-peer counselor (Breastfeeding USA, La Leche League, WIC, ROSE, or local breastfeeding counselor). You call the counselor or visit the local meeting in person. You explain your questions and ask for assistance. The counselors explain the possibilities and options, but you are under no orders to follow this advice. You still retain your ability to make your own choices and find your path. In other words, asking for help in this situation is truly akin to information gathering. Once you have gathered sufficient information, you can still exercise your own will to make choices and decisions.

Another obstacle when it comes to asking for help is the idea of reciprocity. Suppose your neighbor shovels your driveway out of the kindness of his heart on a snowy morning. In that case, you may feel inclined to compensate your neighbor for this kind gesture with some repayment (e.g., some type of nice gesture). The same goes for practical help with breastfeeding, childcare, or picking up something from the store. Specifically, if someone performs these favors, you may feel obligated to repay family, friends, and neighbors for their kind help. For many people, the feeling of owing something to others is too burdensome and uncomfortable.

TRUE STORY

When my sister was pregnant with her third child, she renovated her kitchen. While this sounds like a mistake to some people, she knew that putting it off until after the birth would be a huge miscalculation. She had a make-shift kitchen in the living room during the renovations, but it was hard to cook a full meal for her family. Many friends and neighbors helped her during the renovation and after the birth of her baby. After the chaos of the renovation and early infancy period had passed, she wanted to somehow thank her network of friends and neighbors who had generously helped her with childcare, meal prep, and other chores. So, she organized a large backyard barbeque to thank all of those who had helped over the past months. She was surprised to find that her guest list was over 80 people.

It is not likely that infancy and breastfeeding will require you to rely on 80 friends, family, and neighbors, but you may need to ask for help from a few. Here are a few tips for asking for help if it feels uncomfortable for you:

- Recognize that people genuinely do want to help you.
- Make a list of the people or organizations that you can go to for help.
- Ask at your pediatrician's office about local lactation support groups and parenting support groups.
- Call your insurance company to see what services they cover for lactation and any time limits. (For example, some services only cover services during the first weeks or months after birth.)
- Be sure that the person you ask for help is capable of helping you.
- Identify your needs and be specific about the help you want. If you need someone to help with a chore, keep it simple. This simplicity provides for fewer mistakes.

- Read subtle cues from those who agree to help you. For example, are they eagerly agreeing to help or perhaps hesitantly agreeing to help?
- Thanking your friends and family can be simple. Send an email or text with a genuine note of thanks. If someone went out of their way to help you, send a note in the mail or a small gift of thanks. Sometimes just a genuine, verbal "thank you" is enough.

Resources for Finding Help:

USA

National Women's Health and Breastfeeding Helpline – Call 1-800-994-9662

Help is available from the Office on Women's Health Monday through Friday, 9am to 6pm Eastern Time. They can answer health and infant feeding questions in English or Spanish.

La Leche League operates a 24-hour hotline in the U. S. Call 1-877-4 LALECHE, 1-877-452-5324.

Call La Leche League to speak with a trained peer support volunteer about your breastfeeding questions.

Postpartum Support International

Call for mental health questions and support. 1-800-944-4773. Call or text in English or Spanish, and a trained volunteer will call you back. You can also visit their webpage to find resources.

Lack of Knowledge

Breastfeeding is a skill that people must learn; it is not necessarily innate for parents. Think of other skills acquired throughout a lifetime, such as riding a bike, playing piano, cooking, using the internet, reading, mental math, driving a car, and playing games. We acquire hundreds of skills during a lifetime, and we need to *learn* all of them. Suppose you have never performed a certain skill before, especially something as high stakes as breastfeeding. In that case, it makes sense to take some training to gain the knowledge and skills necessary to perform the task. Breastfeeding is no exception.

The lack of knowledge about breastfeeding, accomplishing it, and why it is optimal is not just an issue for new parents. Our communal knowledge about breastfeeding here in the U.S. is generally lacking across all ages, races, and socioeconomic levels. New parents, their own parents, siblings, cousins, friends, coworkers, and even pediatricians are not always good sources of breastfeeding information unless they have had specific training or many years of experience supporting lactation. Society was not always deficient in breastfeeding wisdom. Unfortunately, decades of formula feeding created a massive deficit in our knowledge base. Even though breastfeeding is making a comeback, we have a long way to go before we have community acceptance of breastfeeding and a high working knowledge of lactation across all sectors of the society. It will likely take several more generations for the learning curve of breastfeeding to reach across all levels of society.

There are many components to the "learning curve" when it comes to breastfeeding. Some of the most significant factors include: 1) prior knowledge and skill level of the parent, 2) knowledge and skill of the health care provider, and 3) protection of the baby's innate skills and the opportunity to learn positive feeding behaviors at the breast.

Many people, especially those living in a formula-feeding culture, have almost no experience with breastfeeding prior to the day we give birth. Taking a breastfeeding education class can certainly help. Still, a lack of depth and experience with breastfeeding is not easy to overcome with a simple 60-minute course on infant feeding.

Ideally, we would grow up learning about breastfeeding by watching other parents, our aunts, friends, cousins, and even strangers feed their babies at the breast. How do animals know how to feed their babies? "Watch and learn" is how other primates gain knowledge and skills about infant feeding. We live in a society that does not usually promote or condone public breastfeeding so witnessing a baby at the breast is a rare sight.

Most of us have grown up without much exposure to breastfeeding. Therefore, we must take steps to educate ourselves about infant feeding and gain the skills required to make breastfeeding work. A study done in 2008 showed that parents who took part in breastfeeding education classes had significantly higher rates of breastfeeding at six months than parents who had prenatal care without breastfeeding education (Rosen et al., 2008). Is it realistic for people to assume they can learn new skills and counteract years of living in a formula-feeding culture in a single prenatal breastfeeding class? Newer research shows that breastfeeding outcomes are higher when prenatal classes are combined with postnatal support than when parents only take a prenatal breastfeeding class. In other words, breastfeeding rates improve when we receive education about breastfeeding before the baby's birth and participate in postnatal breastfeeding groups for support and continued education after the birth (Schreck et al., 2017). Think of it as on the job training.

TRUE STORY

Janet Tamaro, the author of *So That's What They're For*, tells the true story of a gorilla living in an Ohio zoo years ago that demonstrates the power of "watch and learn." The pregnant gorilla lived alone in her enclosure with no exposure to gorilla infant rearing practices. When her baby was born, the gorilla mother had no skills for infant feeding, and unfortunately, the baby died. In time, the gorilla became pregnant again. The zookeepers were anxious to teach this gorilla the skills of infant feeding. They organized an effort to teach these skills by having several human parents who were nursing small babies at that time visit her enclosure. During the gorilla's second pregnancy, the human parents nursed their babies outside the window. The human parents continued to visit and feed their babies once the newborn gorilla arrived. Through careful demonstration from the parents and careful attention from the mother gorilla, the new mother gorilla learned to latch her baby and successfully nurse at the breast. In many ways, this gorilla had prenatal classes and postnatal support to make sense of infant feeding. It was a "watch and learn" situation.

Strategies for Learning About Breastfeeding:

- Take an independent breastfeeding class.
- Take an online breastfeeding class.
- Read about breastfeeding. There are many excellent books on breastfeeding and lots of good information is available online as well.
- Watch videos (remember to watch and learn). Stanford University and Dr. Jack Newman are both excellent video resources. Nancy Mohrbacher's YouTube page has wealth of information and videos about positioning, latch and many other useful topics. Read and learn from reputable websites with no other agenda than to promote breastfeeding.

Breastfeeding in Public: The Infant Feeding Taboo

In many parts of the world, nursing a baby in public will draw unwanted attention from onlookers. It is hard to imagine that, on the one hand, we are a species whose classification (Mammalia) has milk production at the core of its identity. Yet, on the other hand, feeding that milk to infants and toddlers in public spaces is taboo. So, how is it that feeding a baby at the breast is distasteful or even shameful when feeding takes place in the company of strangers?

Of course, it is not distasteful or shameful to feed your baby at any time but societies that are more reliant on artificial infant formula are much less likely to be accepting and open to seeing a baby at the breast. This topic is multifaceted, complex, and has a somewhat perverse history. It is much too broad for me to cover thoroughly in this book.

To be brief, the taboo nature of breastfeeding in public can be linked to several convergent elements of 19th and 20th century society and culture. For example, feeding a baby at the breast in some social classes had been viewed as less-than-civilized. This perception may have had roots (in the distant past) among the royal families in which queens and princesses did not feed their infants but employed wet nurses to do the work of infant feeding instead. If others in high society could afford to emulate the royals, many followed suit and employed wet nurses.

More recently, many other factors contributed to the taboo status of feeding at the breast, including:

- Sexualization of the breast in advertising, movies, clothing styles, and men's magazines
- Industrial production of infant foods: formula, baby food solids, toddler foods
- The elevated status of medical doctors and celebrity doctors advising about infant feeding
- More women entering the workforce in the post-WWII era

Isn't it interesting that the solidification of the "breast as sexual" occurred when artificial formula was becoming increasingly popular in the U.S.? Hugh Hefner published the first edition of *Playboy* magazine in 1953. The 1950s also saw the reformulation of Similac and the introduction of Enfamil. By the 1960s, formula was firmly entrenched in American life. People abandoned the association between breasts and infants in favor of the association of breasts and sex. Because of this shift, society had decidedly adopted the view that nursing an infant in public was objectionable.

Although we have come a long way since the '60s and '70s, and breastfeeding initiation rates have increased dramatically, we are still not a breastfeeding society. Instead, we (in the U.S. and many other Western nations) are predominately a formula-feeding society. Consequently, the taboo of public nursing lives on.

For example, people are still asked to cover up at restaurants, in shopping malls, at swimming pools, and in libraries regularly because the stigma of breastfeeding in public still exists. In addition, many people do not know the law and will assume that breastfeeding is not legal in some public contexts.

TRUE STORIES

A nursing mother near Galveston, Texas, was asked to leave a public pool in 2019 because she would not cover up. When she pushed back, the manager called the police, who instructed the mother to leave. This happened despite Texas having a law that guarantees that anyone may nurse their baby in public as long as they have the legal right to be there. Even the police officer did not know the law.

In Anacortes, Washington, in 2021, a couple with a newborn was meeting family for dinner at a local restaurant. The infant showed feeding cues, and the mother began breastfeeding. The restaurant owner approached after he saw the baby nursing and asked the couple to leave. According to the couple, the owner also asked them never to return to the restaurant and called the mother an animal.

In 2020, during the COVID-19 pandemic, a college student with a 10-month-old baby was asked by her instructor at Fresno City College not to breastfeed during an online class, that she should just do it after class. What is astonishing about this is that the mother and baby were in their own home. Even more bizarre is that this particular instructor then told the entire class that he received a "weird" email from a student, asking about engaging in inappropriate things during the online class. The fact that this instructor characterized infant feeding as inappropriate is telling. This characterization blatantly highlights the taboo nature of breastfeeding.

In 2017, a woman was asked to cover up while feeding her baby at London's Victoria and Albert Museum. She noted the odd nature of such a request in the museum environment. There are dozens of artworks depicting the naked breast.

Will This Taboo Ever Die?

There has been an ongoing campaign among mothers and lactation professionals to "normalize breastfeeding." For the most part, this is an informal movement and a hashtag that does not get the attention it deserves. Truth be told, it is time. It is time for the taboo of public breastfeeding to unravel completely. I tend not to view this taboo as a minor, backward nuisance but as a legitimate human rights issue.

While this may not be preventable, there are some things you can do to ensure that you handle it well, should somebody approach you about breastfeeding in public. First, know your rights. Each Canadian province and each U.S. state have laws protecting your right to breastfeed. If someone asks you to cover or leave, you can cite the local law that protects you (if you have done some research). Second, file a complaint or a grievance. This filing is the only redress you have. By doing so, you will help educate people, so that type of harassment happens less often. Some cities are more prepared for complaints than others. For example, in Canada, the city of Toronto asks that people file a complaint with the Human Rights Tribunal of Ontario if someone violates their right to breastfeed in public. Brilliant! Third, take to social media or organize a nurse-in. In several of the *True Stories* mentioned above, the local breastfeeding group organized a nurse-in to protest the expulsion or harassment while nursing in public. Another posted about her experiences on Twitter. You may be surprised by how quickly shopkeepers, restaurateurs, and pool managers try to rectify their bad behavior when they are outed on social media.

Can the taboo of public breastfeeding be changed overnight? Not likely. But every incident is an opportunity for learning, growth, and change.

EPILOGUE

My Secret Obsession

If you could visit my house, within minutes you would recognize that I love house plants. I usually keep about 17-20 live plants in my home and many more outdoors as well. My latest acquisition is an indoor Audrey Ficus tree. I am excited about the potential for this to become a big, beautiful tree.

House plants create an atmosphere of beauty, brighten up vacant and dark corners; they enhance the aesthetic of kitchen counters, windowsills and even bathrooms. Green is my favorite color and I use house plants to bring in a variety of green shades into my spaces without having to find inspiration to paint every room. I appreciate plants for their ability to instantly bring life to a room, inspire creativity, and enhance the mood of any area of the home.

As a plant owner, I have also learned that decorating with plants is not as simple as using fabric, unique furniture pieces, artwork, or thrown pillows. Plants are very different from these types of décor, specifically because they are living organisms. They require more care and attention than the upkeep for a sofa or maintenance of window coverings. To care for my plants, I have had to learn the subtle nuances and distinctive requirements for each plant I have. Some like low light all day. Others like bright light in the morning with indirect light in the afternoon. All of them require water but in varying amounts. Some plants seem to get used to their place in the home and prefer not to be moved (but luckily, most of them do tolerate my need to move frequently). I would not characterize myself as someone with a "green thumb," but I enjoy the plants to such a degree that I make it a priority to provide them with the best environment and help them to thrive.

There have been times, however, when I've noticed an abundance of dead leaves, wilting fronds, or the rapid decline of what was once a thriving plant. Any time this happens, I try to identify what might be causing the deterioration. Sometimes I can find ways to remedy the situation and sometimes I can't. As a plant owner, I have recognized that even though house plants are hardy, they do require precisely the right care. Occasionally I start plants from seeds, usually for edible garden plants. In this case, it is imperative to get growth off to a good start right from the beginning. Without the proper amount of sunlight, the right soil composition and drainage, protection from frost or cold temps, and optimal water, my house plants and seeds do not grow and thrive.

Cultivating Your Milk Supply

The precise mechanics of protecting and promoting plant life are clearly not the same as those you might use for protecting your milk supply, but the intentions are the same. To cultivate your very best milk supply, you have to optimize the necessary inputs (lactation promotion factors) and remove the all the weeds (lactation interference).

Some people do seem to have an unfailing, robust ability when it comes to lactation. The weeds in the garden of lactation do not seem to impact those with the "green thumb" of lactation. But for many of us who are sensitive, any interference in the lactation garden can cause suboptimal cultivation of the milk supply. Just like plants, each one of us is different, with different body composition and distinct needs for thriving through the season of lactation. But the foundation for cultivating a robust milk supply has commonalities for all of us. Remember to follow an excellent lactation promotion protocol to protect your milk supply. You wouldn't expect to throw a handful of seeds out the back window and find a beautiful garden there a few days later. There are precise rules about gardening that one must follow to optimize the growth of healthy plants. Similarly, as you now know, there are important elements of lactation promotion that are required in order to optimize milk production.

Additional tips to remember:

- Get enough natural sunlight, especially in the morning to optimize circadian rhythms for you and for your baby.
- Get plenty of water. Avoid junk drinks, high sugar soda, high sugar juices and smoothies, too much caffeine and alcohol.

- Remove milk (via baby at the breast, pumping, or hand expression) regularly. Aim for at least nine to ten times per day. Do not skip overnight feedings (or milk removal). If you are struggling with milk production, err on the high side.
- Use the RELAX method steps to help optimize feeding.
- Reach out to your network for support.
- Plant the seeds of good lactation promotion early on and continue to avoid the weeds.

I wish you all the best on your infant feeding journey! May your lactation garden cultivate the milk supply you need to feed your babies!

References

AAP, & ACOG (Eds.). (2017). *Guidelines for perinatal care* (Eighth edition). American Academy of Pediatrics; The American College of Obstetricians and Gynecologists.

Aarts, C., Hörnell, A., Kylberg, E., Hofvander, Y., & Gebre-Medhin, M. (1999). Breastfeeding patterns in relation to thumb sucking and pacifier use. *Pediatrics, 104*(4), e50–e50. https://doi.org/10.1542/peds.104.4.e50

Ainsworth, A. J., Holman, M. A., McGree, M., Weaver, A., Torbenson, V., & Tolcher, M. C. (2017). Risk factors for postpartum hemorrhage following nulliparous induction of labor [3C]. *Obstetrics & Gynecology, 129*(1), 31S-31S. https://doi.org/10.1097/01.AOG.0000514312.69761.62

Amir, L. H., & Donath, S. (2007). A systematic review of maternal obesity and breastfeeding intention, initiation and duration. *BMC Pregnancy and Childbirth, 7*(1), 9. https://doi.org/10.1186/1471-2393-7-9

Amitay, E. L., Dubnov Raz, G., & Keinan-Boker, L. (2016). Breastfeeding, other early life exposures and childhood leukemia and lymphoma. *Nutrition and Cancer, 68*(6), 968–977. https://doi.org/10.1080/01635581.2016.1190020

Antonakou, A., & Papoutsis, D. (2016). The effect of epidural analgesia on the delivery outcome of induced labour: A retrospective case series. *Obstetrics and Gynecology International, 2016*, 1–5. https://doi.org/10.1155/2016/5740534

Armeni, E., Karopoulou, E., & Lambrinoudaki, I. (2019). Obstetric history and cardiovascular disease (CVD) risk. In R. D. Brinton, A. R. Genazzani, T. Simoncini, & J. C. Stevenson (Eds.), *Sex Steroids' Effects on Brain, Heart and Vessels* (pp. 149–160). Springer International Publishing. https://doi.org/10.1007/978-3-030-11355-1_10

Arora, S., McJunkin, C., Wehrer, J., & Kuhn, P. (2000). Major factors influencing breastfeeding rates: Mother's perception of father's attitude and milk supply. *Pediatrics, 106*(5), e67–e67. https://doi.org/10.1542/peds.106.5.e67

ARRWIP. (2019). *Pregnancy in Prison Statistics (PIPS) Project.* Advocacy and Research on Reproductive Wellness of Incarcerated People. https://arrwip.org/projects/pregnancy-in-prison-statistics-pips-project/

Ashwal, E., Melamed, N., Hiersch, L., Wiznitzer, A., Yogev, Y., & Peled, Y. (2014). The incidence and risk factors for retained placenta after vaginal delivery – a single center experience. *The Journal of Maternal-Fetal & Neonatal Medicine, 27*(18), 1897–1900. https://doi.org/10.3109/14767058.2014.883374

Australian Government Department of Health. (2019). *Breastfeeding.* https://www1.health.gov.au/internet/main/publishing.nsf/Content/health-pubhlth-strateg-brfeed-index.htm

Babic, A., Sasamoto, N., Rosner, B. A., Tworoger, S. S., Jordan, S. J., Risch, H. A., Harris, H. R., Rossing, M. A., Doherty, J. A., Fortner, R. T., Chang-Claude, J., Goodman, M. T., Thompson, P. J., Moysich, K. B., Ness, R. B., Kjaer, S. K., Jensen, A., Schildkraut, J. M., Titus, L. J., Terry, K. L. (2020). Association between breastfeeding and ovarian cancer risk. *JAMA Oncology, 6*(6), e200421. https://doi.org/10.1001/jamaoncol.2020.0421

Basree, M. M., Shinde, N., Koivisto, C., Cuitino, M., Kladney, R., Zhang, J., Stephens, J., Palettas, M., Zhang, A., Kim, H. K., Acero-Bedoya, S., Trimboli, A., Stover, D. G., Ludwig, T., Ganju, R., Weng, D., Shields, P., Freudenheim, J., Leone, G. W., Ramaswamy, B. (2019). Abrupt involution induces inflammation, estrogenic signaling, and hyperplasia linking lack of breastfeeding with increased risk of breast cancer. *Breast Cancer Research, 21*(1), 80. https://doi.org/10.1186/s13058-019-1163-7

Bergman, N. (2017). Breastfeeding and perinatal neuroscience. In C. W. Genna (Ed.), *Supporting sucking skills in breastfeeding infants* (Third edition). Jones & Bartlett Learning.

Bergman, N. (2019). Historical background to maternal-neonate separation and neonatal care. *Birth Defects Research, 111*(15), 1081–1086. https://doi.org/10.1002/bdr2.1528

Bergman, N., Linley, L., & Fawcus, S. (2004). Randomized controlled trial of skin-to-skin contact from birth versus conventional incubator for physiological stabilization in 1200- to 2199-gram newborns. *Acta Paediatrica, 93*(6), 779–785. https://doi.org/10.1111/j.1651-2227.2004.tb03018.x

Bettegowda, V. R., Dias, T., Davidoff, M. J., Damus, K., Callaghan, W. M., & Petrini, J. R. (2008). The relationship between cesarean delivery and gestational age among US singleton births. *Clinics in Perinatology, 35*(2), 309–323. https://doi.org/10.1016/j.clp.2008.03.002

Blankenship, S. A., Woolfolk, C. L., Raghuraman, N., Stout, M. J., Macones, G. A., & Cahill, A. G. (2019). First stage of labor progression in women with large-for-gestational age infants. *American Journal of Obstetrics and Gynecology, 221*(6), 640.e1-640.e11. https://doi.org/10.1016/j.ajog.2019.06.042

Boban, M., & Zakarija-Grković, I. (2016). In-hospital formula supplementation of healthy newborns: Practices, reasons, and their medical justification. *Breastfeeding Medicine, 11*(9), 448–454. https://doi.org/10.1089/bfm.2016.0039

Bonifacino, E., Schwartz, E. B., Jun, H., Wessel, C. B., & Corbelli, J. A. (2018). Effect of lactation on maternal hypertension: A systematic review. *Breastfeeding Medicine, 13*(9), 578–588. https://doi.org/10.1089/bfm.2018.0108

Bramson, L., Lee, J. W., Moore, E., Montgomery, S., Neish, C., Bahjri, K., & Melcher, C. L. (2010). Effect of early skin-to-skin mother—Infant contact during the first 3 hours following birth on exclusive breastfeeding during the maternity hospital stay. *Journal of Human Lactation, 26*(2), 130–137. https://doi.org/10.1177/0890334409355779

Brodribb, W. & the Academy of Breastfeeding Medicine. (2018). ABM clinical protocol #9: Use of galactogogues in initiating or augmenting maternal milk production, second revision 2018. *Breastfeeding Medicine, 13*(5), 307–314. https://doi.org/10.1089/bfm.2018.29092.wjb

Brownell, E., Howard, C. R., Lawrence, R. A., & Dozier, A. M. (2012). Delayed onset lactogenesis II predicts the cessation of any or exclusive breastfeeding. *The Journal of Pediatrics, 161*(4), 608–614. https://doi.org/10.1016/j.jpeds.2012.03.035

Buccini, G. dos S., Pérez-Escamilla, R., Paulino, L. M., Araújo, C. L., & Venancio, S. I. (2017). Pacifier use and interruption of exclusive breastfeeding: Systematic review and meta-analysis: Pacifier and exclusive breastfeeding interruption. *Maternal & Child Nutrition, 13*(3), e12384. https://doi.org/10.1111/mcn.12384

Buccini, G. dos S., Pérez-Escamilla, R., & Venancio, S. I. (2016). Pacifier use and exclusive breastfeeding in Brazil. *Journal of Human Lactation, 32*(3), NP52–NP60. https://doi.org/10.1177/0890334415609611

Burris, H. H., & Hacker, M. R. (2017). Birth outcome racial disparities: A result of intersecting social and environmental factors. *Seminars in Perinatology, 41*(6), 360–366. https://doi.org/10.1053/j.semperi.2017.07.002

Cadwell, K., Brimdyr, K., & Phillips, R. (2018). Mapping, measuring, and analyzing the process of skin-to-skin contact and early breastfeeding in the first hour after birth. *Breastfeeding Medicine, 13*(7), 485–492. https://doi.org/10.1089/bfm.2018.0048

California Penal Code 4002.5, 4002.5 (2018). https://leginfo.legislature.ca.gov/faces/codes⊠displaySection.xhtml?sectionNum=4002.5.&lawCode=PEN

Caparros-Gonzalez, R. A., Romero-Gonzalez, B., Gonzalez-Perez, R., Lara-Cinisomo, S., Martin-Tortosa, P. L., Oliver-Roig, A., & Peralta-Ramirez, M. I. (2019). Maternal and neonatal hair cortisol levels and psychological stress are associated with onset of secretory activation of human milk production. *Advances in Neonatal Care, 19*(6), E11–E20. https://doi.org/10.1097/ANC.0000000000000660

Case, T. I., Repacholi, B. M., & Stevenson, R. J. (2006). My baby doesn't smell as bad as yours. *Evolution and Human Behavior, 27*(5), 357–365. https://doi.org/10.1016/j.evolhumbehav.2006.03.003

Casey, T., Sun, H., Burgess, H. J., Crodian, J., Dowden, S., Cummings, S., Plaut, K., Haas, D., Zhang, L., & Ahmed, A. (2019). Delayed lactogenesis II is associated with lower sleep efficiency and greater variation in nightly sleep duration in the third trimester. *Journal of Human Lactation, 35*(4), 713–724. https://doi.org/10.1177/0890334419830991

CDC. (2010). *Clinical Growth Charts.* Centers for Disease Control and Prevention. https://www.cdc.gov/growthcharts/clinical_charts.htm

CDC. (2020a). *Breastfeeding Report Card: United States 2020*. Centers for Disease Control and Prevention. https://www.cdc.gov/breastfeeding/data/reportcard.htm

CDC. (2020b). *National Immunization Survey*. https://www.cdc.gov/vaccines/imz-managers/nis/about.html

Centers for Disease Control. (2020). *Linked Birth/Infant Death Records*. https://wonder.cdc.gov/lbd.html

Channell Doig, A., Jasczynski, M., Fleishman, J. L., & Aparicio, E. M. (2020). Breastfeeding among mothers who have experienced childhood maltreatment: A review. *Journal of Human Lactation*, *36*(4), 710–722. https://doi.org/10.1177/0890334420950257

Chantry, C. J., Dewey, K. G., Peerson, J. M., Wagner, E. A., & Nommsen-Rivers, L. A. (2014). In-hospital formula use increases early breastfeeding cessation among first-time mothers intending to exclusively breastfeed. *The Journal of Pediatrics*, *164*(6), 1339-1345.e5. https://doi.org/10.1016/j.jpeds.2013.12.035

Chantry, C. J., Nommsen-Rivers, L. A., Peerson, J. M., Cohen, R. J., & Dewey, K. G. (2011). Excess weight loss in first-born breastfed newborns relates to maternal intrapartum fluid balance. *Pediatrics*, *127*(1), e171–e179. https://doi.org/10.1542/peds.2009-2663

Cheng, Y. W., Shaffer, B. L., Nicholson, J. M., & Caughey, A. B. (2014). Second stage of labor and epidural use: A larger effect than previously suggested. *Obstetrics & Gynecology*, *123*(3), 527–535. https://doi.org/10.1097/AOG.0000000000000134

Chiruvolu, A., Miklis, K. K., Stanzo, K. C., Petrey, B., Groves, C. G., McCord, K., Qin, H., Desai, S., & Tolia, V. N. (2017). Effects of skin-to-skin care on late preterm and term infants at-risk for neonatal hypoglycemia. *Pediatric Quality & Safety*, *2*(4), e030. https://doi.org/10.1097/pq9.0000000000000030

CHTI. (2021). *Section 4: Breastfeeding Management and Troubleshooting—Growth Charts for Breastfed Babies*. Community Health Training Institute. https://bfcme.hriainstitute.org/breastfeedingcme/cme-1/section-4/growth-charts-for-breastfed-babies

Cohen-Engler, Hadash, A., Shehadeh, N., & Pillar, G. (2012). Breastfeeding may improve nocturnal sleep and reduce infantile colic: Potential role of breast milk melatonin. *European Journal of Pediatrics*, *171*(4), 729–732. https://doi.org/10.1007/s00431-011-1659-3

Colson, S. D., Meek, J. H., & Hawdon, J. M. (2008). Optimal positions for the release of primitive neonatal reflexes stimulating breastfeeding. *Early Human Development*, *84*(7), 441–449. https://doi.org/10.1016/j.earlhumdev.2007.12.003

Conde-Agudelo, A. (2000). Maternal morbidity and mortality associated with interpregnancy interval: Cross sectional study. *BMJ, 321*(7271), 1255–1259. https://doi.org/10.1136/bmj.321.7271.1255

Conde-Agudelo, A., Rosas-Bermúdez, A., & Kafury-Goeta, A. C. (2006). Birth spacing and risk of adverse perinatal outcomes: A meta-analysis. *JAMA, 295*(15), 1809. https://doi.org/10.1001/jama.295.15.1809

Conde-Agudelo, A., Rosas-Bermúdez, A., & Kafury-Goeta, A. C. (2007). Effects of birth spacing on maternal health: A systematic review. *American Journal of Obstetrics and Gynecology, 196*(4), 297–308. https://doi.org/10.1016/j.ajog.2006.05.055

Cotterman, K. J. (2004). Reverse pressure softening: A simple tool to prepare areola for easier latching during engorgement. *Journal of Human Lactation, 20*(2), 227–237. https://doi.org/10.1177/0890334404264224

Coviello, E. M., Grantz, K. L., Huang, C. C., Kelly, T. E., & Landy, H. J. (2016). Risk factors for retained placenta. *Obstetric Anesthesia Digest, 36*(4), 202–203. https://doi.org/10.1097/01.aoa.0000504730.26655.a7

Crenshaw, J. T., Brimdyr, K. H., Champion, J. D., Gilder, R. E., Winslow, E. H., Svennson, K., Widström, A. M., & Cadwell, K. (2012). Use of a video-ethnographic intervention, PRECESS immersion method, to improve skin-to-skin care and breastfeeding rates. *Journal of Obstetric, Gynecologic & Neonatal Nursing, 41*, S149–S150. https://doi.org/10.1111/j.1552-6909.2012.01362_44.x

CRO. (2016). *Labor Induction, Percent by State, 2016.* Cesareanrates.org. https://www.cesareanrates.org/labor-induction-by-state

Davey, M. A., & King, J. (2016). Caesarean section following induction of labour in uncomplicated first births- a population-based cross-sectional analysis of 42,950 births. *BMC Pregnancy and Childbirth, 16*(1), 92. https://doi.org/10.1186/s12884-016-0869-0

Davies, H. A., Clark, J. D., Dalton, K. J., & Edwards, O. M. (1989). Insulin requirements of diabetic women who breast feed. *BMJ, 298*(6684), 1357–1358. https://doi.org/10.1136/bmj.298.6684.1357

Deneux-Tharaux, C., Carmona, E., Bouvier-Colle, M. H., & Bréart, G. (2006). Postpartum maternal mortality and cesarean delivery. *Obstetrics & Gynecology, 108*(3, Part 1), 541–548. https://doi.org/10.1097/01.AOG.0000233154.62729.24

Dennis, C. L., & McQueen, K. (2007). Does maternal postpartum depressive symptomatology influence infant feeding outcomes? *Acta Paediatrica, 96*(4), 590–594. https://doi.org/10.1111/j.1651-2227.2007.00184.x

Dettwyler, K. A. (2004). When to wean: Biological versus cultural perspectives. *Clinical Obstetrics and Gynecology, 47*(3), 712–723. https://doi.org/10.1097/01.grf.0000137217.97573.01

Dewey, K. G., Nommsen-Rivers, L. A., Heinig, M. J., & Cohen, R. J. (2003). Risk factors for suboptimal infant breastfeeding behavior, delayed onset of lactation, and excess neonatal weight loss. *Pediatrics, 112*(3), 607–619. https://doi.org/10.1542/peds.112.3.607

DiGirolamo, A. M., Grummer-Strawn, L. M., & Fein, S. B. (2008). Effect of maternity-care practices on breastfeeding. *Pediatrics, 122*(Supplement_2), S43–S49. https://doi.org/10.1542/peds.2008-1315e

Donaldson-Myles, F. (2012). Can hormones in breastfeeding protect against postnatal depression? *British Journal of Midwifery, 20*(2), 88–93. https://doi.org/10.12968/bjom.2012.20.2.88

Durbin, D. R., Hoffman, B. D., COUNCIL ON INJURY, VIOLENCE, AND POISON PREVENTION, Agran, P. F., Denny, S. A., Hirsh, M., Johnston, B., Lee, L. K., Monroe, K., Schaechter, J., Tenenbein, M., Zonfrillo, M. R., & Quinlan, K. (2018). Child passenger safety. *Pediatrics, 142*(5), e20182460. https://doi.org/10.1542/peds.2018-2460

Elfgen, C., Hagenbuch, N., Görres, G., Block, E., & Leeners, B. (2017). Breastfeeding in women having experienced childhood sexual abuse. *Journal of Human Lactation, 33*(1), 119–127. https://doi.org/10.1177/0890334416680789

Ely, D. M., & Driscoll, A. K. (2021). Infant Mortality in the United States, 2019: Data From the Period Linked Birth/Infant Death File. National Vital Statistics Reports: From the Centers for Disease Control and Prevention, National Center for Health Statistics, National Vital Statistics System, 70(14), 1-18.

Fein, S. B., Labiner-Wolfe, J., Shealy, K. R., Li, R., Chen, J., & Grummer-Strawn, L. M. (2008). Infant feeding practices study II: Study methods. *Pediatrics, 122*(Supplement_2), S28–S35. https://doi.org/10.1542/peds.2008-1315c

Feldman-Winter, L., Grossman, X., Palaniappan, A., Kadokura, E., Hunter, K., Milcarek, B., & Merewood, A. (2012). Removal of industry-sponsored formula sample packs from the hospital: Does it make a difference? *Journal of Human Lactation, 28*(3), 380–388. https://doi.org/10.1177/0890334412444350

Flaherman, V. J., Maisels, M. J., the Academy of Breastfeeding Medicine, Brodribb, W., Noble, L., Brent, N., Bunik, M., Harrel, C., Lawrence, R. A., Marinelli, K. A., Reece-Stremtan, S., Rosen-Carole, C., Seo, T., St. Fleur, R., & Young, M. (2017). ABM clinical protocol #22: Guidelines for management of jaundice in the breastfeeding infant 35 weeks or more of gestation—Revised 2017. *Breastfeeding Medicine, 12*(5), 250–257. https://doi.org/10.1089/bfm.2017.29042.vjf for the TEDDY Study Group

Frank, N. M., Lynch, K. F., Uusitalo, U., Yang, J., Lönnrot, M., Virtanen, S. M., Hyöty, H., & Norris, J. M. (2019). The relationship between breastfeeding and reported respiratory and gastrointestinal infection rates in young children. *BMC Pediatrics, 19*(1), 339. https://doi.org/10.1186/s12887-019-1693-2

Froh, E. B., Cascino, A., Cerreta, S. K., Karsch, E. A., Kornberg, L. F., Lilley, J. E., Welch, L., & Spatz, D. L. (2018). Status of Legislative Efforts to Promote and Protect Breastfeeding and the Provision of Human Milk for Women Returning to Work in the First Postpartum Year. *Breastfeeding Medicine, 13*(7), 506–509. https://doi.org/10.1089/bfm.2018.0092

Ganju, A., Suresh, A., Stephens, J., Palettas, M., Burke, D., Miles, L., Lehman, K., Rudesill, R., Lustberg, M., Bose-Brill, S., & Ramaswamy, B. (2018). Learning, life, and lactation: Knowledge of breastfeeding's impact on breast cancer risk reduction and its influence on breastfeeding practices. *Breastfeeding Medicine, 13*(10), 651–656. https://doi.org/10.1089/bfm.2018.0170

Gardella, C., Taylor, M., Benedetti, T., Hitti, J., & Critchlow, C. (2001). The effect of sequential use of vacuum and forceps for assisted vaginal delivery on neonatal and maternal outcomes. *American Journal of Obstetrics and Gynecology, 185*(4), 896–902. https://doi.org/10.1067/mob.2001.117309

Gatti, L. (2008). Maternal Perceptions of Insufficient Milk Supply in Breastfeeding. *Journal of Nursing Scholarship, 40*(4), 355–363. https://doi.org/10.1111/j.1547-5069.2008.00234.x

Gertz, B., & DeFranco, E. (2019). Predictors of breastfeeding non-initiation in the NICU. *Maternal & Child Nutrition, 15*(3). https://doi.org/10.1111/mcn.12797

Glauber, R. (2018). Trends in the motherhood wage penalty and fatherhood wage premium for low, middle, and high earners. *Demography, 55*(5), 1663–1680. https://doi.org/10.1007/s13524-018-0712-5

Goer, H. (2019). *Parsing the ARRIVE Trial: Should First-Time Parents Be Routinely Induced at 39 Weeks?* https://www.lamaze.org/Connecting-the-Dots/parsing-the-arrive-trial-should-first-time-parents-be-routinely-induced-at-39-weeks

Government of Canada. (2015). *Nutrition for healthy term infants: Recommendations from birth to six months.* https://www.canada.ca/en/health-canada/services/canada-food-guide/resources/infant-feeding/nutrition-healthy-term-infants-recommendations-birth-six-months.html

Grossman, X., Chaudhuri, J. H., Feldman-Winter, L., & Merewood, A. (2012). Neonatal weight loss at a US baby-friendly hospital. *Journal of the Academy of Nutrition and Dietetics, 112*(3), 410–413. https://doi.org/10.1016/j.jada.2011.10.024

Grotegut, C. A., Paglia, M. J., Johnson, L. N., Thames, B., & James, A. H. (2011). Oxytocin exposure during labor among women with postpartum hemorrhage secondary to uterine atony. *Obstetric Anesthesia Digest, 31*(4), 234–235. https://doi.org/10.1097/01.aoa.0000406689.19068.ae

Grubesic, T. H., & Durbin, K. M. (2017). Breastfeeding support: A geographic perspective on access and equity. *Journal of Human Lactation, 33*(4), 770–780. https://doi.org/10.1177/0890334417706361

Grubesic, T. H., & Durbin, K. M. (2020). The complex geographies of telelactation and access to community breastfeeding support in the state of Ohio. *PLOS ONE, 15*(11), e0242457. https://doi.org/10.1371/journal.pone.0242457

Güngör, D., Nadaud, P., LaPergola, C. C., Dreibelbis, C., Wong, Y. P., Terry, N., Abrams, S. A., Beker, L., Jacobovits, T., Järvinen, K. M., Nommsen-Rivers, L. A., O'Brien, K. O., Oken, E., Pérez-Escamilla, R., Ziegler, E. E., & Spahn, J. M. (2019). Infant milk-feeding practices and diabetes outcomes in offspring: A systematic review. *The American Journal of Clinical Nutrition, 109* (Supplement⊠1), 817S-837S. https://doi.org/10.1093/ajcn/nqy311

Güngör, D., Nadaud, P., LaPergola, C. C., Dreibelbis, C., Wong, Y. P., Terry, N., Abrams, S. A., Beker, L., Jacobovits, T., Järvinen, K. M., Nommsen-Rivers, L. A., O'Brien, K. O., Oken, E., Pérez-Escamilla, R., Ziegler, E. E., & Spahn, J. M. (2019b). Infant milk-feeding practices and food allergies, allergic rhinitis, atopic dermatitis, and asthma throughout the life span: A systematic review. *The American Journal of Clinical Nutrition, 109*(Supplement_1), 772S-799S. https://doi.org/10.1093/ajcn/nqy283

Hales, C. M., Carroll, M. D., Fryar, C. D., & Ogden, C. L. (2017). Prevalence of Obesity Among Adults and Youth: United States, 2015-2016. *NCHS Data Brief, 288*, 1–8.

Hall, R. T., Mercer, A. M., Teasley, S. L., McPherson, D. M., Simon, S. D., Santos, S. R., Meyers, B. M., & Hipsh, N. E. (2002). A breast-feeding assessment score to evaluate the risk for cessation of breast-feeding by 7 to 10 days of age. *The Journal of Pediatrics, 141*(5), 659–664. https://doi.org/10.1067/mpd.2002.129081

Hasegawa, J., Farina, A., Turchi, G., Hasegawa, Y., Zanello, M., & Baroncini, S. (2013). Effects of epidural analgesia on labor length, instrumental delivery, and neonatal short-term outcome. *Journal of Anesthesia, 27*(1), 43–47. https://doi.org/10.1007/s00540-012-1480-9

Hastings, G., Angus, K., Eadie, D., & Hunt, K. (2020). Selling second best: How infant formula marketing works. *Globalization and Health, 16*(1), 77. https://doi.org/10.1186/s12992-020-00597-w

Henly, S. J., Anderson, C. M., Avery, M. D., Hills-Bonuyk, S. G., Potter, S., & Duckett, L. J. (1995). Anemia and insufficient milk in first-time mothers. *Birth, 22*(2), 87–92. https://doi.org/10.1111/j.1523-536X.1995.tb00565.x

Hobbs, A. J., Mannion, C. A., McDonald, S. W., Brockway, M., & Tough, S. C. (2016). The impact of caesarean section on breastfeeding initiation, duration and difficulties in the first four months postpartum. *BMC Pregnancy and Childbirth, 16*(1), 90. https://doi.org/10.1186/s12884-016-0876-1

Hodges, E. A., Johnson, S. L., Hughes, S. O., Hopkinson, J. M., Butte, N. F., & Fisher, J. O. (2013). Development of the responsiveness to child feeding cues scale. *Appetite, 65*, 210–219. https://doi.org/10.1016/j.appet.2013.02.010

Holm, J., Eriksson, L., Ploner, A., Eriksson, M., Rantalainen, M., Li, J., Hall, P., & Czene, K. (2017). Assessment of breast cancer risk factors reveals subtype heterogeneity. *Cancer Research, 77*(13), 3708–3717. https://doi.org/10.1158/0008-5472.CAN-16-2574

Holmes, A. V., McLeod, A. Y., & Bunik, M. (2013). ABM clinical protocol #5: Peripartum breastfeeding management for the healthy mother and infant at term, revision 2013. *Breastfeeding Medicine, 8*(6), 469–473. https://doi.org/10.1089/bfm.2013.9979

Hoseth, E. (2000). Blood glucose levels in a population of healthy, breast fed, term infants of appropriate size for gestational age. *Archives of Disease in Childhood - Fetal and Neonatal Edition, 83*(2), 117F - 119. https://doi.org/10.1136/fn.83.2.F117

Howard, C. (2000). Office prenatal formula advertising and its effect on breast-feeding patterns. *Obstetrics & Gynecology, 95*(2), 296–303. https://doi.org/10.1016/S0029-7844(99)00555-4

Hung, K. J., & Berg, O. (2011). Early skin-to-skin after cesarean to improve breastfeeding. *MCN: The American Journal of Maternal/Child Nursing, 36*(5), 318–324. https://doi.org/10.1097/NMC.0b013e3182266314

Hutcheon, J. A., Nelson, H. D., Stidd, R., Moskosky, S., & Ahrens, K. A. (2019). Short interpregnancy intervals and adverse maternal outcomes in high-resource settings: An updated systematic review. *Paediatric and Perinatal Epidemiology, 33*(1). https://doi.org/10.1111/ppe.12518

International Breastfeeding Centre. (2009). *Low blood sugar in the newborn baby.* https://ibconline.ca/information-sheets/hypoglycaemia-of-the-newborn-low-blood-sugar/

Ip, S., Chung, M., Raman, G., Trikalinos, T. A., & Lau, J. (2009). A summary of the agency for healthcare research and quality's evidence report on breastfeeding in developed countries. *Breastfeeding Medicine, 4*(s1), S-17-S-30. https://doi.org/10.1089/bfm.2009.0050

Jackson, R. L. (1988). Ecological breastfeeding and child spacing. *Clinical Pediatrics, 27*(8), 373–377. https://doi.org/10.1177/000992288802700804

Jamieson, D. (2019). How employers make it impossible for working women to breastfeed. *Huffington Post.* https://tinyurl.com/yc6zxkuk

Johns, M. (2018). Abbott Labs to pay $50,000 for alleged deceptive survey marketing of new parents. *Legal Newsline.* https://legalnewsline.com/stories/511637566-abbott-labs-to-pay-50-000-for-alleged-deceptive-survey-marketing-of-new-parents

Jordan, S. J., Na, R., Johnatty, S. E., Wise, L. A., Adami, H. O., Brinton, L. A., Chen, C., Cook, L. S., Dal Maso, L., De Vivo, I., Freudenheim, J. L., Friedenreich, C. M., La Vecchia, C., McCann, S. E., Moysich, K. B., Lu, L., Olson, S. H., Palmer, J. R., Petruzella, S., & Webb, P. M. (2017). Breastfeeding and endometrial cancer risk: An analysis from the epidemiology of endometrial cancer consortium. *Obstetrics & Gynecology, 129*(6), 1059–1067. https://doi.org/10.1097/AOG.0000000000002057

Jou, J., Kozhimannil, K. B., Johnson, P. J., & Sakala, C. (2015). Patient-perceived pressure from clinicians for labor induction and cesarean delivery: A population-based survey of U.S. women. *Health Services Research, 50*(4), 961–981. https://doi.org/10.1111/1475-6773.12231

Kair, L. R., & Colaizy, T. T. (2016). Obese mothers have lower odds of experiencing pro-breastfeeding hospital practices than mothers of normal weight: CDC pregnancy risk assessment monitoring system (PRAMS), 2004–2008. *Maternal and Child Health Journal, 20*(3), 593–601. https://doi.org/10.1007/s10995-015-1858-z

Kellams, A., Harrel, C., Omage, S., Gregory, C., Rosen-Carole, C., & the Academy of Breastfeeding Medicine. (2017). ABM clinical protocol #3: Supplementary feedings in the healthy term breastfed neonate, revised 2017. *Breastfeeding Medicine*, *12*(4), 188–198. https://doi.org/10.1089/bfm.2017.29038.ajk

Kelleher, J., Bhat, R., Salas, A. A., Addis, D., Mills, E. C., Mallick, H., Tripathi, A., Pruitt, E. P., Roane, C., McNair, T., Owen, J., Ambalavanan, N., & Carlo, W. A. (2013). Oronasopharyngeal suction versus wiping of the mouth and nose at birth: A randomised equivalency trial. *The Lancet*, *382*(9889), 326–330. https://doi.org/10.1016/S0140-6736(13)60775-8

Kendall-Tackett, K. (2007). A new paradigm for depression in new mothers: The central role of inflammation and how breastfeeding and anti-inflammatory treatments protect maternal mental health. *International Breastfeeding Journal*, *2*(1), 6. https://doi.org/10.1186/1746-4358-2-6

Kent, J., Ashton, E., Hardwick, C., Rowan, M., Chia, E., Fairclough, K., Menon, L., Scott, C., Mather-McCaw, G., Navarro, K., & Geddes, D. (2015). Nipple pain in breastfeeding mothers: Incidence, causes and treatments. *International Journal of Environmental Research and Public Health*, *12*(10), 12247–12263. https://doi.org/10.3390/ijerph121012247

King, V. J., Pilliod, R., & LIttle, A. (2010). *Rapid review: Elective induction of labor.* Center for Evidence-based Policy. . https://www.nationalpartnership.org/our-work/resources/health-care/maternity/quick-facts-about-labor-induction.pdf

Kirkegaard, H., Bliddal, M., Støvring, H., Rasmussen, K. M., Gunderson, E. P., Køber, L., Sørensen, T. I. A., & Nohr, E. A. (2018). Breastfeeding and later maternal risk of hypertension and cardiovascular disease – The role of overall and abdominal obesity. *Preventive Medicine*, *114*, 140–148. https://doi.org/10.1016/j.ypmed.2018.06.014

Kozhimannil, K. B., Jou, J., Gjerdingen, D. K., & McGovern, P. M. (2016). Access to workplace accommodations to support breastfeeding after passage of the affordable care act. *Women's Health Issues*, *26*(1), 6–13. https://doi.org/10.1016/j.whi.2015.08.002

Kumar, R. K., Singhal, A., Vaidya, U., Banerjee, S., Anwar, F., & Rao, S. (2017). Optimizing nutrition in preterm low birth weight infants—Consensus summary. *Frontiers in Nutrition*, *4*, 20. https://doi.org/10.3389/fnut.2017.00020

Lamaze. (2021). *Lamaze Healthy Birth Practices*. https://www.lamaze.org/childbirth-practices

Lamaze International. (2007). Position paper: Promoting, supporting, and protecting normal birth. *Journal of Perinatal Education*, *16*(3), 11–15. https://doi.org/10.1624/105812407X217084

Lawrence, R. A., & Lawrence, R. M. (2016). *Breastfeeding: A guide for the medical profession* (Eighth edition). Elsevier.

Leahy-Warren, P., Creedon, M., O'Mahony, A., & Mulcahy, H. (2017). Normalising breastfeeding within a formula feeding culture: An Irish qualitative study. *Women and Birth*, *30*(2), e103–e110. https://doi.org/10.1016/j.wombi.2016.10.002

Lewallen, L. P., Dick, M. J., Flowers, J., Powell, W., Zickefoose, K. T., Wall, Y. G., & Price, Z. M. (2006). Breastfeeding support and early cessation. *Journal of Obstetric, Gynecologic & Neonatal Nursing*, *35*(2), 166–172. https://doi.org/10.1111/j.1552-6909.2006.00031.x

Ley, S. H., Chavarro, J. E., Li, M., Bao, W., Hinkle, S. N., Wander, P. L., Rich-Edwards, J., Olsen, S., Vaag, A., Damm, P., Grunnet, L. G., Mills, J. L., Hu, F. B., & Zhang, C. (2020). Lactation duration and long-term risk for incident type 2 diabetes in women with a history of gestational diabetes mellitus. *Diabetes Care*, *43*(4), 793–798. https://doi.org/10.2337/dc19-2237

Little, E., Legare, C., & Carver, L. (2018). Mother–infant physical contact predicts responsive feeding among U.S. breastfeeding mothers. *Nutrients*, *10*(9), 1251. https://doi.org/10.3390/nu10091251

Liu, B., Jorm, L., & Banks, E. (2010). Parity, breastfeeding, and the subsequent risk of maternal type 2 diabetes. *Diabetes Care*, *33*(6), 1239–1241. https://doi.org/10.2337/dc10-0347

Ludington-Hoe, S. M., Lewis, T., Morgan, K., Cong, X., Anderson, L., & Reese, S. (2006). Breast and infant temperatures with twins during shared kangaroo care. *Journal of Obstetric, Gynecologic & Neonatal Nursing*, *35*(2), 223–231. https://doi.org/10.1111/j.1552-6909.2006.00024.x

Lund-Blix, N. A., Dydensborg Sander, S., Størdal, K., Nybo Andersen, A.-M., Rønningen, K. S., Joner, G., Skrivarhaug, T., Njølstad, P. R., Husby, S., & Stene, L. C. (2017). Infant feeding and risk of type 1 diabetes in two large scandinavian birth cohorts. *Diabetes Care*, *40*(7), 920–927. https://doi.org/10.2337/dc17-0016

Lundström, J. N., Boyle, J. A., Zatorre, R. J., & Jones-Gotman, M. (2009). The neuronal substrates of human olfactory based kin recognition. *Human Brain Mapping*, *30*(8), 2571–2580. https://doi.org/10.1002/hbm.20686

MacDorman, M. F., Declercq, E., Menacker, F., & Malloy, M. H. (2006). Infant and neonatal mortality for primary cesarean and vaginal births to women with "no indicated risk," United States, 1998–2001 birth cohorts. *Birth*, *33*(3), 175–182. https://doi.org/10.1111/j.1523-536X.2006.00102.x

Martin, J. A., Hamilton, B. E., Osterman, M. J. K., & Driscoll, A. K. (2019). Births: Final data for 2018. *National Vital Statistics Reports: From the Centers for Disease Control and Prevention, National Center for Health Statistics, National Vital Statistics System*, *68*(13), 1–47.

Martin, J. A., Hamilton, B. E., Osterman, M. J. K., Driscoll, A. K., & Mathews, T. J. (2017). Births: Final data for 2015. *National Vital Statistics Reports: From the Centers for Disease Control and Prevention, National Center for Health Statistics, National Vital Statistics System*, *66*(1), 1.

McClellan, H. L., Hepworth, A. R., Garbin, C. P., Rowan, M. K., Deacon, J., Hartmann, P. E., & Geddes, D. T. (2012). Nipple pain during breastfeeding with or without visible trauma. *Journal of Human Lactation*, *28*(4), 511–521. https://doi.org/10.1177/0890334412444464

McCormick, D. P., Sarpong, K., Jordan, L., Ray, L. A., & Jain, S. (2010). Infant obesity: Are we ready to make this diagnosis? *The Journal of Pediatrics*, *157*(1), 15–19. https://doi.org/10.1016/j.jpeds.2010.01.028

McInerney, C. M., & Gupta, A. (2015). Delaying the first bath decreases the incidence of neonatal hypoglycemia. *Journal of Obstetric, Gynecologic & Neonatal Nursing*, *44*, S73–S74. https://doi.org/10.1111/1552-6909.12650

McKinney, C. O., Hahn-Holbrook, J., Chase-Lansdale, P. L., Ramey, S. L., Krohn, J., Reed-Vance, M., Raju, T. N. K., Shalowitz, M. U., & on behalf of the Community Child Health Research Network. (2016). Racial and Ethnic Differences in Breastfeeding. *Pediatrics*, *138*(2), e20152388. https://doi.org/10.1542/peds.2015-2388

McNally, J., Hugh-Jones, S., Caton, S., Vereijken, C., Weenen, H., & Hetherington, M. (2016). Communicating hunger and satiation in the first 2 years of life: A systematic review: Hunger and satiation in the first 2 years of life. *Maternal & Child Nutrition*, *12*(2), 205–228. https://doi.org/10.1111/mcn.12230

MDH. (2018). *Mississippi Vital Statistics Report 2010*. Mississippi Department of Health. http://www.msdh.state.ms.us/msdhsite/_static/resources/8015.pdf

Meek, J. Y., & Noble, L. (2022). Policy statement: breastfeeding and the use of human milk. Pediatrics, 150(1).

Merewood, A., Mehta, S. D., Chamberlain, L. B., Philipp, B. L., & Bauchner, H. (2005). Breastfeeding rates in US baby-friendly hospitals: Results of a national survey. *Pediatrics*, *116*(3), 628–634. https://doi.org/10.1542/peds.2004-1636

Mikiel-Kostyra, K., Mazur, J., & Boltruszko, I. (2007). Effect of early skin-to-skin contact after delivery on duration of breastfeeding: A prospective cohort study. *Acta Paediatrica*, *91*(12), 1301–1306. https://doi.org/10.1111/j.1651-2227.2002.tb02824.x

Miller, E. K., Bugna, J., Libster, R., Shepherd, B. E., Scalzo, P. M., Acosta, P. L., Hijano, D., Reynoso, N., Batalle, J. P., Coviello, S., Klein, M. I., Bauer, G., Benitez, A., Kleeberger, S. R., & Polack, F. P. (2012). Human rhinoviruses in severe respiratory disease in very low birth weight infants. *Pediatrics*, *129*(1), e60–e67. https://doi.org/10.1542/peds.2011-0583

Miralles, O., Sánchez, J., Palou, A., & Picó, C. (2006). A physiological role of breast milk leptin in body weight control in developing infants*. *Obesity*, *14*(8), 1371–1377. https://doi.org/10.1038/oby.2006.155

Mitro, S., Gordon, A. R., Olsson, M. J., & Lundström, J. N. (2012). The smell of age: Perception and discrimination of body odors of different ages. *PLoS ONE*, *7*(5), e38110. https://doi.org/10.1371/journal.pone.0038110

Mizuno, K., Mizuno, N., Shinohara, T., & Noda, M. (2007). Mother-infant skin-to-skin contact after delivery results in early recognition of own mother's milk odour. *Acta Paediatrica, 93*(12), 1640–1645. https://doi.org/10.1111/j.1651-2227.2004.tb00856.x

Moon, R. Y., & Hauck, F. R. (2016). SIDS risk: It's more than just the sleep environment. *Pediatrics, 137*(1), e20153665. https://doi.org/10.1542/peds.2015-3665

Moore, E. R., & Anderson, G. C. (2007). Randomized controlled trial of very early mother-infant skin-to-skin contact and breastfeeding status. *Journal of Midwifery & Women's Health, 52*(2), 116–125. https://doi.org/10.1016/j.jmwh.2006.12.002

Morley, R., Fewtrell, M. S., A. Abbott, R., Stephenson, T., MacFadyen, U., & Lucas, A. (2004). Neurodevelopment in children born small for gestational age: A randomized trial of nutrient-enriched versus standard formula and comparison with a reference breastfed group. *Pediatrics, 113*(3), 515–521. https://doi.org/10.1542/peds.113.3.515

Much, D., Beyerlein, A., Roßbauer, M., Hummel, S., & Ziegler, A. G. (2014). Beneficial effects of breastfeeding in women with gestational diabetes mellitus. *Molecular Metabolism, 3*(3), 284–292. https://doi.org/10.1016/j.molmet.2014.01.002

Murtagh, L., & Moulton, A. D. (2011). Working mothers, breastfeeding, and the law. *American Journal of Public Health, 101*(2), 217–223. https://doi.org/10.2105/AJPH.2009.185280

Negin, J., Coffman, J., Vizintin, P., & Raynes-Greenow, C. (2016). The influence of grandmothers on breastfeeding rates: A systematic review. *BMC Pregnancy and Childbirth, 16*(1), 91. https://doi.org/10.1186/s12884-016-0880-5

Neifert, M., & Bunik, M. (2013). Overcoming clinical barriers to exclusive breastfeeding. *Pediatric Clinics of North America, 60*(1), 115–145. https://doi.org/10.1016/j.pcl.2012.10.001

New York Times. (2018). *Opposition to Breast-Feeding Resolution by U.S. Stuns World Health Officials.* https://www.nytimes.com/2018/07/08/health/world-health-breastfeeding-ecuador-trump.html

Newman, J. (1990). Breastfeeding problems associated with the early introduction of bottles and pacifiers. *Journal of Human Lactation, 6*(2), 59–63. https://doi.org/10.1177/089033449000600214

Newnham, E. C., Moran, P. S., Begley, C. M., Carroll, M., & Daly, D. (2021). Comparison of labour and birth outcomes between nulliparous women who used epidural analgesia in labour and those who did not: A prospective cohort study. *Women and Birth, 34*(5), e435–e441. https://doi.org/10.1016/j.wombi.2020.09.001

Noel-Weiss, J., Woodend, A. K., Peterson, W. E., Gibb, W., & Groll, D. L. (2011). An observational study of associations among maternal fluids during parturition, neonatal output, and breastfed newborn weight loss. *International Breastfeeding Journal, 6*(1), 9. https://doi.org/10.1186/1746-4358-6-9

Oddy, W. H. (2017). Breastfeeding, childhood asthma, and allergic disease. *Annals of Nutrition and Metabolism*, *70*(Suppl. 2), 26–36. https://doi.org/10.1159/000457920

Office of the Surgeon General (US), Centers for Disease Control and Prevention (US), & Office on Women's Health (US). (2011). *The Surgeon General's Call to Action to Support Breastfeeding*. Office of the Surgeon General (US). http://www.ncbi.nlm.nih.gov/books/NBK52682/

Olaiya, O., Dee, D. L., Sharma, A. J., & Smith, R. A. (2016). Maternity care practices and breastfeeding among adolescent mothers aged 12–19 years—United States, 2009–2011. *MMWR. Morbidity and Mortality Weekly Report*, *65*(2), 17–22. https://doi.org/10.15585/mmwr.mm6502a1

Olsson, M. J., Lundström, J. N., Kimball, B. A., Gordon, A. R., Karshikoff, B., Hosseini, N., Sorjonen, K., Olgart Höglund, C., Solares, C., Soop, A., Axelsson, J., & Lekander, M. (2014). The scent of disease: Human body odor contains an early chemosensory cue of sickness. *Psychological Science*, *25*(3), 817–823. https://doi.org/10.1177/0956797613515681

Oommen, H., Oddbjørn Tveit, T., Eskedal, L. T., Myr, R., Swanson, D. M., & Vistad, I. (2021). The association between intrapartum opioid fentanyl and early breastfeeding: A prospective observational study. *Acta Obstetricia et Gynecologica Scandinavica*, *100*(12), 2294–2302. https://doi.org/10.1111/aogs.14268

Orbach-Zinger, S., Landau, R., Davis, A., Oved, O., Caspi, L., Fireman, S., Fein, S., Ioscovich, A., Bracco, D., Hoshen, M., & Eidelman, L. A. (2019). The effect of labor epidural analgesia on breastfeeding outcomes: A prospective observational cohort study in a mixed-parity cohort. *Anesthesia & Analgesia*, *129*(3), 784–791. https://doi.org/10.1213/ANE.0000000000003442

Oribhabor, G. I., Nelson, M. L., Buchanan-Peart, K.-A. R., & Cancarevic, I. (2020). A mother's cry: A race to eliminate the influence of racial disparities on maternal morbidity and mortality rates among black women in America. *Cureus*. https://doi.org/10.7759/cureus.9207

Palou, A., & Picó, C. (2009). Leptin intake during lactation prevents obesity and affects food intake and food preferences in later life. *Appetite*, *52*(1), 249–252. https://doi.org/10.1016/j.appet.2008.09.013

Pavill, B. C. (2002). Fathers & breastfeeding. *AWHONN Lifelines*, *6*(4), 324–331. https://doi.org/10.1111/j.1552-6356.2002.tb00497.x

Paynter, M. J. (2018). Policy and legal protection for breastfeeding and incarcerated women in Canada. *Journal of Human Lactation*, *34*(2), 276–281. https://doi.org/10.1177/0890334418758659

Peevy, K. J., Landaw, S. A., & Gross, S. J. (1980). Hyperbilirubinemia in infants of diabetic mothers. *Pediatrics*, *66*(3), 417–419.

Preer, G. L., Newby, P. K., & Philipp, B. L. (2012). Weight loss in exclusively breastfed infants delivered by cesarean birth. *Journal of Human Lactation, 28*(2), 153–158. https://doi.org/10.1177/0890334411434177

Procaccini, D., Curley, A. L. C., & Goldman, M. (2018). Baby-friendly practices minimize newborn infants weight loss. *Breastfeeding Medicine, 13*(3), 189–194. https://doi.org/10.1089/bfm.2017.0182

Public Health Agency of Canada. (2018). *Chapter 4: Care during labour and birth*. https://www.canada.ca/en/public-health/services/publications/healthy-living/maternity-newborn-care-guidelines-chapter-4.html

Qu, G., Wang, L., Tang, X., Wu, W., & Sun, Y. (2018). Association between duration of breastfeeding and maternal hypertension: A systematic review and meta-analysis. *Breastfeeding Medicine, 13*(5), 318–326. https://doi.org/10.1089/bfm.2017.0180

Quigley, M. A., Kelly, Y. J., & Sacker, A. (2007). Breastfeeding and hospitalization for diarrheal and respiratory infection in the United Kingdom millennium cohort study. *Pediatrics, 119*(4), e837–e842. https://doi.org/10.1542/peds.2006-2256

Radzyminski, S., & Callister, L. C. (2016). Mother's beliefs, attitudes, and decision making related to infant feeding choices. *The Journal of Perinatal Education, 25*(1), 18–28. https://doi.org/10.1891/1058-1243.25.1.18

Ramakrishnan, R., Oberg, C. N., & Kirby, R. S. (2014). The association between maternal perception of obstetric and pediatric care providers' attitudes and exclusive breastfeeding outcomes. *Journal of Human Lactation, 30*(1), 80–87. https://doi.org/10.1177/0890334413513072

Rameez, R. M., Sadana, D., Kaur, S., Ahmed, T., Patel, J., Khan, M. S., Misbah, S., Simonson, M. T., Riaz, H., & Ahmed, H. M. (2019). Association of maternal lactation with diabetes and hypertension: A systematic review and meta-analysis. *JAMA Network Open, 2*(10), e1913401. https://doi.org/10.1001/jamanetworkopen.2019.13401

Ransjo-Arvidson, A. B., Matthiesen, A. S., Lilja, G., Nissen, E., Widstrom, A. M., & Uvnas-Moberg, K. (2001). Maternal analgesia during labor disturbs newborn behavior: Effects on breastfeeding, temperature, and crying. *Birth, 28*(1), 5–12. https://doi.org/10.1046/j.1523-536x.2001.00005.x

Rasmussen, K. M., & Kjolhede, C. L. (2004). Prepregnant overweight and obesity diminish the prolactin response to suckling in the first week postpartum. *Pediatrics, 113*(5), e465–e471. https://doi.org/10.1542/peds.113.5.e465

Rasmussen, K. M., Lee, V. E., Ledkovsky, T. B., & Kjolhede, C. L. (2006). A description of lactation counseling practices that are used with obese mothers. *Journal of Human Lactation, 22*(3), 322–327. https://doi.org/10.1177/0890334406290177

Ravelli, A. C. J., Eskes, M., Groot, C. J. M., Abu-Hanna, A., & Post, J. A. M. (2020). Intrapartum epidural analgesia and low Apgar score among singleton infants born at term: A propensity score matched study. *Acta Obstetricia et Gynecologica Scandinavica*, *99*(9), 1155–1162. https://doi.org/10.1111/aogs.13837

Rayburn, W. F., & Zhang, J. (2002). Rising rates of labor induction: Present concerns and future strategies. *Obstetrics & Gynecology*, *100*(1), 164–167. https://doi.org/10.1097/00006250-200207000-00024

Rempel, L. A., & Rempel, J. K. (2011). The breastfeeding team: The role of involved fathers in the breastfeeding family. *Journal of Human Lactation*, *27*(2), 115–121. https://doi.org/10.1177/0890334410390045

Righard, L., & Alade, M. O. (1990). Effect of delivery room routines on success of first breast-feed. *The Lancet*, *336*(8723), 1105–1107. https://doi.org/10.1016/0140-6736(90)92579-7

Rippey, P. L. F., & Noonan, M. C. (2012). Is breastfeeding truly cost free? Income consequences of breastfeeding for women. *American Sociological Review*, *77*(2), 244–267. https://doi.org/10.1177/0003122411435477

Riviello, C., Mello, G., & Jovanovic, L. G. (2009). Breastfeeding and the basal insulin requirement in type 1 diabetic women. *Endocrine Practice*, *15*(3), 187–193. https://doi.org/10.4158/EP.15.3.187

Rocha, B. de O., Machado, M. P., Bastos, L. L., Barbosa Silva, L., Santos, A. P., Santos, L. C., & Ferrarez Bouzada, M. C. (2020). Risk factors for delayed onset of lactogenesis II among primiparous mothers from a Brazilian baby-friendly hospital. *Journal of Human Lactation*, *36*(1), 146–156. https://doi.org/10.1177/0890334419835174

Rosen, H., Shmueli, A., Ashwal, E., Hiersch, L., Yogev, Y., & Aviram, A. (2018). Delivery outcomes of large-for-gestational-age newborns stratified by the presence or absence of gestational diabetes mellitus. *International Journal of Gynaecology and Obstetrics: The Official Organ of the International Federation of Gynaecology and Obstetrics*, *141*(1), 120–125. https://doi.org/10.1002/ijgo.12387

Rosen, I. M., Krueger, M. V., Carney, L. M., & Graham, J. A. (2008). Prenatal breastfeeding education and breastfeeding outcomes. *MCN: The American Journal of Maternal/Child Nursing*, *33*(5), 315–319. https://doi.org/10.1097/01.NMC.0000334900.22215.ec

Ryan, A. S., Pratt, W. F., Wysong, J. L., Lewandowski, G., McNally, J. W., & Krieger, F. W. (1991). A comparison of breast-feeding data from the national surveys of family growth and the ross laboratories mothers surveys. *American Journal of Public Health*, *81*(8), 1049–1052. https://doi.org/10.2105/AJPH.81.8.1049

Sadacharan, R., Grossman, X., Matlak, S., & Merewood, A. (2014). Hospital discharge bags and breastfeeding at 6 months: Data from the infant feeding practices study II. *Journal of Human Lactation*, *30*(1), 73–79. https://doi.org/10.1177/0890334413513653

Sankar, M. J., Sinha, B., Chowdhury, R., Bhandari, N., Taneja, S., Martines, J., & Bahl, R. (2015). Optimal breastfeeding practices and infant and child mortality: A systematic review and meta-analysis. *Acta Paediatrica*, *104*, 3–13. https://doi.org/10.1111/apa.13147

Sasamoto, N., Babic, A., Jordan, S., Risch, H., Harris, H., Rossing, M. A., Doherty, J., Goodman, M., Thompson, P., Kjær, S. K., Jensen, A., Schildkraut, J., Titus, L., Cramer, D., Bandera, E., Sieh, W., McGuire, V., Sutphen, R., Pearce, C. L., & Terry, K. (2019). Abstract 640: Breastfeeding pattern and ovarian cancer risk: Results from the Ovarian Cancer Association Consortium. *Epidemiology*, 640–640. https://doi.org/10.1158/1538-7445.AM2019-640

Saxton, A., Fahy, K., Rolfe, M., Skinner, V., & Hastie, C. (2015). Does skin-to-skin contact and breast feeding at birth affect the rate of primary postpartum haemorrhage: Results of a cohort study. *Midwifery*, *31*(11), 1110–1117. https://doi.org/10.1016/j.midw.2015.07.008

Schreck, P. K., Solem, K., Wright, T., Schulte, C., Ronnisch, K. J., & Szpunar, S. (2017). Both prenatal and postnatal interventions are needed to improve breastfeeding outcomes in a low-income population. *Breastfeeding Medicine*, *12*(3), 142–148. https://doi.org/10.1089/bfm.2016.0131

Scott, V. C., Taylor, Y. J., Basquin, C., & Venkitsubramanian, K. (2019). Impact of key workplace breastfeeding support characteristics on job satisfaction, breastfeeding duration, and exclusive breastfeeding among health care employees. *Breastfeeding Medicine*, *14*(6), 416–423. https://doi.org/10.1089/bfm.2018.0202

Sexton, S., & Natale, R. (2009). Risks and benefits of pacifiers. *American Family Physician*, *79*(8), 681–685.

Signore, C., & Klebanoff, M. (2008). Neonatal morbidity and mortality after elective cesarean delivery. *Clinics in Perinatology*, *35*(2), 361–371. https://doi.org/10.1016/j.clp.2008.03.009

Smillie, C. M. (2017). How infants learn to feed: A neurobehavioral model. In C. W. Genna (Ed.), *Supporting Sucking Skills in Breastfeeding Infants* (Third edition). Jones & Bartlett Learning.

Stock, S. J., Josephs, K., Farquharson, S., Love, C., Cooper, S. E., Kissack, C., Akolekar, R., Norman, J. E., & Denison, F. C. (2013). Maternal and neonatal outcomes of successful Kielland's rotational forceps delivery. *Obstetrics & Gynecology*, *121*(5), 1032–1039. https://doi.org/10.1097/AOG.0b013e31828b72cb

Strathearn, L., Li, J., Fonagy, P., & Montague, P. R. (2008). What's in a smile? Maternal brain responses to infant facial cues. *Pediatrics*, *122*(1), 40–51. https://doi.org/10.1542/peds.2007-1566

Stuebe, A. M., Bryant, A. G., Lewis, R., & Muddana, A. (2016). Association of etonogestrel-releasing contraceptive implant with reduced weight gain in an exclusively breastfed infant: Report and literature review. *Breastfeeding Medicine*, *11*(4), 203–206. https://doi.org/10.1089/bfm.2016.0017

Stuebe, A. M., Grewen, K., & Meltzer-Brody, S. (2013). Association between maternal mood and oxytocin response to breastfeeding. *Journal of Women's Health, 22*(4), 352–361. https://doi.org/10.1089/jwh.2012.3768

Taylor, R. W., Grant, A. M., Goulding, A., & Williams, S. M. (2005). Early adiposity rebound: Review of papers linking this to subsequent obesity in children and adults. *Current Opinion in Clinical Nutrition and Metabolic Care, 8*(6), 607–612. https://doi.org/10.1097/01.mco.0000168391.60884.93

Tedder, J. (2015). The roadmap to breastfeeding success: Teaching child development to extend breastfeeding duration. *The Journal of Perinatal Education, 24*(4), 239–248. https://doi.org/10.1891/1058-1243.24.4.239

Thavarajah, H., Flatley, C., & Kumar, S. (2018). The relationship between the five minute Apgar score, mode of birth and neonatal outcomes. *The Journal of Maternal-Fetal & Neonatal Medicine, 31*(10), 1335–1341. https://doi.org/10.1080/14767058.2017.1315666

Thompson, J. F., Heal, L. J., Roberts, C. L., & Ellwood, D. A. (2010). Women's breastfeeding experiences following a significant primary postpartum haemorrhage: A multicentre cohort study. *International Breastfeeding Journal, 5*(1), 5. https://doi.org/10.1186/1746-4358-5-5

Thompson, J. M. D., Tanabe, K., Moon, R. Y., Mitchell, E. A., McGarvey, C., Tappin, D., Blair, P. S., & Hauck, F. R. (2017). Duration of breastfeeding and risk of SIDS: An individual participant data meta-analysis. *Pediatrics, 140*(5), e20171324. https://doi.org/10.1542/peds.2017-1324

Tromp, I., Kiefte-de Jong, J., Raat, H., Jaddoe, V., Franco, O., Hofman, A., de Jongste, J., & Moll, H. (2017). Breastfeeding and the risk of respiratory tract infections after infancy: The Generation R Study. *PLOS ONE, 12*(2), e0172763. https://doi.org/10.1371/journal.pone.0172763

Twells, L., Anne, L., & Ludlow, V. (2012). Can breastfeeding reduce the risk of childhood obesity? In S. Ari Yuca (Ed.), *Childhood Obesity*. InTech. https://doi.org/10.5772/33112

Unar-Munguía, M., Torres-Mejía, G., Colchero, M. A., & González de Cosío, T. (2017). Breastfeeding mode and risk of breast cancer: A dose–response meta-analysis. *Journal of Human Lactation, 33*(2), 422–434. https://doi.org/10.1177/0890334416683676

UNICEF (Ed.). (2019). *Children, food and nutrition*. UNICEF.

UNICEF. (2021). *Infant and Young Child Feeding*. https://www1.health.gov.au/internet/main/publishing.nsf/Content/health-pubhlth-strateg-brfeed-index.htm

Uvnas-Moberg, K., & Kendall-Tackett, K. (2018). The mystery of D-MER: What can hormonal research tell us about dysphoric milk-ejection reflex? *Clinical Lactation, 9*(1), 23–29. https://doi.org/10.1891/2158-0782.9.1.23

Uwaezuoke, S. N., Eneh, C. I., & Ndu, I. K. (2017). Relationship between exclusive breastfeeding and lower risk of childhood obesity: A narrative review of published evidence. *Clinical Medicine Insights: Pediatrics, 11*, 117955651769019. https://doi.org/10.1177/1179556517690196

Valdes, E. G. (2021). Examining cesarean delivery rates by race: A population-based analysis using the Robson ten-group classification system. *Journal of Racial and Ethnic Health Disparities, 8*(4), 844–851. https://doi.org/10.1007/s40615-020-00842-3

Vanguri, S., Rogers-McQuade, H., Sriraman, N. K., the Academy of Breastfeeding Medicine, Young, M., Noble, L., Bartick, M., Calhoun, S., Feldman-Winter, L., Kair, L. R., Lappin, S., Larson, I., Lawrence, R. A., Lefort, Y., Marinelli, K. A., Marshall, N., Mitchell, K., Murak, C., Myers, E., & Wonodi, A. (2021). ABM clinical protocol #14: Breastfeeding-friendly physician's office—Optimizing care for infants and children. *Breastfeeding Medicine, 16*(3), 175–184. https://doi.org/10.1089/bfm.2021.29175.sjv

Vennemann, M. M., Bajanowski, T., Brinkmann, B., Jorch, G., Yücesan, K., Sauerland, C., Mitchell, E. A., & and the GeSID Study Group. (2009). Does breastfeeding reduce the risk of sudden infant death syndrome? *Pediatrics, 123*(3), e406–e410. https://doi.org/10.1542/peds.2008-2145

Vestermark, V., Høgdall, C. K., Birch, M., Plenov, G., & Toftager-Larsen, K. (1991). Influence of the mode of delivery on initiation of breast-feeding. *European Journal of Obstetrics & Gynecology and Reproductive Biology, 38*(1), 33–38. https://doi.org/10.1016/0028-2243(91)90204-X

Visuthranukul, C., Abrams, S. A., Hawthorne, K. M., Hagan, J. L., & Hair, A. B. (2019). Premature small for gestational age infants fed an exclusive human milk-based diet achieve catch-up growth without metabolic consequences at 2 years of age. *Archives of Disease in Childhood - Fetal and Neonatal Edition, 104*(3), F242–F247. https://doi.org/10.1136/archdischild-2017-314547

Walker, M. (2017). *Breastfeeding management for the clinician: Using the evidence* (Fourth edition). Jones & Bartlett Learning.

Wallenborn, J. T., & Masho, S. W. (2018). Association between Breastfeeding Duration and Type of Birth Attendant. *Journal of Pregnancy, 2018*, 1–7. https://doi.org/10.1155/2018/7198513

Wambach, K. A., Aaronson, L., Breedlove, G., Domian, E. W., Rojjanasrirat, W., & Yeh, H. W. (2011). A randomized controlled trial of breastfeeding support and education for adolescent mothers. *Western Journal of Nursing Research, 33*(4), 486–505. https://doi.org/10.1177/0193945910380408

Wambach, K. A., & Cohen, S. M. (2009). Breastfeeding experiences of urban adolescent mothers. *Journal of Pediatric Nursing, 24*(4), 244–254. https://doi.org/10.1016/j.pedn.2008.03.002

Wambach, K. A., & Koehn, M. (2004). Experiences of infant-feeding decision-making among urban economically disadvantaged pregnant adolescents. *Journal of Advanced Nursing, 48*(4), 361–370. https://doi.org/10.1111/j.1365-2648.2004.03205.x

Wambach, K., & Riordan, J. (2016). *Breastfeeding and human lactation.*

Wang, K. L., Liu, C. L., Zhuang, Y., & Qu, H. Y. (2013). Breastfeeding and the risk of childhood hodgkin lymphoma: A systematic review and meta-analysis. *Asian Pacific Journal of Cancer Prevention, 14*(8), 4733–4737. https://doi.org/10.7314/APJCP.2013.14.8.4733

Watchmaker, B., Boyd, B., & Dugas, L. (2020). *Newborn feeding recommendations and practices increase the risk of development of overweight and obesity* [Preprint]. In Review. https://doi.org/10.21203/rs.2.20437/v4

Watkins, A. L., Dodgson, J. E., & McClain, D. B. (2017). Online lactation education for healthcare providers: A theoretical approach to understanding learning outcomes. *Journal of Human Lactation, 33*(4), 725–735. https://doi.org/10.1177/0890334417724348

Weisfeld, G. E., Czilli, T., Phillips, K. A., Gall, J. A., & Lichtman, C. M. (2003). Possible olfaction-based mechanisms in human kin recognition and inbreeding avoidance. *Journal of Experimental Child Psychology, 85*(3), 279–295. https://doi.org/10.1016/S0022-0965(03)00061-4

Wetzl, R. G., Delfino, E., Peano, L., Gogna, D., Vidi, Y., Vielmi, F., Bianquin, E., Cerioli, S., Bettinelli, M. E., Giannì, M. L., Frassy, G., Boris, E., & Arioni, C. (2019). A priori choice of neuraxial labour analgesia and breastfeeding initiation success: A community-based cohort study in an Italian baby-friendly hospital. *BMJ Open, 9*(3), e025179. https://doi.org/10.1136/bmjopen-2018-025179

WHO. (2000). *Child Growth Standards*. World Health Organization. https://www.who.int/toolkits/child-growth-standards

WHO. (2018). *WHO recommendations: Intrapartum care for a positive childbirth experience.* World Health Organization. https://apps.who.int/iris/bitstream/handle/10665/260178/9789241550215-eng.pdf

Widström, A.-M., Lilja, G., Aaltomaa-Michalias, P., Dahllöf, A., Lintula, M., & Nissen, E. (2011). Newborn behaviour to locate the breast when skin-to-skin: A possible method for enabling early self-regulation: Newborns' location of the breast. *Acta Paediatrica, 100*(1), 79–85. https://doi.org/10.1111/j.1651-2227.2010.01983.x

Wiessinger, D., West, D., & Pitman, T. (2010). *The womanly art of breastfeeding* (8th ed). Ballantine Books.

Wight, N., & Marinelli, K. A. (2014). ABM Clinical Protocol #1: Guidelines for blood glucose monitoring and treatment of hypoglycemia in term and late-preterm neonates, revised 2014. *Breastfeeding Medicine, 9*(4), 173–179. https://doi.org/10.1089/bfm.2014.9986

Wolfberg, A. J., Michels, K. B., Shields, W., O'Campo, P., Bronner, Y., & Bienstock, J. (2004). Dads as breastfeeding advocates: Results from a randomized controlled trial of an educational intervention. *American Journal of Obstetrics and Gynecology, 191*(3), 708–712. https://doi.org/10.1016/j.ajog.2004.05.019

Wood, C. T., Skinner, A. C., Yin, H. S., Rothman, R. L., Sanders, L. M., Delamater, A., Ravanbakht, S. N., & Perrin, E. M. (2016). Association between bottle size and formula intake in 2-month-old infants. *Academic Pediatrics, 16*(3), 254–259. https://doi.org/10.1016/j.acap.2015.08.001

Woods, N. K., Chesser, A. K., & Wipperman, J. (2013). Describing adolescent breastfeeding environments through focus groups in an urban community. *Journal of Primary Care & Community Health, 4*(4), 307–310. https://doi.org/10.1177/2150131913487380

World Health Organization. (1997). *Thermal Protection of the Newborn: A Practical Guide* (WHO/RHT/MSM/97.2). World Health Organization. https://apps.who.int/iris/bitstream/handle/10665/63986/WHO_RHT_MSM_97.2.pdf?sequence=1

World Health Organization. (2018a). *Births by cesarean section: Data by country.* https://apps.who.int/gho/data/node.main.BIRTHSBYCAESAREAN?lang=en

World Health Organization. (2018b). *Ten steps to successful breastfeeding.* World Health Organization. https://www.who.int/teams/nutrition-and-food-safety/food-and-nutrition-actions-in-health-systems/ten-steps-to-successful-breastfeeding

World Health Organization. (2021). *The World Health Organization's infant feeding recommendation.* https://www.who.int/news-room/fact-sheets/detail/infant-and-young-child-feeding

Xu, L., Lochhead, P., Ko, Y., Claggett, B., Leong, R. W., & Ananthakrishnan, A. N. (2017). Systematic review with meta-analysis: Breastfeeding and the risk of Crohn's disease and ulcerative colitis. *Alimentary Pharmacology & Therapeutics, 46*(9), 780–789. https://doi.org/10.1111/apt.14291

Yu, J., Pudwell, J., Dayan, N., & Smith, G. (2019). Postpartum breastfeeding and cardiovascular risk assessment in women following pregnancy complications. *Journal of Obstetrics and Gynaecology Canada, 41*(5), 737. https://doi.org/10.1016/j.jogc.2019.02.247

Yu, Z., Sun, S., & Zhang, Y. (2018). High-risk factors for suppurative mastitis in lactating women. *Medical Science Monitor: International Medical Journal of Experimental and Clinical Research, 24*, 4192–4197. https://doi.org/10.12659/MSM.909394

Zhang, Y., Zhou, J., Ma, Y., Liu, L., Xia, Q., Fan, D., & Ai, W. (2019). Mode of delivery and preterm birth in subsequent births: A systematic review and meta-analysis. *PLOS ONE, 14*(3), e0213784. https://doi.org/10.1371/journal.pone.0213784

Zmora, I., Bas-Lando, M., Armon, S., Farkash, R., Ioscovich, A., Samueloff, A., & Grisaru-Granovsky, S. (2019). Risk factors, early and late postpartum complications of retained placenta: A case control study. *European Journal of Obstetrics & Gynecology and Reproductive Biology, 236*, 160–165. https://doi.org/10.1016/j.ejogrb.2019.03.024

www.ingramcontent.com/pod-product-compliance
Lightning Source LLC
Chambersburg PA
CBHW052118270326
41930CB00012B/2672

* 9 7 8 1 9 4 6 6 6 5 6 6 9 *